ACSM's GUIDELINES FOR EXERCISE TESTING AND PRESCRIPTION

Sixth Edition

SENIOR EDITOR
Barry A. Franklin, PhD, FACSM
Director, Cardiac Rehabilitation and Exercise Laboratories
William Beaumont Hospital
Royal Oak, Michigan
Professor of Physiology
Wayne State University
Detroit, Michigan

ASSOCIATE EDITOR—CLINICAL
Mitchell H. Whaley, PhD, FACSM
Associate Professor
School of Physical Education
Ball State University
Muncie, Indiana

ASSOCIATE EDITOR—FITNESS
Edward T. Howley, PhD, FACSM
Department of Exercise Science
University of Tennessee
Knoxville, Tennessee

AUTHORS
Gary J. Balady, MD
Kathy A. Berra, MSN, ANP
Lawrence A. Golding, PhD, FACSM
Neil F. Gordon, MD, PhD, MPH, FACSM
Donald A. Mahler, MD, FACSM
Jonathan N. Myers, PhD, FACSM
Lois M. Sheldahl, PhD, FACSM

SPECIAL CONTRIBUTORS
I. Martin Grais, MD, FACC, FACP
David L. Herbert, Esq.
William G. Herbert, PhD, FACSM
David P. Swain, PhD, FACSM
Sheri L. Tokarczyk, MS, PA-C
Andrew J. Young, PhD, FACSM

ACSM's
GUIDELINES
FOR
EXERCISE TESTING
AND
PRESCRIPTION

Sixth Edition

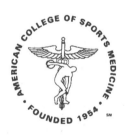

AMERICAN COLLEGE
OF SPORTS MEDICINE

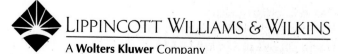

LIPPINCOTT WILLIAMS & WILKINS
A **Wolters Kluwer** Company

Philadelphia · Baltimore · New York · London
Buenos Aires · Hong Kong · Sydney · Tokyo

Editor: Eric P. Johnson
Managing Editor: Linda S. Napora
Marketing Manager: Chris Kushner
Production Editor: Bill Cady

351 West Camden Street
Baltimore, Maryland 21201-2436 USA

530 Walnut Street
Philadelphia, Pennsylvania 19106

Printed in the United States of America

First Edition 1975   *Third Edition* 1986   *Fifth Edition* 1995
Second Edition 1980   *Fourth Edition* 1991

Library of Congress Cataloging-in-Publication Data

American College of Sports Medicine.
    ACSM's guidelines for exercise testing and prescription   /   American College of Sports-
Medicine; senior editor, Barry A. Franklin, associate editor (clinical) Mitchell H. Whaley, associate editor (fitness) Edward T. Howley; authors, Gary J. Balady . . . [et al.].—6th ed.
        p.   ; cm.
    Includes bibliographical references and index.
      ISBN 0-683-30355-4 (spiral bound)
      ISBN 0-7817-2735-9 (perfect bound)
      1. Exercise therapy. 2. Heart—Diseases—Exercise therapy. I. Title: Guidelines for exer-
cise testing and prescription. II. Franklin, Barry A. III. Whaley, Mitchell H., 1955–   . IV.
Howley, Edward T., 1943–   V. Title.
    [DNLM: 1. Exertion. 2. Exercise Test—standards. 3. Exercise Therapy—standards. WE 103
A514a 2000]
RC684.E9 A45 2000
615.8'24—dc21

                                                                    99-059386

*The publishers have made every effort to trace the copyright holders for borrowed material. If they
have inadvertently overlooked any, they will be pleased to make the necessary arrangements at the
first opportunity.*

To purchase additional copies of this book, call our customer service department at **(800)
638-3030** or fax orders to **(301) 824-7390**. International customers should call **(301) 714-2324**.
Or visit **Lippincott Williams & Wilkins on the Internet: http://www.lww.com**.

For more information concerning American College of Sports Medicine certification and suggested preparatory materials, call **(800) 486-5643** or visit the American College of Sports
Medicine Website at **www.acsm.org**.

                                                        02 03 04
                                                    3 4 5 6 7 8 9 10

Dedicated to Michael L. Pollock, PhD, FACSM (1936–1998), preeminent scientist, clinician, researcher, teacher, and friend. His tireless pursuit of the optimal frequency, intensity, duration, and modes of physical conditioning, including aerobic, resistance, and flexibility training, contributed immensely to the refinement and evolution of exercise prescription as it exists today. Many of the concepts and ideas in the sixth edition of the *Guidelines* are based on his pioneering scientific work.

Sir Isaac Newton said, "If I have seen further . . . it is by standing upon the shoulders of giants." *ACSM's Guidelines for Exercise Testing and Prescription* has been written by representatives of the Certification and Education Committee (formerly called the Preventive and Rehabilitative Exercise Committee) of the American College of Sports Medicine. Several individuals on the committee and others from the College contributed to each edition. The primary responsibility for writing and editing each edition was assumed by the following individuals:

First Edition, 1975
  Karl G. Stoedefalke, PhD,
    Co-Chair
  John A. Faulkner, PhD,
    Co-Chair
  Samuel M. Fox, MD
  Henry S. Miller, Jr., MD
  Bruno Balke, MD

Second Edition, 1980
  R. Anne Abbott, PhD, Chair
  Karl G. Stoedefalke, PhD
  N. Blythe Runsdorf, PhD
  John A. Faulkner, PhD

Third Edition, 1986
  Steven N. Blair, PED, Chair
  Larry W. Gibbons, MD
  Patricia Painter, PhD
  Russell R. Pate, PhD
  C. Barr Taylor, MD
  Josephine Will, MS

Fourth Edition, 1991
  Russell R. Pate, PhD, Chair
  Steven N. Blair, PED
  J. Larry Durstine, PhD
  Duane O. Eddy, PhD
  Peter Hanson, MD
  Patricia Painter, PhD
  L. Kent Smith, MD
  Larry A. Wolfe, PhD

Fifth Edition, 1995
  W. Larry Kenney, PhD,
    Senior Editor
  Reed H. Humphrey, PhD, PT
    Associate Editor—Clinical
  Cedric X. Bryant, PhD,
    Associate Editor—Fitness
  Donald A. Mahler, MD
  Victor F. Froelicher, MD
  Nancy Houston Miller, RN
  Tracy D. York, MS

PREFACE

This sixth edition of *ACSM's Guidelines for Exercise Testing and Prescription* represents another step in the evolution of this manual first published by the American College of Sports Medicine in 1975. A volume that began as a concise summary of recommendations for exercise testing and prescription, primarily in cardiac patients, has now become one of the single most widely read and referenced texts of its kind in the world (~100,000 copies of the fifth edition have been sold), and a virtual pharmacopoeia of exercise guidelines for a broad spectrum of patients. The aim of this revision was to present the most current information in a usable form for physicians and allied health professionals, including fitness and clinical exercise professionals, nurses, physician assistants, physical and occupational therapists, dietitians, and health care administrators. This edition also places heightened emphasis on preventing illness in apparently healthy persons and those "at risk" as well as on treating patients with chronic disease.

There are now several ACSM texts that complement and expand upon this book. The unique role of the sixth edition of the *Guidelines* is to present the value and application of exercise testing and prescription in persons with and without chronic disease. For more detailed treatment of topics covered in the *Guidelines*, the reader is directed to its companion publication, *ACSM's Resource Manual for Guidelines for Exercise Testing and Prescription, Third Edition*. This textual compendium of individual chapters and accompanying appendices largely represents the fundamental knowledge that must be mastered by candidates applying for ACSM's certifications in preventive and rehabilitative exercise programming. For special populations not covered in the *Guidelines*, the reader is referred to *Exercise Management for Persons with Chronic Diseases and Disabilities*. Finally, the *ACSM Fitness Book* provides self-assessment tests and an easy-to-use progressive exercise program for use by the apparently healthy adult.

Since publication of the fifth edition of the *Guidelines*, several scientific statements, position stands, and consensus development conferences have emphasized the following points:

- Physical inactivity is a major health problem in the United States. More than 60% of American adults are not regularly physically active. In fact, 25% of all adults are not active at all.
- People of all ages, both male and female, benefit from regular physical activity.
- Physical activity is highly beneficial in the treatment of persons with chronic disease and disabilities.

- People who are habitually sedentary can improve their health, fitness, and well-being by becoming even moderately active.
- Physical activity need not be vigorous to achieve health benefits.
- Greater health benefits may be achieved by increasing the amount (intensity, frequency, or duration) of physical activity.
- Physical activity reduces the risk of all-cause and cardiovascular mortality and of coronary heart disease, obesity, hypertension, breast and colon cancer, and diabetes mellitus in particular.
- Physical activity improves mental health and is important for the health of muscles, bones, and joints.
- Exercise testing provides invaluable information in assessing functional capacity, the safety of physical exertion, and the effect of various interventions. Moreover, the results have long-term prognostic significance in regard to morbidity and mortality.
- Vigorous physical activity can precipitate musculoskeletal complications, cardiovascular events, or other adverse responses in certain individuals.

Accordingly, the sixth edition has expanded its focus to include several new topic areas: cardiovascular screening, staffing, and emergency policies at health and/or fitness facilities; implications of the Surgeon General's report; recommendations to reduce the risks associated with exercise; upper body exercise testing and training; ramp testing; activity programming for health versus fitness; exercise training for return to work; supervision of exercise tests; exercise testing with concomitant myocardial perfusion imaging; pharmacologic testing and exercise echocardiography; complementary lifestyle changes (e.g., smoking cessation, stress management); absolute versus relative exercise intensity; advances in exercise prescription (e.g., concept of $\dot{V}O_2$ reserve, resistance and/or flexibility training); and special patient populations (e.g., patients with angina or silent ischemia, congestive heart failure, pacemakers, implantable cardioverter defibrillators, and cardiac transplant recipients).

This sixth edition of the *Guidelines* has two new chapters: "Methods for Changing Exercising Behaviors" and "Legal Issues." It is hoped that these additions will enhance the value of the book, particularly for those who may be challenged by suboptimal client or patient compliance rates and/or liability issues. Substantive revisions have been made in these chapters: "Benefits and Risks Associated With Exercise," "Pretest Clinical Evaluation," "Physical Fitness Testing and Interpretation," "Interpretation of Clinical Test Data," "Exercise Prescription for Cardiac Patients," "General Principles of Exercise Prescription," and "Other Clinical Conditions Influencing Exercise Prescription." The changes have been directed toward incorporating the most current clinical practices and state-of-the-art, research-based recommendations.

A decision was made to largely maintain the additional quantitative data—threshold values, clinical laboratory cutoffs considered "abnormal," normative fitness data—that were included in the fifth edition. Where appropriate, those values are referenced to reports or publications prepared by other professional organizations or national associations. In addition, a conscious effort was made to increase the number of figures and boxes to highlight key or salient points in the text, to set off information that merited special attention with colored screening, to more clearly designate subheadings in a descending order of importance, and to minimize the number of abbreviations in each chapter.

An important modification evident in this edition is a thorough updating of the user-friendly appendices. The tables in the section on electrocardiography (Appendix C) have been expanded to provide a quick reference guide to ECG interpretation, including a sequential approach to evaluating heart rate, rhythm, axis, hypertrophy, and infarction. Appendix D (Metabolic Calculations) has been rewritten to improve its clarity and accuracy, with specific reference to the calculation of energy expenditure for cycle ergometry and stepping. Appendix F presents information about ACSM Certification Programs™, including revised knowledge, skills, and abilities (KSAs) underlying each level of certification. The latter was largely based on input from the Committee on Certification and Education, selected ACSM members, and the results of a role delineation survey of certified exercise professionals.

This edition has been prepared by a volunteer writing team and special contributors with representative expertise in physiology, fitness, cardiology, pulmonary medicine, nursing, and physical therapy. Our acknowledgments begin with Brenda White who meticulously orchestrated the word processing and editing of this book with a unique sense of pride, perfection, and perseverance. Special thanks also go to our Associate Editors, Edward T. Howley, PhD, FACSM, and Mitchell H. Whaley, PhD, FACSM, for their chapter contributions, editorial expertise, and unwavering commitment to this herculean endeavor, and to Jeffrey L. Roitman, EdD, FACSM, for his invaluable assistance with Appendix F. Further, we express our gratitude to Linda Napora and Bill Cady, our managing and production editors, respectively, for their ongoing patience, encouragement, and expertise. Appreciation also goes to the authors of the previous editions of the *Guidelines*; much of their innovative and enduring work remains in the sixth edition.

This text has undergone an extensive review process by external and internal experts; the latter include many members of the American College of Sports Medicine. The College and authors wish to express their thanks to those individuals who contributed ideas, comments, critical reviews, and editorial assistance.

Barry A. Franklin, PhD, FACSM
Senior Editor

Note Bene

The views and information contained in the sixth edition of *ACSM's Guidelines for Exercise Testing and Prescription* are provided as *guidelines* as opposed to *standards of practice*. This distinction is an important one, since specific legal connotations may be attached to such terminology. The distinction is also critical inasmuch as it gives the exercise professional the freedom to deviate from these guidelines when necessary and appropriate in the course of exercising independent and prudent judgment. *ACSM's Guidelines for Exercise Testing and Prescription* presents a framework whereby the professional may certainly–and in some cases has the obligation to–tailor to individual client or patient needs and alter to meet institutional or legislated requirements.

CONTRIBUTORS

AUTHORS

Gary J. Balady, MD
Professor of Medicine
Director, Preventive Cardiology
Boston University Medical
    Center
Boston, Massachusetts

Kathy A. Berra, MSN, ANP
Clinical Trial Coordinator
Stanford Center for Research in
    Disease Prevention
Stanford University
Palo Alto, California

**Lawrence A. Golding, PhD,
    FACSM**
Distinguished University Professor
Department of Kinesiology
University of Nevada–Las Vegas
Las Vegas, Nevada

**Neil F. Gordon, MD, PhD,
    MPH, FACSM**
Medical Director
Center for Heart Disease Prevention
St Joseph's/Candler Health System
Savannah, Georgia

**Donald A. Mahler, MD,
    FACSM**
Professor of Medicine
Department of Medicine
Dartmouth Medical School
Lebanon, New Hampshire

**Jonathan N. Myers, PhD,
    FACSM**
Clinical Assistant Professor of
    Medicine
Cardiology Division
Stanford University/Palo Alto
    VAHCS
Palo Alto, California

**Lois M. Sheldahl, PhD,
    FACSM**
Director, Cardiopulmonary
    Prevention and Rehabilitation
    Clinic
Department of Medicine/
    Cardiology
VA Medical Center
Milwaukee, Wisconsin

SPECIAL CONTRIBUTORS

**I. Martin Grais, MD, FACC,
    FACP**
Assistant Professor of Clinical
    Medicine
Section of Cardiology
Northwestern University Medical
    School
Chicago, Illinois

David L. Herbert, Esq.
Attorney at Law and Partner
Herbert, Benson, Attorneys at Law
Vice President, Medical Risk
Management Services, Inc.
Canton, Ohio

**William G. Herbert, PhD,
    FACSM**
Virginia Tech
Laboratory for Health and Exercise
    Science
Blacksburg, Virginia

David P. Swain, PhD, FACSM
Associate Professor, Exercise
Director, Wellness Institute and
    Research Center
Old Dominion University
Norfolk, Virginia

Sheri L. Tokarczyk, MS, PA-C
Physician Assistant
Department of Surgery
Evanston Northwestern Healthcare
Evanston, Illinois

Andrew J. Young, PhD
Research Physiologist
Thermal and Mountain Medicine
    Division
U.S. Army Research Institute of
    Environmental Medicine
Natick, Massachusetts

CONTENTS

Abbreviations

AACVPR American Association of Cardiovascular and Pulmonary Rehabilitation

ABI ankle/brachial systolic pressure index

ACE angiotensin-converting enzyme

ACGIH American Conference of Governmental Industrial Hygienists

ACOG American College of Obstetricians and Gynecologists

ACP American College of Physicians

ACSM American College of Sports Medicine

ADL activities of daily living

AHA American Heart Association

AIHA American Industrial Hygiene Association

AMA American Medical Association

AMS acute mountain sickness

AICD automatic implantable cardioverter defibrillator

AST aspartate aminotransferase

AV atrioventricular

BIA bioelectrical impedance analysis

BLS basic life support

BMI body mass index

BP blood pressure

BR breathing reserve

BUN blood urea nitrogen

C ceiling (heat stress) limit

CABG(S) coronary artery bypass graft (surgery)

CAD coronary artery disease

CDC Centers for Disease Control and Prevention

CHF congestive heart failure

CHO carbohydrate

CI cardiac index

COPD chronic obstructive pulmonary disease

CPAP continuous positive airway pressure

CPR cardiopulmonary resuscitation

CPK creatine phosphokinase

CRQ Chronic Respiratory Questionnaire

DBP diastolic blood pressure

DOMS delayed onset muscle soreness

DVR dynamic variable resistance

ECG electrocardiogram (electrocardiographic)

EF ejection fraction

EIB exercise-induced bronchoconstriction

EIH exercise-induced hypotension

EL Exercise Leader®

ERV expiratory reserve volume

ES Exercise Specialist®

FC functional capacity

FEV$_{1.0}$ forced expiratory volume in one second

FFM fat-free mass

F$_I$O$_2$ fraction of inspired oxygen

F$_I$CO$_2$ fraction of inspired carbon dioxide

FN false negative

FP false positive

FRV functional residual volume

FVC forced vital capacity

GXT graded exercise test

HAPE high-altitude pulmonary edema

HDL high-density lipoprotein

HFD Health/Fitness Director®

HFI Health/Fitness Instructor$_{SM}$

HR heart rate

HR$_{max}$ maximal heart rate

HR$_{rest}$ resting heart rate

HRR heart rate reserve

IC inspiratory capacity

ICD implantable cardioverter defibrillator

IDDM insulin-dependent diabetes mellitus

KSAs knowledge, skills, and abilities

LAD	left axis deviation	**RIMT**	resistive inspiratory muscle training
LBBB	left bundle-branch block		
LDH	lactate dehydrogenase	**1-RM**	one repetition maximum
LDL	low-density lipoprotein	**RQ**	respiratory quotient
L-G-L	Lown-Ganong-Levine	**RPE**	rating of perceived exertion
LLN	lower limit of normal	**RV**	residual volume
LV	left ventricle (left ventricular)	**RVG**	radionuclide ventriculography
		RVH	right ventricular hypertrophy
MCHC	mean corpuscular hemoglobin concentration		
MET	metabolic equivalent	S_aO_2	percent saturation of arterial oxygen
MI	myocardial infarction	**SBP**	systolic blood pressure
MUGA	multigated acquisition (scan)	**SEE**	standard error of estimate
MVC	maximal voluntary contraction	**SPECT**	single photon emission computed tomography
MVV	maximal voluntary ventilation	**SVT**	supraventricular tachycardia
NCEP	National Cholesterol Education Program	**THR**	target heart rate
		TLC	total lung capacity
NIDDM	non–insulin-dependent diabetes mellitus	**TN**	true negative
		TP	true positive
NIH	National Institutes of Health	**TPR**	total peripheral resistance
		TV	tidal volume
NIOSH	National Institute for Occupational Safety and Health		
		VC	vital capacity
NYHA	New York Heart Association	$\dot{V}CO_2$	volume of carbon dioxide per minute
P_aO_2	partial pressure of arterial oxygen	$\dot{V}_E$	expired ventilation per minute
PAC	premature atrial contraction	$\dot{V}_{Emax}$	maximal exercise ventilation
PAR-Q	Physical Activity Readiness Questionnaire	$\dot{V}_I$	inspired ventilation per minute
PD	Program Director$_{SM}$	**VMT**	ventilatory muscle training
PE_{max}	maximal expiratory pressure	$\dot{V}O_2$	volume of oxygen consumed per minute
PI_{max}	maximal inspiratory pressure	$\dot{V}O_{2max}$	maximal oxygen uptake
PNF	proprioceptive neuromuscular facilitation	$\dot{V}O_{2peak}$	peak oxygen uptake
		$\dot{V}O_2R$	oxygen uptake reserve
PO_2	partial pressure of oxygen	$\%\dot{V}O_2R$	percentage of oxygen uptake reserve
PTCA	percutaneous transluminal coronary angioplasty	**VT**	ventilatory threshold
PVC	premature ventricular contraction		
PVD	peripheral vascular disease	**WBGT**	wet-bulb globe temperature
		WHR	waist-to-hip ratio
R	respiratory exchange ratio	**W-P-W**	Wolff-Parkinson-White
RAD	right axis deviation		
RAL	recommended alert limit	**YMCA**	Young Men's Christian Association
RBBB	right bundle-branch block		
rep	repetition	**YWCA**	Young Women's Christian Association

SECTION I

Health Appraisal, Risk Assessment, and Safety of Exercise

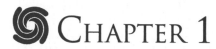 CHAPTER 1

Benefits and Risks Associated With Exercise

This chapter reviews the health and fitness benefits of regular physical activity and/or exercise, reviews the risks associated with exercise testing and training, and provides recommendations to reduce the incidence and severity of exercise-related complications in adult fitness and exercise-based rehabilitation programs.

PUBLIC HEALTH PERSPECTIVE

An important mission of the American College of Sports Medicine (ACSM) is to promote increased physical activity and fitness to the public. While previous editions of this text focused on supervised *exercise* programs, recent physical activity recommendations from the Centers for Disease Control and Prevention and the ACSM (1) and the U.S. Surgeon General (2) have amended and expanded the traditional emphasis on formal exercise prescriptions to include a broader public health perspective on *physical activity.* The intent of these reports was twofold: 1) to increase both professional and public awareness of the health benefits associated with daily participation in physical activity, and 2) to draw attention to the amounts and intensities of physical activity necessary to achieve these benefits, levels lower than those thought to be necessary for the traditional physiological training effect associated with exercise (3). A major theme running through both of the recent public health reports (1,2) is that more traditional exercise recommendations (3) have overlooked the numerous health benefits associated with regular participation in intermittent, moderate-intensity physical activity (e.g., less than 20 minutes per session and less than 50% of maximal aerobic power [$\dot{V}O_{2max}$]).

The Surgeon General's report, *Physical Activity and Health* (2), stated two conclusions that merit attention here:

"Significant health benefits can be obtained by including a moderate amount of physical activity (e.g., 30 minutes of brisk walking or raking leaves, 15 minutes of running, or 45 minutes of playing volleyball) on most, if not all, days of the week. Through a modest increase in daily activity, most Americans can improve their health and quality of life."

"Additional health benefits can be gained through greater amounts of physical activity. People who can maintain a regular regimen of activity that is of longer duration or of more vigorous intensity are likely to derive greater benefit."

Implicit within this report is the notion that the health and fitness benefits associated with physical activity most likely follow a dose–response relationship. In other words, some activity is better than none, and more activity—up to a point—is better than less. Although the optimal dose of physical activity has yet to be defined, the dose–response relationship between physical activity and various health benefits clearly supports the need for professionals to encourage the public to engage in at least moderate amounts and moderate intensities of daily physical activity (i.e., activities that are approximately 3 to 6 metabolic equivalents [METs] or the equivalent of walking at 3 to 4 mph [15 to 20 minutes to walk 1 mile] for most healthy adults) (1). The public health benefits of increasing physical activity within the general population are potentially enormous due to both the high prevalence of a sedentary lifestyle and the impact increased physical activity has on disease risk (4). Therefore, exercise program professionals must know existing public health statements pertaining to physical activity and must stay abreast of the evolving scientific literature related to these physical activity recommendations. When knowledge of the additional health and fitness benefits associated with greater quantities and intensities of physical activity (i.e., exercise) is combined with the fact that the list of chronic diseases favorably affected by exercise continues to grow, there remains a clear need for medically—and scientifically—sound preventive and rehabilitative exercise programs. These exercise programs should be designed, supervised, and conducted by qualified personnel.

Several key terms defined elsewhere (5) are reviewed here due to their importance in understanding the relationship between this text and recent public health statements on physical activity (1,2). *Physical activity* is defined as bodily movement that is produced by the contraction of skeletal muscle and that substantially increases energy expenditure. *Exercise*, a subclass of physical activity, is defined as planned, structured, and repetitive bodily movement done to improve or maintain one or more components of physical fitness. *Physical fitness* is defined as a set of attributes that people have or achieve that relates to the ability to perform physical activity. Professionals should recognize that both the quality and quantity of physical activity recommended within later chapters of this text relate to *exercise* recommendations and should not be viewed as inconsistent or contrary to recent physical activity recommendations for the general public (1,2).

BENEFITS OF REGULAR PHYSICAL ACTIVITY AND/OR EXERCISE

Numerous laboratory-based studies have quantified the many health and fitness benefits (e.g., physiologic, metabolic, and psychological) associated with endurance exercise training (Box 1-1) (2,3,6-8). In addition, an ever-increasing number of prospective epidemiologic studies supports the notion that both a physically active lifestyle and a moderate-to-high level of cardio-respiratory fitness independently lower the risk for various chronic diseases (Table 1-1) (9). Inverse dose–response relationships for physical activity or cardiorespiratory fitness are strongest for all-cause and cardiovascular mortality; however, lower incidence rates for hypertension, obesity, cancer of the colon, type 2 diabetes, and osteoporosis have also been consistently reported in the literature. The bulk of the epidemiologic evidence supporting the health benefits of a more active lifestyle has been based on studies using single assessments of physical activity or fitness. However, results from recent studies correlating *increases* in physical activity or fitness in initially sedentary or unfit adults with subsequent reductions in mortality support the hypothesis that regular activity increases longevity (10,11). Although increased physical activity or fitness may yet prove beneficial in reducing risk for the other chronic diseases listed in Table 1-1, more research is needed to firmly establish these relationships. Moreover, because of the multifactorial nature of the chronic diseases associated with a sedentary lifestyle, there may well be no single minimal dose of physical activity that yields protection from all of the diseases and conditions listed in Table

---

BOX 1-1. Benefits of Regular Physical Activity and/or Exercise*

Improvement in Cardiovascular and Respiratory Function
- Increased maximal oxygen uptake due to both central and peripheral adaptations
- Lower minute ventilation at a given submaximal intensity
- Lower myocardial oxygen cost for a given absolute submaximal intensity
- Lower heart rate and blood pressure at a given submaximal intensity
- Increased capillary density in skeletal muscle
- Increased exercise threshold for the accumulation of lactate in the blood
- Increased exercise threshold for the onset of disease signs or symptoms (e.g., angina pectoris, ischemic ST-segment depression, claudication)

Reduction in Coronary Artery Disease Risk Factors
- Reduced resting systolic/diastolic pressures
- Increased serum high-density lipoprotein cholesterol and decreased serum triglycerides
- Reduced total body fat, reduced intra-abdominal fat
- Reduced insulin needs, improved glucose tolerance

BOX 1-1. *(continued)*

Decreased Mortality and Morbidity
- Primary prevention (i.e., interventions to prevent an acute cardiac event)
    1. Higher activity and/or fitness levels are associated with lower death rates from coronary artery disease
    2. Higher activity and/or fitness levels are associated with lower incidence rates for combined cardiovascular diseases, coronary artery disease, cancer of the colon, and type 2 diabetes
- Secondary prevention (i.e., interventions after a cardiac event [to prevent another])
    1. Based on meta-analyses (pooled data across studies), cardiovascular and all-cause mortality are reduced in post-myocardial infarction patients who participate in cardiac rehabilitation exercise training, especially as a component of multifactorial risk factor reduction
    2. Randomized controlled trials of cardiac rehabilitation exercise training involving post-myocardial infarction patients do not support a reduction in the rate of nonfatal reinfarction

Other Postulated Benefits
- Decreased anxiety and depression
- Enhanced feelings of well-being
- Enhanced performance of work, recreational, and sport activities

*Adapted from United States Department of Health and Human Services. Physical activity and health: a report of the Surgeon General. Atlanta, GA: US Department of Health and Human Services, Centers for Disease Control and Prevention, National Center for Chronic Disease Prevention and Health Promotion, 1996; Pollock ML, Gaesser GA, Butcher JD. The recommended quantity and quality of exercise for developing and maintaining cardiorespiratory and muscular fitness, and flexibility in healthy adults. Med Sci Sports Exerc 1998;30:975–991; Franklin BA, Roitman JL. Cardiorespiratory adaptations to exercise. In: Roitman JL, ed. ACSM's Resource Manual for Guidelines for Exercise Testing and Prescription. Baltimore: Williams & Wilkins, 1998:156–163; Wenger NK, Froelicher ES, Smith LK, et al. Cardiac rehabilitation. Clinical practice guidelines No. 17. Rockville, MD: US Department of Health and Human Services, Public Health Service, Agency for Health Care Policy and Research and the National Heart, Lung and Blood Institute, AHCPR Publication No. 96-0672, October 1995; and Whaley MH, Kaminsky LA. Epidemiology of physical activity, physical fitness and selected chronic diseases. In: Roitman JL, ed. ACSM's Resource Manual for Guidelines for Exercise Testing and Prescription. Baltimore: Williams & Wilkins, 1998:13–26.

1-1 (9). Further research is needed to more clearly define the minimal dose of physical activity associated with primary prevention of various chronic diseases.

Risks Associated With Exercise Testing

Although the complications associated with exercise testing appear to be relatively low, the ability to maintain a high degree of safety depends on knowing when not to perform the test, when to terminate the test, and being prepared for any emergency that might arise (12). In one widely

TABLE 1-1. Results of Studies Investigating the Relationship Between Physical Activity or Physical Fitness and Incidences of Selected Chronic Diseases

Disease or Condition	Number of Studies	Trends Across Activity or Fitness Categories and Strength of Evidence
All-cause mortality	***	↓ ↓ ↓
Coronary artery disease	***	↓ ↓ ↓
Hypertension	**	↓ ↓
Obesity	***	↓ ↓
Stroke	***	↓
Peripheral vascular disease	*	→
Cancer		
Colon	***	↓ ↓ ↓
Rectal	***	→
Stomach	*	→
Breast	**	↓
Prostate	***	↓
Lung	*	↓
Pancreatic	*	→
Type 2 diabetes mellitus	**	↓ ↓
Osteoarthritis	*	→
Osteoporosis	**	↓ ↓

*Few studies, probably less than 5; **approximately 5 to 10 studies; ***more than 10 studies.

→ No apparent difference in disease rates across activity or fitness categories; ↓ some evidence of reduced disease rates across activity or fitness categories; ↓ ↓ good evidence of reduced disease rates across activity or fitness categories, control of potential confounders, good methods, some evidence of biological mechanisms; ↓ ↓ ↓ excellent evidence of reduced disease rates across activity or fitness categories, good control of potential confounders, excellent methods, extensive evidence of biological mechanisms, relationship is considered causal.

Modified with permission from Blair SN. Physical activity, physical fitness, and health. Res Q Exerc Sport 1993;64:365-376.

quoted study (13) involving 170,000 exercise stress tests performed in 73 medical centers, the mortality rate was 1 death per 10,000 tests (0.01%), and the combined morbidity/mortality rate was 4/10,000 (0.04%). A 1980 survey (14) of 518,448 exercise stress tests conducted in 1375 centers revealed a 50% lower mortality rate of 0.5 deaths per 10,000 tests (0.005%) but a higher combined complication rate of 8.86/10,000 tests (0.09%). However, applying these widely cited survey results to contemporary exercise laboratories is tenuous at best because of the varied testing modalities, protocols, and end points employed, the mix of submaximal and maximal tests, the differences in exclusion criteria and types of patients studied, and the emphasis on direct physician supervision. Current thrombolytic and revascularization procedures (which markedly decrease early postinfarction mortality) and pharmacotherapeutic advances may also alter the risk of exercise testing in some patient subsets.

Additional investigators have reported the cardiovascular complication rates of exercise testing by physicians. In one series (15), 263 patients with a history of malignant ventricular arrhythmias (high-risk patients) underwent a total of 1377 maximal exercise tests. Of the 263 patients, 24 (9%) experienced a "complication," defined as a threatening arrhythmia that mandated immediate medical treatment (cardioversion, use of intravenous drugs, or closed-chest compression); however, there were no deaths or myocardial infarctions (MIs). In the largest experience to date, involving more than 1 million exercise tests, there were no fatal or nonfatal complications in athletes, whereas coronary patients demonstrated morbidity and mortality rates of 1.4 and 0.2 per 10,000 tests, respectively (16). A Swedish prospective study (50,000 tests) reported a morbidity rate of 5.2 per 10,000 tests and a mortality rate of 0.4 per 10,000 tests (17). In more than 70,000 tests in one preventive medicine clinic there were 6 major cardiac complications (e.g., ventricular tachycardia, ventricular fibrillation, MI), including 1 death (18).

Over the past two decades, cost containment initiatives and time constraints on physicians have encouraged the use of specially trained health care professionals (e.g., nurses, exercise physiologists, physician assistants, and physical therapists) to conduct exercise tests, with a physician immediately available for preliminary consultation or management of emergencies that may arise. The safety of this practice has now been substantiated. One study evaluated the safety of diagnostic exercise testing by physical therapists and reported morbidity and mortality rates of 3.8 and 0.9 per 10,000 tests, respectively (19,20). Using a nurse-supervised exercise stress testing laboratory, there were 12 complications and no deaths during 4050 tests (21); however, another series reported 3 deaths in more than 12,000 exercise tests conducted by specially trained nurses (22). A 13-year experience using exercise physiologists for the supervision of exercise stress tests revealed no deaths, 4 MIs, and 5 episodes of ventricular fibrillation in 28,133 exercise tests (23). Of 58,047 tests supervised by specially trained physiologists or nurses, including a significant subset of high-risk patients (approximately 15 to 20%), there were 14 complications (event rate of 1 per 4146 exercise tests); 2 of these were fatal (24).

A summary of 12 different reports involving nearly 2 million exercise tests is shown in Table 1-2, with specific reference to morbidity and mortality rates, total complications, and supervision (i.e., physician versus nonphysician) (13–24). Comparison of the results is difficult because of the inclusion of both diagnostic and fitness tests, the wide variety of healthy and diseased populations and associated comorbid conditions, and the multitude of test modalities, protocols, and end points employed. Although it is not possible to stratify risk by population or testing method, the rate of complications appears higher in populations undergoing diagnostic exercise testing, as compared with persons being tested for athletics or as part of a preventive medical examination. Moreover, the incidence of cardiovascular events seems to be no higher with nonphysician than with physician supervision of exercise testing. Based on these data, including a subset of patients with

TABLE 1-2. Complication Rates of Exercise Testing (1969–1995)

Investigator (ref. #)	Number of Tests	Morbidity Rate (per 10,000)	Mortality Rate (per 10,000)	Total Complications (per 10,000)	Physician Supervised?
Rochmis & Blackburn (13)	170,000	2.4	1.0	3.4	Yes*
Stuart & Ellestad (14)	518,448	8.4	0.5	8.9	Yes*
Scherer & Kaltenbach (16)	353,638[†]	0	0	0	Yes*
	712,285[‡]	1.4	0.2	1.6	Yes*
Young et al. (15)	1,377[§]	232	0	232	Yes*
Atterhog et al. (17)	50,000	5.2	0.4	5.6	Yes*
Cahalin/Blessey (19,20)	18,707	3.8	0.9	4.7	No
DeBusk (22)	>12,000	—	2.5	—	No
Gibbons et al. (18)	71,914	0.7	0.1	0.8	Yes*
Lem et al. (21)	4,050	0.3	0	0.3	No
Knight et al. (23)	28,133	3.2	0	3.2	No
Franklin et al. (24)	58,047	2.1	0.3	2.4	No

*More than 85% of these tests were directly supervised by physicians; †athletes; ‡coronary patients; §patients with a history of malignant ventricular arrhythmias; complications were defined as the occurrence of serious arrhythmias during exercise testing (i.e., ventricular fibrillation, ventricular tachycardia, or bradycardia) that mandated immediate medical treatment (cardioversion, use of intravenous drugs, or closed-chest compression).

malignant ventricular arrhythmias (15), the following general statements can be made regarding the safety of peak or symptom-limited graded exercise testing:

- The risk of death during or immediately after an exercise test is less than or equal to 0.01%.
- The risk of acute MI during or immediately after an exercise test is less than or equal to 0.04%.
- The risk of a complication requiring hospitalization (including acute MI and/or serious arrhythmias) is less than or equal to 0.2%.

The risks associated with submaximal physical fitness testing appear to be even lower. The submaximal cycle ergometer test described in Chapter 4 has been administered to thousands of adults (ages 18 to 65 years) in worksite health promotion programs and community health and fitness centers, with no reported deaths, MIs, or lasting morbid events. Pretest screening and submaximal exercise testing were performed by nurses or ACSM Certified Exercise Test Technologists$_{SM}$ (25). The Canadian Aerobics Fitness Test has been used worldwide by an estimated 1 million people with no reported untoward events other than minor musculoskeletal injuries and isolated syncopal episodes (26). Thus, submaximal physical fitness testing can be administered safely by qualified personnel in nonmedical settings when prefaced by appropriate pretest screening such as the Physical Activity Readiness Questionnaire (PAR-Q; see Chapter 2). Nevertheless, the limitations of using arbitrary submaximal heart rates (e.g., 70 or 85% of age-predicted maximal heart rate) as end points for exercise testing are well documented, in view of the variation in measured maximal heart rate for any given age (standard deviation $\pm$ 10 to 12 beats·min^{-1}). Consequently, a calculated "submaximal" heart rate for fitness testing may evoke maximal effort in some cases, but only modest aerobic demands in other similarly aged persons.

RISKS ASSOCIATED WITH VIGOROUS EXERCISE

Pathophysiologic evidence suggests that the increased myocardial demands of vigorous exercise may precipitate cardiovascular events in persons with known or occult heart disease. By increasing myocardial oxygen consumption and simultaneously shortening diastole and coronary perfusion time, exercise may evoke a transient oxygen deficiency in the subendocardial tissue, which may be exacerbated by a decrease in venous return secondary to an abrupt cessation of exercise. Symptomatic or silent myocardial ischemia, sodium-potassium imbalance, increased catecholamine excretion, and circulating free fatty acids may all be arrhythmogenic (Fig. 1-1). Moreover, several hypotheses have been advanced to explain how vigorous physical activity can provoke plaque rupture and acute coronary thrombosis. These events may occur with abrupt increases in heart rate and blood pressure,

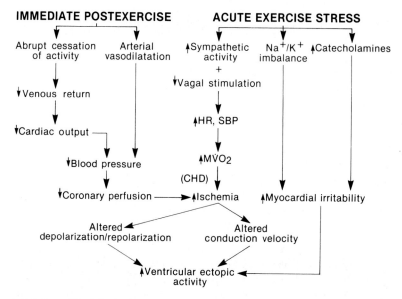

FIGURE 1-1. Physiologic alterations accompanying acute exercise and recovery, and their possible sequelae. CHD, coronary heart disease; HR, heart rate; MV̇O$_2$, myocardial oxygen uptake; Na$^+$/K$^+$, sodium/potassium ion; SBP, systolic blood pressure.

induced coronary artery spasm in diseased artery segments, or via twisting of the epicardial coronary arteries, leading to disruption of vulnerable atherosclerotic plaque and thrombotic occlusion of a coronary vessel (27). An increase in platelet activation and hyperreactivity, which could contribute to (or even initiate) coronary thrombosis, has also been reported in sedentary subjects who engaged in sporadic high-intensity exercise, but not physically conditioned ones (28).

The risk of cardiovascular complications appears to be transiently increased during vigorous exercise compared with that observed at other times. One survey reported 1 jogging death per year for every 7620 joggers in Rhode Island, corresponding to 1 death per 396,000 man-hours of jogging (29). This rate was 7 times the estimated death rate from heart disease during more sedentary activities (30). For patients with coronary artery disease, the relative risk of developing cardiac arrest during vigorous exercise may be more than 100-fold greater than what might be expected to occur spontaneously (31). The relative risk of acute MI is also 2 to 6 times higher during vigorous physical exertion (6 or more metabolic equivalents [METs]) than during other activities; however, the risk varies greatly depending on the patient's usual frequency of physical activity (32,33).

These data seem to contradict the widely held belief that regular exercise reduces the risk of cardiovascular events. The critical question, however, is whether or not the overall cardiovascular benefits of regular exercise outweigh the transient, additional risk. The relative risk of cardiac arrest during exercise compared with that observed at other times is 56 times greater among sedentary men but only 5 times greater among men with high levels of habitual physical activity (34). However, the overall risk of cardiac arrest among habitually active men is only 40% of that for sedentary men. The risk of acute MI during physical exertion also varies inversely with the individual's usual frequency of exercise. In one study, patients who exercised less than 4 and 4 or more times per week had relative risks of 6.9 and 1.3, respectively (33). Another investigation revealed that among persons who usually exercised less than 1, 1 to 2, 3 to 4, and 5 or more times per week, the respective relative risks were 107, 19.4, 8.6, and 2.4, respectively (32). Collectively, these findings suggest that regular exercise provides protection against the triggering of cardiac arrest and acute MI during vigorous exertion and at other times.

Incidence of Cardiovascular Complications

In the absence of significant cardiac pathology, the risk of exercise is extremely low. One retrospective survey of YMCA sports centers revealed 1 death and 1 cardiac arrest per 2,897,057 and 2,253,267 person-hours, respectively (35). A slightly higher rate of cardiovascular complications was reported in a 5-year retrospective survey of cardiac events that occurred during or immediately after exercise in community recreation centers. Forty-eight facilities reported 30 nonfatal and 38 fatal cardiovascular complications in 33,726,000 participant hours of exposure; the resultant mortality and morbidity rates were 1/887,526 person-hours and 1/1,124,200 person-hours of participation, respectively (36). One preventive medicine center had 2 nonfatal complications during a total of 374,798 person-hours of exercise, equivalent to maximum risk estimates (upper 95% confidence limits) ranging from 0.3 to 2.7 and 0.6 to 6.0 events per 10,000 person-hours for men and women, respectively (37). A recent review concluded that approximately 0.75 and 0.13 per 100,000 young male and female athletes and 6 per 100,000 middle-aged men die during vigorous exertion per year (27).

The incidence of cardiovascular complications during exercise is considerably greater among persons with cardiovascular disease than among presumably healthy adults. An early survey of 30 cardiac rehabilitation programs in North America revealed an average of 1 nonfatal and 1 fatal cardiovascular complication every 34,673 and 116,402 participant-hours, respectively (38). In 1986, investigators reported 29 cardiovascular events (21 cardiac arrests and 8 MIs), including 3 fatal events, during 2,351,916 hours of outpatient cardiac exercise therapy (39). Accordingly, the incidence of complications was 1 cardiac arrest per 111,996 patient hours, 1 MI per 293,990 patient-hours, and 1 fatality per 783,972 patient-hours of exercise. Unfortunately, the data from both surveys antedate the current use of risk stratification procedures, revascularization, and newer pharmacotherapies for coronary patients. Thus, these complication rates may not necessarily be extrapolated to contemporary cardiac patients. More recent studies suggest 1 major cardiovascular complication in every 60,000 participant-hours of outpatient cardiac exercise therapy (40–42). At this rate, a typical rehabilitation program with 95 patients exercising 3 hours per week could expect 1 cardiovascular event every 4 years. Finally, the risk of exercise in the morning appears to be no greater than that in the afternoon (42,43).

It remains difficult to identify persons who may be predisposed to cardiovascular complications during exercise. In general, the risk is lowest among healthy young adults and nonsmoking women, greater for those with symptoms and multiple risk factors, and highest in those with established cardiac disease. Although a profile of the "high-risk" patient has emerged (Box 1-2), one or more of these widely varied characteristics may pertain to a significant number of cardiac patients who will never experience an exercise-related cardiovascular complication. Regardless of the presence or absence of heart disease, the overall absolute risk of cardiovascular complications during exercise is low, especially when weighed against the associated health benefits.

Issues Regarding Preliminary Screening

Lack of uniformity in guidelines and policies for exercise testing and participation has led to much discussion and concern among exercise program

---

BOX 1-2. Characteristics Associated With Exercise-Related Cardiovascular Complications*

Clinical Status
- Multiple myocardial infarctions
- Impaired left ventricular function (ejection fraction of <30%)
- Rest or unstable angina pectoris
- Serious arrhythmias at rest
- High-grade left anterior descending lesions and/or significant (≥70% occlusion) multivessel atherosclerosis on angiography
- Low serum potassium

Exercise Training Participation
- Disregard for appropriate warm-up and cool-down
- Consistently exceeds prescribed training heart rate (i.e., intensity violators)

Exercise Test Data
- Low or high exercise tolerance (≤4 METs or ≥10 METs)
- Chronotropic impairment of drugs (<120 beats·min^{-1})
- Inotropic impairment (exertional hypotension with increasing workloads)
- Myocardial ischemia (angina and/or ST-depression of ≥0.2 mV)
- Malignant cardiac arrhythmias (especially in patients with impaired left ventricular function)

Other
- Cigarette smoker
- Male gender

*Adapted from Haskell WL. Cardiovascular complications during exercise training of cardiac patients. Circulation 1978;57:920–924; VanCamp SP, Peterson RA. Cardiovascular complications of outpatient cardiac rehabilitation programs. JAMA 1986;256:1160–1163; and Haskell WL. The efficacy and safety of exercise programs in cardiac rehabilitation. Med Sci Sports Exerc 1994;26:815–823.

personnel. Issues of primary concern include who should be tested, physician attendance during the test, use of maximal versus submaximal testing, how to risk stratify individuals before and after testing, and defining the appropriate level of supervision for exercise training.

No matter how rigid or conservative guidelines and policies might be, due to the vagaries of the atherosclerotic process, the accuracy in predicting which persons will have a cardiovascular complication during exercise remains imperfect. Some data are available to estimate the likelihood of such an event, but clinical and legal judgment, as well as common sense, must be used to make policy decisions involving the safety of participants.

Although diagnostic exercise testing is widely recommended to establish the safety of participation in vigorous exercise, "normal" electrocardiographic (ECG) responses have been observed in persons who subsequently experienced cardiovascular complications during exercise (44). Factors that may contribute to the apparently normal ECG responses include inadequate cardiac stress, insufficient ECG lead monitoring, drug therapy that masks anginal pain and/or ischemic ST-segment depression, and baseline ECG anomalies (e.g., substantial ST-segment depression at rest, left ventricular hypertrophy, left bundle-branch block) that make the exercise ECG uninterpretable with respect to evidence of myocardial ischemia. Recent studies have also shown that most acute MIs occur at sites in coronary arteries that previously had less than 70% obstruction on a recent angiogram (45). Apparently, a series of triggering events (called plaque rupture) can cause abrupt occlusion of a coronary artery, even at modest obstructions. Exercise testing is largely ineffective in detecting mild-to-moderate coronary lesions (i.e., less than 70% occlusion); in contrast, significant obstructions are often manifested as ischemic ST-segment depression, angina pectoris, or both. It is impractical to use diagnostic exercise testing to prevent untoward events because of the extremely low rate of cardiovascular complications in asymptomatic adults who exercise (35), the high rate of abnormal ECGs among physically active people (46), the exorbitant costs of mass exercise testing and follow-up of abnormal studies with expensive additional evaluations, and the uncertainties associated with exercise-induced ST-segment depression in persons with a low likelihood of heart disease (47).

Exercise testing is performed in many settings for nondiagnostic purposes, such as worksite health promotion programs, YMCAs and YWCAs, Jewish Community Centers, health clubs, and other community recreation centers. This testing tends to be functional (in many cases the ECG is not monitored) and is aimed at assessing physical fitness, providing a basis for the exercise prescription, or monitoring progress in an exercise program. The ACSM believes that this type of exercise testing is appropriate for fitness appraisal in conjunction with appropriate screening and when performed by qualified personnel. Such testing programs may be useful in educating participants about exercise and physical fitness and in helping to motivate sedentary individuals to exercise.

Recommendations to Reduce the Incidence and Severity of Complications During Exercise

Recommendations to reduce the incidence of musculoskeletal and cardiovascular complications during adult fitness and exercise-based cardiac rehabilitation programs include the following:

ENSURE MEDICAL CLEARANCE AND FOLLOW-UP

Medical clearance and follow-up, including maximal exercise testing, are essential screening components in physical conditioning programs for older adults (men 45 years or older, women 55 years or older), those at increased risk for cardiovascular events (e.g., 2 or more risk factors or 1 or more major signs or symptoms of coronary heart disease), and those with known cardiac, pulmonary, or metabolic disease, especially when vigorous exercise (more than 60% $\dot{V}O_{2max}$) is contemplated. Although routine exercise testing to forestall exercise-related cardiovascular complications has been questioned (35,44), exercise testing clearly aids in identifying the individual who is at increased risk for symptomatic or asymptomatic myocardial ischemia, malignant ventricular arrhythmias, or both. Exercise testing has the greatest diagnostic impact in symptomatic persons and those with an intermediate likelihood of coronary artery disease (i.e., a pretest probability of 10 to 90%) (see Chapter 5).

PROVIDE ON-SITE MEDICAL SUPERVISION, IF NECESSARY

The degree of medical supervision should be linked inversely with the stability of the client. Although traditional, medically supervised group programs are associated with increased cost and extended travel time, such programs are more appropriate for the growing medical complexity of candidates who may be at increased risk for exercise-induced complications. Medically supervised programs that are equipped with a defibrillator and appropriate emergency drugs act to reduce complications during exercise therapy. Recent reports indicate that approximately 80% of all patients with cardiac arrest occurring under such conditions are successfully resuscitated (40). Moreover, one 16-year experience (42) and the results of others (41) suggest that acute cardiac events can be treated successfully by nursing staff, assisted by exercise physiologists/technologists and emergency medical service backup, without direct gymnasium supervision by a physician (i.e., in the exercise room).

ESTABLISH AN EMERGENCY PLAN

Exercise program staff should be prepared to handle musculoskeletal and cardiovascular complications. This includes performing cardiopulmonary resuscitation (CPR), attending to orthopedic injuries (e.g., having ice immediately available), and stabilizing the participant for transport to an emergency center, if necessary. To this end, emergency drills and CPR mannequin practice should be conducted regularly. Cardiac rehabilitation programs should be medically supervised and equipped with a defibrillator and appropriate emergency drugs. The defibrillator should be charged and checked daily, and outdated drugs should be discarded and replaced. A "plan of action" should be established whereby specific responsibilities are assigned (e.g., perform CPR, call emergency medical services, transport crash ["code"] cart and defibrillator to the victim, clear other participants from the immediate area, wait for and direct the emergency medical service to the victim). Finally, telephone numbers for emergency assistance should be clearly labeled on all telephones; if possible, a direct line (e.g., "red phone") should be established.

PROMOTE PARTICIPANT EDUCATION

Exercisers should know their prescribed heart rate range for exercise training, how to take their pulse accurately, and the work rates that are compatible with their aerobic requirements for training. Rating of perceived exertion is strongly recommended as a useful and important adjunct to heart rate as an intensity guide (48). Participants should be strongly encouraged to remain at or below the prescribed intensity and counseled to discontinue exercise and seek medical advice if they experience major warning signs or symptoms (e.g., chest pain, light-headedness, abdominal discomfort, unusual fatigue or shortness of breath, palpitations) that may suggest a deterioration in their clinical status or impending cardiovascular complications. They should be educated to alert staff as to changes in their medication regimen because an updated target heart rate may be warranted.

INITIALLY ENCOURAGE MILD-TO-MODERATE EXERCISE INTENSITY

The lower the intensity, the less likely that an exercise-related complication will occur (40). Victims of exercise-related sudden cardiac death often have a history of poor compliance to the prescribed training heart rate range (i.e., exercise intensity violators) (49,50). These and other recent data suggest that unconventionally vigorous exercise is associated with an increased risk of musculoskeletal (51) and cardiovascular complications (52). The exercise leader should recognize that excessive frequency (>5 d·wk^{-1}) and duration (>45 min·session^{-1}) of training offer the participant little additional gain in aerobic capacity, yet the incidence of orthopedic injury increases disproportionately (53). However, it appears that formerly overweight or obese patients may need to expend the caloric equivalent of more than 60 minutes of moderate-to-vigorous activity on most or all days of the week to maintain their weight loss.

USE CONTINUOUS OR INSTANTANEOUS ECG MONITORING FOR SELECTED PARTICIPANTS

Unfortunately, heart disease may progress even among persons who maintain vigorous risk factor modification and exercise training programs (54). The cardiac response to physical stress may deteriorate over time. As an alternative to costly continuous or transtelephonic ECG monitoring, instantaneous electrocardiography (recording ECG rate, rhythm, and repolarization through defibrillator paddles) may be used to screen for ischemic ST-segment depression, threatening ventricular arrhythmias, and exercise intensity violators (55). Participants at increased risk and those with documented disease should be encouraged to practice frequent self-monitoring of pulse rate and to obtain instant ECGs when heart rate or rhythm irregularities are detected.

EMPHASIZE APPROPRIATE WARM-UP AND COOL-DOWN PROCEDURES BEFORE AND AFTER VIGOROUS EXERCISE, INCLUDING STRETCHING

A disproportionate number of cardiovascular complications have been reported during the warm-up and cool-down phases of cardiac exercise training (38). A progressive warm-up that includes both musculoskeletal (e.g., stretching, flexibility exercises) and cardiorespiratory activities may prevent musculoskeletal injuries (3) and decrease the occurrence of ECG and wall motion abnormalities that are suggestive of myocardial ischemia and/or ventricular irritability—abnormalities that may be provoked by sudden strenuous exertion (56,57). A cool-down enhances venous return during recovery, reducing the possibility of postexercise hypotension and related sequelae. Moreover, it ameliorates the potential deleterious effects of the postexercise rise in plasma catecholamines (58). Flexibility exercises can be done as part of the warm-up, cool-down, or both. In contrast, intermittent mild-to-moderate intensity activity can generally be performed without a warm-up or cool-down.

MODIFY RECREATIONAL GAME RULES AND MINIMIZE COMPETITION

The ability of the participant to regulate exercise intensity is easier during walking, jogging, or stationary cycle ergometry as compared with recreational games. However, recreational games provide a varied exercise stimulus and are popular among participants. Nonetheless, somatic and myocardial aerobic demands during game activities are influenced, to a large extent, by team members and opponent expertise. Also, the excitement of competition may increase sympathetic activity and catecholamine levels, lowering the threshold to ventricular fibrillation (59). The exercise leader should minimize competition and modify game rules to control the energy cost and heart rate response to play.

MAINTAIN SUPERVISION DURING THE RECOVERY PERIOD

Because cardiovascular complications often occur after exercise in the vulnerable tapering-off period, staff should remain "on-site" until all clients or patients have exited the shower and changing areas.

TAKE PRECAUTIONS IN THE COLD

Dynamic exercise in cold weather is relatively safe if proper clothing is worn and the wind chill factor is considered (see Appendix E) (60). For example, at 10°F in a 20 mi·hr^{-1} wind, the cooling effect is equivalent to calm air at −25°F. Inhalation of or exposure to cold air may increase stroke volume and cardiac work, activate the thermoregulatory reflex which causes cutaneous systemic vasoconstriction to conserve body heat, and trigger reflex spasm or constriction of the coronary arteries (61). The consequent increases in peripheral vascular resistance and arterial pressure coupled with a reduction in coronary blood flow can precipitate symptomatic or silent myocardial ischemia, which may be arrhythmogenic (62). Recommendations for exercising in cold weather are summarized in Appendix E and include the following: change wet clothing, particularly socks and gloves; wear several layers of light clothing that can be shed or replaced as needed; stay moving to increase body heat production; wear a hat or cap; and protect body areas that have a large surface area-to-mass ratio—for example, the hands and feet. For those who suffer from angina when inhaling cold air, discomfort can be reduced or alleviated by wearing a face mask to warm the inspired air (63).

CONSIDER ADDED CARDIAC DEMANDS IN THE HEAT

Exercise in hot and humid weather may constitute an even greater hazard for the exercisers with documented or occult coronary disease. Heart rate and myocardial oxygen demands increase disproportionately to keep up with increasing aerobic requirements. Persons who are not acclimated to heat and who are exposed to temperatures greater than 24°C experience added heart rate increases of 1 beat·min⁻ per °C (Fig. 1-2) and 2 to 4 beats · min⁻ per °C with concomitant increased humidity (64). Recommendations for exercising in hot and/or humid weather are summarized in Appendix E and include the following: maintain hydration by drinking fluids before, during, and after activity; decrease the exercise dosage (e.g., speed, duration, resistance) at temperatures greater than 27°C and/or greater than 75% relative humidity; exercise during the cooler parts of the day; wear light

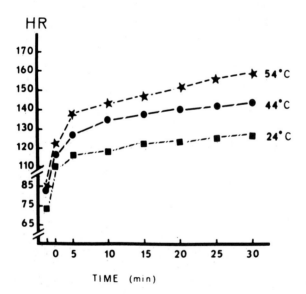

FIGURE 1-2. Influence of environmental temperature on heart rate responses at a constant work rate over time. Heart rate (HR) increases approximately 1 beat·min⁻¹ for each degree Celsius increment in ambient temperature above 24°C. (Adapted from Pandolf KB, Cafarelli E, Noble BJ, et al. Hyperthermia: effect on exercise prescription. Arch Phys Med Rehabil 1975;56:524–526.)

clothing and shorts to facilitate cooling by evaporation; and start gradually to allow the body at least 4 to 14 days to acclimatize to the heat (65).

References

1. Pate RR, Pratt M, Blair SN, et al. Physical activity and public health: a recommendation from the Centers for Disease Control and Prevention and the American College of Sports Medicine. JAMA 1995;273:402–407.
2. United States Department of Health and Human Services. Physical activity and health: a report of the Surgeon General. Atlanta, GA: US Department of Health and Human Services, Centers for Disease Control and Prevention, National Center for Chronic Disease Prevention and Health Promotion, 1996.
3. Pollock ML, Gaesser GA, Butcher JD. The recommended quantity and quality of exercise for developing and maintaining cardiorespiratory and muscular fitness, and flexibility in healthy adults. Med Sci Sports Exerc 1998;30:975–991.
4. Hahn RA, Teutsch SM, Rothenberg RB, et al. Excess death from nine chronic diseases in the United States, 1986. JAMA 1990;264:2654–2659.
5. Caspersen CJ, Powell KE, Christenson GM. Physical activity, exercise, and physical fitness. Public Health Rep 1985;100:125–131.
6. Franklin BA, Roitman JL. Cardiorespiratory adaptations to exercise. In: Roitman JL, ed. ACSM's Resource Manual for Guidelines for Exercise Testing and Prescription. Baltimore: Williams & Wilkins, 1998:156–163.
7. Wenger NK, Froelicher ES, Smith LK, et al. Cardiac rehabilitation. Clinical practice guidelines No. 17. Rockville, MD: US Department of Health and Human Services, Public Health Service, Agency for Health Care Policy and Research and the National Heart, Lung and Blood Institute, AHCPR Publication No. 96-0672, October 1995.
8. Whaley MH, Kaminsky LA. Epidemiology of physical activity, physical fitness and selected chronic diseases. In: Roitman JL, ed. ACSM's Resource Manual for Guidelines for Exercise Testing and Prescription. Baltimore: Williams & Wilkins, 1998:13–26.
9. Blair SN. Physical activity, physical fitness, and health. Res Q Exerc Sport 1993;64:365–376.
10. Paffenbarger RS, Kampert JB, Lee IM, et al. Changes in physical activity and other lifeway patterns influencing longevity. Med Sci Sports Exerc 1994;26:857–865.
11. Blair SN, Kohl HW, Barlow CE, et al. Changes in physical fitness and all-cause mortality: a prospective study of healthy and unhealthy men. JAMA 1995;273:1093–1098.
12. Fuller T, Movahed A. Current review of exercise testing: application and interpretation. Clin Cardiol 1987;10:189–200.
13. Rochmis P, Blackburn H. Exercise tests: a survey of procedures, safety, and litigation experience in approximately 170,000 tests. JAMA 1971;217:1061–1066.
14. Stuart RJ Jr, Ellestad MH. National survey of exercise stress testing facilities. Chest 1980;77:94–97.
15. Young DZ, Lampert S, Graboys TB, et al. Safety of maximal exercise testing in patients at high risk for ventricular arrhythmia. Circulation 1984;70:184–191.
16. Scherer D, Kaltenbach M. Frequency of life-threatening complications associated with exercise testing. Dtsch Med Wochenschr 1979;33:1161–1165.
17. Atterhog JH, Jonsson B, Samuelsson R. Exercise testing: a prospective study of complication rates. Am Heart J 1979;98:572–579.
18. Gibbons L, Blair SN, Kohl HW, et al. The safety of maximal exercise testing. Circulation 1989;80:846–852.
19. Cahalin LP, Blessey RL, Kummer D, et al. The safety of exercise testing performed independently by physical therapists. J Cardiopulm Rehabil 1987;7:269–276.
20. Blessey RL. Exercise testing by non-physician health care professionals: complication rates, clinical competencies and future trends. Exercise Standards and Malpractice Reporter 1989;3:69–74.
21. Lem V, Krivokapich J, Child JS. A nurse-supervised exercise stress testing laboratory. Heart Lung 1985;14:280–284.
22. DeBusk RF. Exercise test supervision: time for a reassessment. Exercise Standards and Malpractice Reporter 1988;2:65–70.
23. Knight JA, Laubach CA, Butcher RJ, et al. Supervision of clinical exercise testing by exercise physiologists. Am J Cardiol 1995;75:390–391.
24. Franklin BA, Gordon S, Timmis GC, et al. Is direct physician supervision of exercise stress testing routinely necessary? Chest 1997;111:262–265.
25. Blair SN. How to assess exercise habits and physical fitness. In: Matarazzo JD, Weiss SM, Herd JA, et al, eds. Behavioral Health: A Handbook of Health Enhancement and Disease Prevention. New York: John Wiley & Sons, 1984:424–447.

26. Shephard RJ. Can we identify those for whom exercise is hazardous? Sports Med 1984;1:75–86.
27. Thompson PD. The cardiovascular complications of vigorous physical activity. Arch Intern Med 1996;156:2297–2302.
28. Kestin AS, Ellis PA, Barnard MR, et al. Effect of strenuous exercise on platelet activation state and reactivity. Circulation 1993;88:1502–1511.
29. Thompson PD, Funk EJ, Carleton RA, et al. Incidence of death during jogging in Rhode Island from 1975 to 1980. JAMA 1982;247:2535–2538.
30. Koplan JP. Cardiovascular deaths while running. JAMA 1979;242:2578–2579.
31. Cobb LA, Weaver WD. Exercise: a risk for sudden death in patients with coronary heart disease. J Am Coll Cardiol 1986;7:215–219.
32. Mittleman MA, Maclure M, Tofler GH, et al. Triggering of acute MI by heavy physical exertion: protection against triggering by regular exertion. N Engl J Med 1993;329:1677–1683.
33. Willich SN, Lewis M, Löwel H, et al. Physical exertion as a trigger of acute myocardial infarction. N Engl J Med 1993;329:1684–1690.
34. Siscovick DS, Weiss NS, Fletcher RH, et al. The incidence of primary cardiac arrest during vigorous exercise. N Engl J Med 1984;311:874–877.
35. Malinow MR, McGarry DL, Kuehl KS. Is exercise testing indicated for asymptomatic active people? J Cardiac Rehabil 1984;4:376–379.
36. Vander L, Franklin, B, Rubenfire M. Cardiovascular complications of recreational physical activity. Physician Sportsmed 1982;10:89–94.
37. Gibbons LW, Cooper KH, Meyer BM, et al. The acute cardiac risk of strenuous exercise. JAMA 1980;244:1799–1801.
38. Haskell WL. Cardiovascular complications during exercise training of cardiac patients. Circulation 1978;57:920–924.
39. VanCamp SP, Peterson RA. Cardiovascular complications of outpatient cardiac rehabilitation programs. JAMA 1986;256:1160–1163.
40. Haskell WL. The efficacy and safety of exercise programs in cardiac rehabilitation. Med Sci Sports Exerc 1994;26:815–823.
41. Vongvanich P, Paul-Labrador MJ, Merz CNB. Safety of medically supervised exercise in a cardiac rehabilitation center. Am J Cardiol 1996;77:1383–1385.
42. Franklin BA, Bonzheim K, Gordon S, et al. Safety of medically supervised outpatient cardiac rehabilitation exercise therapy: a 16-year follow-up. Chest 1998;114:902–906.
43. Murray PM, Herrington DM, Pettus CW, et al. Should patients with heart disease exercise in the morning or afternoon? Arch Intern Med 1993;153:833–836.
44. Thompson PD, Stern MP, Williams P, et al. Death during jogging or running: a study of 18 cases. JAMA 1979;242:1265–1267.
45. Smith SC. Risk-reduction therapy: the challenge to change. Circulation 1996;93:2205–2211.
46. Spirito P, Maron BJ, Bonow RO, et al. Prevalence and significance of an abnormal ST-segment response to exercise in a young athletic population. Am J Cardiol 1983;51:1663–1666.
47. Blair SN, Kohl HW, Barlow CE. Cardiovascular fitness and cardiovascular disease. In: Fletcher GF, ed. Cardiovascular Responses to Exercise. Mt. Kisco, NY: Futura Publishing Co., 1994.
48. Borg G. Borg's Perceived Exertion and Pain Scales. Champaign, IL: Human Kinetics, 1998.
49. Mead WF, Pyfer HR, Trombold JC, et al. Successful resuscitation of two near simultaneous cases of cardiac arrest with a review of fifteen cases occurring during supervised exercise. Circulation 1976;53:187–189.
50. Hossack KF, Hartwig R. Cardiac arrest associated with supervised cardiac rehabilitation. J Cardiac Rehab 1982;2:402–408.
51. Kilbom A, Hartley L, Saltin B, et al. Physical training in sedentary middle-aged and older men. I. Medical evaluation. Scand J Clin Lab Invest 1969;24:315–322.
52. Friedwald VE Jr, Spence DW. Sudden cardiac death associated with exercise: the risk-benefit issue. Am J Cardiol 1990;66:183–188.
53. Pollock ML, Gettman LR, Milesis CA, et al. Effects of frequency and duration of training on attrition and incidence of injury. Med Sci Sports 1977;9:31–36.
54. Haskell WL, Alderman EL, Fair JM, et al. Effects of intensive multiple risk factor reduction on coronary atherosclerosis and clinical cardiac events in men and women with coronary artery disease: The Stanford Coronary Risk Intervention Project (SCRIP). Circulation 1994;89:975–990.
55. Franklin BA, Reed PS, Gordon S, et al. Instantaneous electrocardiography: a simple screening technique for cardiac exercise programs. Chest 1989;96:174–177.
56. Barnard RJ, MacAlpin R, Kattus AA, et al. Ischemic response to sudden strenuous exercise in healthy men. Circulation 1973;48:936–942.
57. Foster C, Anholm JD, Hellman CK, et al. Left ventricular function during sudden strenuous exercise. Circulation 1981;63:592–596.
58. Dimsdale JE, Hartley H, Guiney T, et al. Postexercise peril: plasma catecholamines and exercise. JAMA 1984;25:630–632.
59. Lown B, Verrier RL, Rabinowitz SH. Neural and psychologic mechanisms and the problem of sudden cardiac death. Am J Cardiol 1977;39:890-902.

60. Pollock ML, Wilmore JH, Fox SM. Exercise in Health and Disease: Evaluation and Prescription for Prevention and Rehabilitation. Philadelphia: WB Saunders, 1984:384.
61. Hattenhauer M, Neill WA. The effect of cold air inhalation on angina pectoris and myocardial oxygen supply. Circulation 1975;51:1053–1058.
62. Hoberg E, Schuler G, Kunze B, et al. Silent myocardial ischemia as a potential link between lack of premonitoring symptoms and increased risk of cardiac arrest during physical stress. Am J Cardiol 1990;65:583–589.
63. Kavanagh T. A cold weather "jogging mask" for angina patients. Can Med Assoc J 1970;103:1290–1291.
64. Pandolf KB, Cafarelli E, Noble BJ, et al. Hyperthermia: effect on exercise prescription. Arch Phys Med Rehabil 1975;56:524–526.
65. Lamb DR. Physiology of Exercise: Responses and Adaptations. New York: Macmillan, 1978.

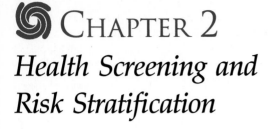

CHAPTER 2
Health Screening and Risk Stratification

This chapter contains guidelines related to preparticipation health screening and risk stratification for both preventive and rehabilitative exercise program professionals. To this end, the American College of Sports Medicine (ACSM) recognizes other published guidelines by the American Heart Association (AHA) and the American Association of Cardiovascular and Pulmonary Rehabilitation (AACVPR) (1–3). Exercise program professionals are encouraged to review each of these other documents when establishing program-specific policies for preparticipation health screening and medical clearance.

PREPARTICIPATION HEALTH SCREENING

It is important to provide an initial screening of participants relative to risk factors and/or symptoms for various chronic cardiovascular, pulmonary, and metabolic diseases to optimize safety during exercise testing and participation and to develop a sound and effective exercise prescription. The purposes of the preparticipation health screening include the following:

- Identification and exclusion of individuals with medical contraindications to exercise.
- Identification of individuals at increased risk for disease because of age, symptoms, and/or risk factors who should undergo a medical evaluation and exercise testing before starting an exercise program.
- Identification of persons with clinically significant disease who should participate in a medically supervised exercise program.
- Identification of individuals with other special needs.

Health screening procedures must be valid, cost-effective, and time-efficient. Procedures range from self-administered questionnaires to sophisticated diagnostic tests. Exercise program professionals should establish pre-participation screening procedures that are appropriate for their clients or a facility's target population. The Physical Activity Readiness Questionnaire (PAR-Q) (4) has been recommended as a minimal standard for entry into moderate-intensity exercise programs (Fig. 2-1). The PAR-Q was designed

Physical Activity Readiness
Questionnaire - PAR-Q
(revised 1994)

PAR - Q & YOU
(A Questionnaire for People Aged 15 to 69)

Regular physical activity is fun and healthy, and increasingly more people are starting to become more active every day. Being active is very safe for most people. However, some people should check with their doctor before they start becoming much more physically active.

If you are planning to become much more physically active than you are now, start by answering the seven questions in the box below. If you are between the ages of 15 and 69, the PAR-Q will tell you if you should check with your doctor before you start. If you are over 69 years of age, and you are not used to being very active, check with your doctor.

Common sense is your best guide when you answer these questions. Please read the questions carefully and answer each one honestly: check YES or NO.

YES	NO		
☐	☐	1.	Has you doctor ever said that you have a heart condition <u>and</u> that you should only do physical activity recommended by a doctor?
☐	☐	2.	Do you feel pain in your chest when you do physical activity?
☐	☐	3.	In the past month, have you had chest pain when you were not doing physical activity?
☐	☐	4.	Do you lose your balance because of dizziness or do you ever lose consciousness?
☐	☐	5.	Do you have a bone or joint problem that could be made worse by a change in your physical activity?
☐	☐	6.	Is your doctor currently prescribing drugs (for example, water pills) for your blood pressure or heart condition?
☐	☐	7.	Do you know of <u>any other reason</u> why you should not do physical activity?

If
you
answered

YES to one or more questions

Talk with your doctor by phone or in person BEFORE you start becoming much more physically active or BEFORE you have a fitness appraisal. Tell your doctor about the PAR-Q and which questions you answered YES.

- You may be able to do any activity you want—as long as you start slowly and build up gradually. Or, you may need to restrict your activities to those which are safe for you. Talk with your doctor about the kinds of activities you wish to participate in and follow his/her advice.
- Find out which community programs are safe and helpful for you.

NO to all questions

If you answered NO honestly to <u>all</u> PAR-Q questions, you can be reasonably sure that you can:

- start becoming much more physically active—begin slowly and build up gradually. This is the safest and easiest way to go.
- take part in a fitness appraisal—this is an excellent way to determine your basic fitness so that you can plan the best way for you to live actively.

DELAY BECOMING MUCH MORE ACTIVE:
- if you are not feeling well because of a temporary illness such as a cold or a fever—wait until you feel better; or
- if you are or may be pregnant—talk to your doctor before you start becoming more active.

Please note: If your health changes so that you then answer YES to any of the above questions, tell your fitness or health professional. Ask whether you should change your physical activity plan.

<u>Informed Use of the PAR-Q:</u> The Canadian Society for Exercise Physiology, Health Canada, and their agents assume no liability for persons who undertake physical activity, and if in doubt after completing this questionnaire, consult your doctor prior to physical activity.

You are encouraged to copy the PAR-Q but only if you use the entire form

NOTE: If the PAR-Q is being given to a person before he or she participates in a physical activity program or a fitness appraisal, this section may be used for legal or administrative purposes.

I have read, understood and completed this questionnaire. Any questions I had were answered to my full satisfaction.

NAME _____

SIGNATURE _____   DATE _____

SIGNATURE OF PARENT _____   WITNESS _____
or GUARDIAN (for participants under the age of majority)

© *Canadian Society for Exercise Physiology*
Société canadienne de physiologie de l'exercice

Supported by: Health   Santé
Canada   Canada

FIGURE 2-1. PAR-Q form. (Reprinted with permission from the Canadian Society for Exercise Physiology, Inc., 1994.)

TABLE 2-1. Coronary Artery Disease Risk Factor Thresholds for Use With ACSM Risk Stratification*

Risk Factors	Defining Criteria
Positive	
Family history	Myocardial infarction, coronary revascularization, or sudden death before 55 years of age in father or other male first-degree relative (i.e., brother or son), or before 65 years of age in mother or other female first-degree relative (i.e., sister or daughter)
Cigarette smoking	Current cigarette smoker or those who quit within the previous 6 months
Hypertension	Systolic blood pressure of ≥140 mm Hg or diastolic ≥90 mm Hg, confirmed by measurements on at least 2 separate occasions, or on antihypertensive medication
Hypercholesterolemia	Total serum cholesterol of >200 mg/dL (5.2 mmol/L) or high-density lipoprotein cholesterol of <35 mg/dL (0.9 mmol/L), or on lipid-lowering medication. If low-density lipoprotein cholesterol is available, use >130 mg/dL (3.4 mmol/L) rather than total cholesterol of >200 mg/dL
Impaired fasting glucose	Fasting blood glucose of ≥110 mg/dL (6.1 mmol/L) confirmed by measurements on at least 2 separate occasions (7)
Obesity[†]	Body Mass Index of ≥30 kg/m² (8), or waist girth of >100 cm (9)
Sedentary lifestyle	Persons not participating in a regular exercise program or meeting the minimal physical activity recommendations[‡] from the U.S. Surgeon General's report (10)
Negative	
High serum HDL cholesterol[§]	>60 mg/dL (1.6 mmol/L)

*Adapted from Expert Panel on Detection, Evaluation, and Treatment of High Blood Cholesterol in Adults. Summary of the second report of the National Cholesterol Education Program (NCEP) expert panel on detection, evaluation, and treatment of high blood cholesterol in adults (Adult Treatment Panel II). JAMA 1993;269:3015–3023.

†Professional opinions vary regarding the most appropriate markers and thresholds for obesity; therefore, exercise professionals should use clinical judgment when evaluating this risk factor.

‡Accumulating 30 minutes or more of moderate physical activity on most days of the week.

§It is common to sum risk factors in making clinical judgments. If high-density lipoprotein (HDL) cholesterol is high, subtract one risk factor from the sum of positive risk factors because high HDL decreases CAD risk.

BOX 2-1. Major Signs or Symptoms Suggestive of Cardiovascular and Pulmonary Disease*

- Pain, discomfort (or other anginal equivalent) in the chest, neck, jaw, arms, or other areas that may be due to ischemia
- Shortness of breath at rest or with mild exertion
- Dizziness or syncope
- Orthopnea or paroxysmal nocturnal dyspnea
- Ankle edema
- Palpitations or tachycardia
- Intermittent claudication
- Known heart murmur
- Unusual fatigue or shortness of breath with usual activities

*These symptoms must be interpreted in the clinical context in which they appear because they are not all specific for cardiovascular, pulmonary, or metabolic disease. For clarification and discussion of the clinical significance of the signs or symptoms, see reference 11.

to identify the small number of adults for whom physical activity might be inappropriate or those who should receive medical advice concerning the most suitable type of activity (5). In addition, the ACSM and the AHA have copublished a preparticipation screening questionnaire specifically designed for health/fitness facilities (2). Regardless of the type of preparticipation screening employed, information should be interpreted by qualified staff, and results should be documented (2). Exercise professionals should recognize that many sedentary individuals can safely begin a moderate-intensity physical activity program without the need for extensive medical screening.

However, it is recommended that persons interested in participating in organized exercise programs be evaluated for selected risk factors associated with the development of coronary artery disease (CAD) (Table 2-1) (6–10) and for signs or symptoms suggestive of cardiovascular, pulmonary, or metabolic disease (Box 2-1) (11). The risk factor list presented in Table 2-1 should not be viewed as an all-inclusive list of risk factors for CAD, but rather as a list of risk factors with clinically relevant thresholds which should be considered collectively when making decisions about the level of medical clearance, the need for exercise testing prior to program entry, and the level of supervision for both exercise testing and exercise program participation. Other variables (e.g., major depression) have also been suggested as positive risk factors in the primary and secondary prevention of CAD (3).

ACSM RISK STRATIFICATION

Once symptom and risk factor screening has occurred, it is recommended that individuals being considered for exercise testing or who plan to increase their physical activity be stratified based on the likelihood of untoward events. This stratification becomes increasingly important as disease prevalence increases in the population under consideration. Using age, health status, symptom, and risk factor information, participants and patients can be initially classified into one of three risk strata (Box 2-2) for triage and preliminary decision making.

No set of guidelines for exercise testing and participation can cover all situations. Local circumstances and policies vary, and specific program procedures are also properly diverse. To provide some general guidance on the need for a medical examination and exercise testing prior to participation in a moderate-to-vigorous exercise program, ACSM suggests the recommendations presented in Table 2-2 for determining when a diagnostic medical examination and exercise test are appropriate and when physician supervision is recommended. Although the testing guidelines are less rigorous for those individuals considered to be low risk, the information gathered from an exercise test may be useful in establishing a safe and effective exercise prescription for these individuals. The exercise testing recommendations reflect the notion that the risk of untoward events increases as a function of exercise intensity (e.g., moderate versus vigorous). Although several descriptions of "moderate" and "vigorous" exercise are listed in Table 2-2, exercise professionals should choose the most applicable definition for their setting when making decisions about the level of screening prior to exercise training and physician supervision during exercise testing. The degree of medical supervision of exercise tests varies appropriately from physician-supervised tests to situations in which there may be no physician present. The degree of physician supervision may vary with local policies and circumstances, the health status of the patient, and the experience of the laboratory staff. The appropriate protocol should be based

---

BOX 2-2. Initial ACSM Risk Stratification

Low risk
    Younger individuals* who are asymptomatic and meet no more than one risk factor threshold from Table 2-1
Moderate risk
    Older individuals (men $\geq$ 45 years of age; women $\geq$ 55 years of age) or those who meet the threshold for two or more risk factors from Table 2-1
High risk
    Individuals with one or more signs/symptoms listed in Box 2-1 or known cardiovascular,† pulmonary,‡ or metabolic§ disease

*Men < 45 years of age; women < 55 years of age.

†Cardiac, peripheral vascular, or cerebrovascular disease.

‡Chronic obstructive pulmonary disease, asthma, interstitial lung disease, or cystic fibrosis (see reference 12).

§Diabetes mellitus (types 1 and 2), thyroid disorders, renal or liver disease.

TABLE 2-2. ACSM Recommendations for (A) Current Medical Examination* and Exercise Testing Prior to Participation and (B) Physician Supervision of Exercise Tests

	Low Risk	Moderate Risk	High Risk
A.			
Moderate exercise[†]	Not necessary[‡]	Not necessary	Recommended
Vigorous exercise[§]	Not necessary	Recommended	Recommended
B.			
Submaximal test	Not necessary	Not necessary	Recommended
Maximal test	Not necessary	Recommended[‖]	Recommended

*Within the past year (see reference 2).

†Absolute moderate exercise is defined as activities that are approximately 3–6 METs or the equivalent of brisk walking at 3 to 4 mph for most healthy adults (13). Nevertheless, a pace of 3 to 4 mph might be considered to be "hard" to "very hard" by some sedentary, older persons. Moderate exercise may alternatively be defined as an intensity well within the individual's capacity, one which can be comfortably sustained for a prolonged period of time (~45 min), which has a gradual initiation and progression, and is generally noncompetitive. If an individual's exercise capacity is known, relative moderate exercise may be defined by the range 40–60% maximal oxygen uptake.

‡The designation of "Not necessary" reflects the notion that a medical examination, exercise test, and physician supervision of exercise testing would not be essential in the preparticipation screening; however, they should not be viewed as inappropriate.

§Vigorous exercise is defined as activities of >6 METs. Vigorous exercise may alternatively be defined as exercise intense enough to represent a substantial cardiorespiratory challenge. If an individual's exercise capacity is known, vigorous exercise may be defined as an intensity of >60% maximal oxygen uptake.

‖When physician supervision of exercise testing is "Recommended," the physician should be in close proximity and readily available should there be an emergent need.

on the age, health status, and physical activity level of the person to be tested.

In all situations where exercise testing is performed, site personnel should be trained and certified in cardiopulmonary resuscitation. Whenever possible, testing should be performed by ACSM-certified personnel because these certifications evaluate knowledge, skills, and abilities directly related to exercise testing.

RISK STRATIFICATION FOR CARDIAC PATIENTS

For cardiac populations, patients may be further stratified regarding safety during exercise using published guidelines (3). Risk stratification criteria from the AACVPR are presented in Table 2-3 (3). Recommendations for the

TABLE 2-3. American Association of Cardiovascular and Pulmonary Rehabilitation (AACVPR) Risk Stratification Criteria for Cardiac Patients*

Low Risk	Moderate Risk	High Risk
• No significant left ventricular dysfunction (ejection fraction of >50%) • No resting or exercise-induced complex arrhythmias • Uncomplicated MI; CABG; angioplasty, atherectomy, or stent: — Absence of CHF or signs/symptoms of postevent ischemia • Normal hemodynamics with exercise or recovery • Asymptomatic including absence of angina with exertion or recovery • Functional capacity of ≥7 METs[†] • Absence of clinical depression **Low-risk classification is assumed when each of the descriptors in the category is present.**	• Moderately impaired left ventricular function (ejection fraction = 40–49%) • Signs/symptoms including angina at moderate levels of exercise (5–6.9 METs) or in recovery **Moderate risk is assumed for patients who do not meet the classification of either high or low risk.**	• Decreased left ventricular function (ejection fraction of <40%) • Survivor of cardiac arrest or sudden death • Complex ventricular arrhythmias at rest or with exercise • MI or cardiac surgery complicated by cardiogenic shock, CHF, and/or signs/symptoms of post-event/procedure ischemia • Abnormal hemodynamics with exercise (especially flat or decreasing systolic blood pressure or chronotropic incompetence with increasing workload) • Signs/symptoms including angina pectoris at low levels of exercise (<5.0 METs) or in recovery • Functional capacity of <5.0 METs[†] • Clinically significant depression **High-risk classification is assumed with the presence of any one of the descriptors included in this category.**

*Adapted from American Association of Cardiovascular and Pulmonary Rehabilitation. Guidelines for Cardiac Rehabilitation and Secondary Prevention Programs. 3rd ed. Champaign, IL: Human Kinetics, 1999.

†Note: If *measured* functional capacity is not available, this variable is not considered in the risk-stratification process.

Abbreviations: MI, myocardial infarction; CABG, coronary artery bypass graft surgery; CHF, congestive heart failure; METs, metabolic equivalents (1 MET = 3.5 mL·kg⁻¹·min⁻¹; resting oxygen consumption).

duration of monitored exercise training and/or education based on the risk factor profile have now been suggested (14). The AHA has developed a more extensive risk classification system for medical clearance of cardiac patients (1) (Box 2-3). The AHA guidelines provide recommendations for participant and/or patient monitoring and supervision and for activity restriction. Exercise program professionals should recognize that the AHA guidelines do not consider comorbidities (e.g., type 1 diabetes mellitus, morbid obesity, severe pulmonary disease, or debilitating neurologic or orthopedic conditions) that could result in modification of the recommendations for monitoring and supervision during exercise training.

Modifying Coronary Risk Status

Although the degree of left ventricular dysfunction and residual myocardial ischemia, manifested as significant ST-segment depression, angina pectoris, or both, largely determines the risk of future cardiac events, risk status can be influenced by several interventions and lifestyle changes (Fig. 2-2). Multicenter trials have confirmed that mortality from acute myocardial infarction can be decreased by approximately 25% with early thrombolytic reperfusion or emergent percutaneous transluminal angioplasty. Patients

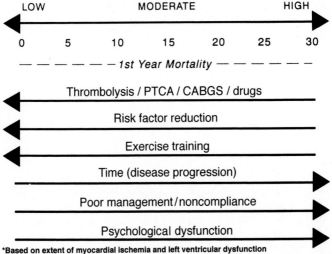

FIGURE 2-2. Variables that may potentially influence the patient's risk status. PTCA, percutaneous transluminal coronary angioplasty; CABGS, coronary artery bypass graft surgery.

BOX 2-3. American Heart Association (AHA) Risk Stratification Criteria*

Class A: Apparently Healthy
- (1) Individuals < age 40 who have no symptoms of or known presence of heart disease or major coronary risk factors and (2) individuals of any age without known heart disease or major risk factors and who have a normal exercise test
- Activity guidelines: No restrictions other than basic guidelines
- ECG and blood pressure monitoring: Not required
- Supervision required: None

Class B: Documented, stable cardiovascular disease with low risk for vigorous exercise but slightly greater than for apparently healthy individuals
- Moderate activity is not believed to be associated with increased risk in this group
- Includes individuals with (1) CAD (MI, CABGS, PTCA, angina pectoris, abnormal exercise test, and abnormal coronary angiograms) whose condition is stable and who have the clinical characteristics outlined below; (2) valvular heart disease; (3) congenital heart disease; (4) cardiomyopathy; and (5) exercise test abnormalities that do not meet the criteria outlined in Class C below
- Clinical characteristics: (1) New York Heart Association (NYHA) class 1 or 2; (2) exercise capacity of >6 METs; (3) no evidence of heart failure; (4) free of ischemia or angina at rest or on the exercise test at or below 6 METs; (5) appropriate rise in systolic blood pressure during exercise; (6) no sequential ectopic ventricular contractions; and (7) ability to satisfactorily self-monitor intensity of activity
- Activity guidelines: Activity should be individualized with exercise prescription by qualified personnel trained in basic CPR or with electronic monitoring at home
- ECG and blood pressure monitoring: Only during the early prescription phase of training, usually 6 to 12 sessions
- Supervision required: Medical supervision during prescription sessions and nonmedical supervision for other exercise sessions until the individual understands how to monitor his or her activity

Class C: Those at moderate-to-high risk for cardiac complications during exercise and/or unable to self-regulate activity or to understand recommended activity level
- Includes individuals with (1) CAD with the clinical characteristics outlined below; (2) cardiomyopathy; (3) valvular heart disease; (4) exercise test abnormalities not directly related to ischemia; (5) previous episode of ventricular fibrillation or cardiac arrest that did not occur in the presence of an acute ischemic event or cardiac procedure; (6) complex ventricular arrhythmias that are uncontrolled at mild to moderate work intensities with medication; (7) three-vessel disease or left main disease; and (8) low ejection fraction (<30%)

- Clinical characteristics: (1) Two or more MIs; (2) NYHA class 3 or greater; (3) exercise capacity of <6 METs; (4) ischemic horizontal or downsloping ST depression of 4 mm or more or angina during exercise; (5) fall in systolic blood pressure with exercise; (6) a medical problem that the physician believes may be life-threatening; (7) previous episode of primary cardiac arrest; and (8) ventricular tachycardia at a workload of <6 METs
- Activity guidelines: Activity should be individualized with exercise prescription by qualified personnel
- ECG and blood pressure monitoring: Continuous during exercise sessions until safety is established, usually in 6 to 12 sessions or more
- Supervision required: Medical supervision during all exercise sessions until safety is established

Class D: Unstable disease with activity restriction

- Includes individuals with (1) unstable ischemia; (2) heart failure that is not compensated; (3) uncontrolled arrhythmias; (4) severe and symptomatic aortic stenosis; and (5) other conditions that could be aggravated by exercise
- Activity guidelines: No activity is recommended for conditioning purposes. Attention should be directed to treating the subject and restoring him or her to class C or higher. Daily activities must be prescribed based on individual assessment by the subject's personal physician

*Modified from Fletcher GA, Balady G, Froelicher VF, et al. Exercise standards: a statement for health care professionals from the American Heart Association. Circulation 1995;91:580–615.

at moderate risk may experience a reduction in ischemic signs or symptoms and recurrent coronary events from elective coronary revascularization. Aggressive risk factor interventions aimed at smoking cessation and cholesterol reduction, and efficacious drugs, including β-blockers, aspirin or other antiplatelet agents/anticoagulants, angiotensin-converting enzyme inhibitors, and lipid-lowering agents, have produced regression or limitation of progression of angiographically documented coronary atherosclerosis and significant reductions in recurrent cardiac events (15). Meta-analyses of randomized, controlled clinical trials on post-myocardial infarction patients showed that exercise-based cardiac rehabilitation decreased cardiovascular mortality and all-cause mortality by 20 to 24% (16–18), especially as a component of multifactorial rehabilitation (i.e., 26% reduction in mortality versus 15% in exercise-only trials), with no significant difference in the rate of nonfatal recurrent cardiac events (19). However, these antedated results (including many studies in the 1970s) cannot necessarily be extrapolated to survival of patients following coronary artery bypass graft surgery or percutaneous transluminal coronary angioplasty (20), or to patients who have undergone contemporary thrombolytic, revascularization, and/or pharmacotherapies. On the other hand, time (disease progression), poor patient management or compliance, and psychological dysfunction, manifested as anger, depression, hostility, or social isolation, can lead to increased risk and an adverse prognosis (21).

References

1. Fletcher GA, Balady G, Froelicher VF, et al. Exercise standards: a statement for health care professionals from the American Heart Association. Circulation 1995;91:580–615.
2. Balady GJ, Chaitman B, Driscoll D, et al. American College of Sports Medicine and American Heart Association Joint Position Statement: Recommendations for cardiovascular screening, staffing, and emergency policies at health/fitness facilities. Med Sci Sports Exerc 1998;30: 1009–1018.
3. American Association of Cardiovascular and Pulmonary Rehabilitation. Guidelines for Cardiac Rehabilitation and Secondary Prevention Programs. 3rd ed. Champaign, IL: Human Kinetics, 1999.
4. Canadian Society for Exercise Physiology. PAR-Q and You. Gloucester, Ontario: Canadian Society for Exercise Physiology, 1994:1–2.
5. Shephard RJ, Thomas S, Weller I. The Canadian home fitness test. 1991 Update. Sports Med 1991;11:358–366.
6. Expert Panel on Detection, Evaluation, and Treatment of High Blood Cholesterol in Adults. Summary of the second report of the National Cholesterol Education Program (NCEP) expert panel on detection, evaluation, and treatment of high blood cholesterol in adults (Adult Treatment Panel II). JAMA 1993;269:3015–3023.
7. American Diabetes Association. Report of the expert committee on the diagnosis and classification of diabetes mellitus. Diabetes Care 1998;21(suppl 1):S5–S19.
8. Eckel RH, Krauss RM, for the AHA Nutrition Committee. American Heart Association Call to Action: obesity as a major risk factor for coronary heart disease. Circulation 1998;97:2099–2100.
9. Pouliot MC, Despres JP, Lemieux S, et al. Waist circumference and abdominal sagittal diameter: best simple anthropometric indexes of abdominal visceral adipose tissue accumulation and related cardiovascular risk in men and women. Am J Cardiol 1995;273:460–468.
10. US Department of Health and Human Services. Physical activity and health: a report of the Surgeon General. Atlanta: US Department of Health and Human Services, Centers for Disease Control and Prevention, National Center for Chronic Disease Prevention and Health Promotion, 1996.
11. Gordon NF, Mitchell BS. Health appraisal in the nonmedical setting. In: Durstine JL, King AC, Painter PL, et al., eds. ACSM's Resource Manual for Guidelines for Exercise Testing and Prescription. 2nd ed. Philadelphia: Lea & Febiger, 1993:219–228.
12. American Association of Cardiovascular and Pulmonary Rehabilitation. Guidelines for Pulmonary Rehabilitation Programs. 2nd ed. Champaign, IL: Human Kinetics, 1998:97–112.
13. Pate RR, Pratt M, Blair SN, et al. Physical activity and public health: a recommendation from the Centers for Disease Control and Prevention and the American College of Sports Medicine. JAMA 1995;273:402–407.
14. Roitman JL, LaFontaine T, Drimmer AM. A new model for risk stratification and delivery of cardiovascular rehabilitation services in the long-term clinical management of patients with coronary artery disease. J Cardiopulmonary Rehabil 1998;18:113–123.
15. Franklin BA, Bonzheim K, Gordon S, et al. Rehabilitation of cardiac patients in the twenty-first century: changing paradigms and perceptions. J Sports Sci 1998;16:S57–S70.
16. Oldridge NB, Guyatt GH, Fisher ME, et al. Cardiac rehabilitation after myocardial infarction: combined experience of randomized clinical trials. JAMA 1988;260:945–950.
17. O'Connor GT, Buring JE, Yusuf S, et al. An overview of randomized trials of rehabilitation with exercise after myocardial infarction. Circulation 1989;80:234–244.
18. Lau J, Antman EM, Jimenez-Silva J, et al. Cumulative meta-analysis of therapeutic trials for myocardial infarction. N Engl J Med 1992;327:248–254.
19. Wenger NK, Froelicher ES, Smith LK, et al. Cardiac Rehabilitation. Clinical Practice Guideline No. 17. Rockville, MD: US Department of Health and Human Services, Public Health Service, Agency for Health Care Policy and Research and the National Heart, Lung, and Blood Institute, AHCPR Publication No. 96-0672, October 1995.
20. American College of Sports Medicine Position Stand. Exercise for patients with coronary artery disease. Med Sci Sports Exerc 1994;26:i–v.
21. Williams RB, Califf RM, Barefoot JC, et al. Prognostic importance of social and economic resources among medically treated patients with angiographically documented coronary artery disease. JAMA 1992;267:520–524.

SECTION II

Exercise Testing

⑨ CHAPTER 3
Pretest Clinical Evaluation

The extent to which medical evaluation is necessary prior to exercise testing depends on the assessment of risk as determined from the procedures outlined in Chapters 1 and 2. For many persons, especially those with coronary artery disease (CAD) and other cardiac disorders, the exercise test and accompanying physical examination are critical to the development of a safe and effective exercise program. In today's health care environment, not all persons will be approved for routine exercise testing. However, it is important to work with health care providers in understanding the importance of the baseline exercise evaluation. This evaluation provides for greater assurance of exercise safety by identifying residual myocardial ischemia, significant arrhythmias, and the effect of certain medical therapies.

A comprehensive pretest evaluation includes a medical history, physical examination, and laboratory tests. These laboratory tests may include, but are not limited to, serum chemistries, complete blood count, comprehensive lipoprotein profile, and pulmonary function. The goal of this chapter is not to be totally inclusive or to supplant more specific references on each subject, but rather to provide a concise set of guidelines for preexercise test patient assessment.

MEDICAL HISTORY, PHYSICAL EXAMINATION, AND LABORATORY TESTS

The pretest medical history should be thorough and include both past and current information. Components of a patient history are presented in Box 3-1.

For some, but not all types of exercise testing, a preliminary physical examination should be performed by a physician or other qualified personnel prior to testing (see Table 2-2). Essential components of a physical examination specific to subsequent exercise testing are found in Box 3-2.

Identification and risk stratification of persons with CAD and those at high risk of developing CAD are facilitated by review of previous test results, such as coronary angiography or exercise radionuclide or echocardiography

BOX 3-1. Components of the Medical History

Medical diagnosis—cardiovascular disease including myocardial infarction; percutaneous coronary artery procedures including angioplasty, coronary stent(s), and atherectomy; coronary artery bypass surgery; valvular surgery(s) and valvular dysfunction (e.g., aortic stenosis/mitral valve disease); other cardiac surgeries such as left ventricular aneurysmectomy and cardiac transplantation; pacemaker and/or implantable cardioverter defibrillator; presence of aortic aneurysm; ablation procedures for arrhythmias; symptoms of ischemic coronary syndrome (angina pectoris); peripheral vascular disease; hypertension; diabetes; obesity; pulmonary disease including asthma, emphysema, and bronchitis; cerebrovascular disease, including stroke and transient ischemic attacks; anemia and other blood dyscrasias (e.g., lupus erythematosis); phlebitis, deep vein thrombosis or emboli; cancer; pregnancy; osteoporosis; musculoskeletal disorders; emotional disorders; eating disorders.

Previous physical examination findings—murmurs, clicks, gallop rhythms, other abnormal heart sounds, and other unusual cardiac and vascular findings; abnormal pulmonary findings (e.g., wheezes, rales, crackles); abnormal blood sugar, blood lipids and lipoproteins, or other significant laboratory abnormalities; high blood pressure; edema.

History of symptoms—discomfort (pressure, tingling, pain, heaviness, burning, tightness, squeezing, numbness) in the chest, jaw, neck, back, or arms; light-headedness, dizziness, or fainting; temporary loss of visual acuity or speech, transient unilateral numbness or weakness; shortness of breath; rapid heart beats or palpitations, especially if associated with physical activity, eating a large meal, emotional upset, or exposure to cold (or any combination of these activities).

Recent illness, hospitalization, new medical diagnoses or surgical procedures.

Orthopedic problems, including arthritis, joint swelling, any condition that would make ambulation or use of certain test modalities difficult.

Medication use, drug allergies.

Other habits, including caffeine, alcohol, tobacco, or recreational (illicit) drug use.

Exercise history—information on readiness for change and habitual level of activity: type of exercise, frequency, duration, and intensity.

Work history with emphasis on current or expected physical demands, noting upper and lower extremity requirements.

Family history of cardiac, pulmonary, or metabolic disease, stroke, sudden death.

BOX 3-2. Components of the Physical Examination

Body weight; in many instances, determination of body mass index (BMI), waist-to-hip ratio, waist girth, and/or body composition (percent body fat) is desirable

Apical pulse rate and rhythm

Resting blood pressure, seated, supine, and standing

Auscultation of the lungs with specific attention to uniformity of breath sounds in all areas (absence of rales, wheezes, and other breathing sounds)

Palpation of the cardiac apical impulse—PMI (point of maximal impulse)

Auscultation of the heart with specific attention to murmurs, gallops, clicks, and rubs

Palpation and auscultation of carotid, abdominal, and femoral arteries

Evaluation of the abdomen for bowel sounds, masses, visceromegaly, tenderness

Palpation and inspection of lower extremities for edema and presence of arterial pulses

Absence or presence of tendon xanthoma and skin xanthelasma

Follow-up examination related to orthopedic or other medical conditions that would limit exercise testing

Tests of neurologic function, including reflexes and cognition (as indicated)

Inspection of the skin, especially of the lower extremities in known diabetics

---

studies (1). Additional testing may include ambulatory ECG (Holter) monitoring and pharmacologic stress testing to clarify further the need for and extent of intervention, assess response to treatment such as medical therapies and revascularization procedures, or determine the need for further assessment.

Alternative Stress Tests

Exercise echocardiography compares rest and exercise myocardial contractility. Ischemia is present in those segments of myocardium that do not demonstrate expected hypercontractility with exercise or show a hypocontractile response to exercise (2,3). Nuclear testing with the injection of thallous (thallium) chloride-201 or technetium-Tc99m sestamibi (Cardiolite, Dupont Medical, North Billerica, MA) (radionuclide substances that are taken up by oxygenated myocardium) during stress testing with post-stress test scintillation imaging compares rest and exercise perfusion. A set of resting images taken before or after exercise stress helps to differentiate regions of decreased isotope uptake as being either a manifestation of exercise-induced ischemia or scar tissue from a previous myocardial infarction (2,3). Pharmacologic stress testing is useful for those patients who are unable to perform a sign or symptom-limited exercise stress test. Patients generally considered

BOX 3-3. Recommended Laboratory Tests by Level of Risk and Clinical Assessment

Apparently healthy or individuals at increased risk, but without known disease

- Total serum cholesterol and HDL cholesterol; other lipoproteins as indicated (see Fig. 3-1)
- Fasting blood glucose, especially in individuals ≥45 y and younger individuals who are obese (BMI of ≥30 kg/m^2), have a first-degree relative with diabetes, are members of a high-risk ethnic population (e.g., African-American, Hispanic, Native American), have delivered a baby weighing >9 lbs, or have been diagnosed with gestational diabetes, are hypertensive, have an HDL cholesterol of ≤35 mg/dL, or on a previous test have had impaired glucose tolerance
- Fasting triglycerides, if individual has an elevated total cholesterol, two or more CAD risk factors, diabetes, central obesity, hypertension, chronic renal failure, or suspected familial dyslipidemia. Also consider measuring triglycerides in women on hormone replacement therapy and in persons reporting or known to have a high alcohol intake
- Thyroid function, as a screening evaluation especially if dyslipidemia is present

Patients with cardiovascular disease

- Above tests plus pertinent previous cardiovascular laboratory tests (e.g., resting 12-lead ECG, Holter monitoring, coronary angiography, radionuclide or echocardiography studies, previous exercise tests)
- Carotid ultrasound and other peripheral vascular studies
- Consider measures of homocysteine, Lp(a), fibrinogen, LDL particle size (especially in young persons with a strong family history of CAD and in those persons without traditional coronary risk factors)
- Chest radiograph, if congestive heart failure is present or suspected
- Comprehensive blood chemistry panel and complete blood count as indicated by history and physical examination (see Table 3-5)

Patients with pulmonary disease

- Chest radiograph
- Pulmonary function tests (see Tables 3-6 and 3-7)
- Other specialized pulmonary studies (e.g., oximetry or blood gas analysis)

for pharmacologic testing are those with significant musculoskeletal or neurologic limitations, those with moderate to severe peripheral vascular disease, those who have other limiting medical conditions, and those who are severely deconditioned and older. Pharmacologic stress tests are done in conjunction with echocardiography or radionuclide imaging and are associated with high levels of sensitivity and specificity. The most commonly used pharmacologic agents include dobutamine (synthetic catecholamine, which increases heart rate) and dipyridamole or adenosine (vasodilators). Dobutamine increases heart rate and contractility, which may provoke an ischemic response in the presence of CAD. Dipyridamole and adenosine cause coronary artery vasodilatation in nondiseased arteries. Comparisons of the blood flow to normal and blocked arteries can then be made (2,3). The decision to use these additional modalities should be based on findings from the history and physical examination. Box 3-3 identifies recommended laboratory tests based on level of risk and clinical status.

Blood Pressure

Measurement of resting blood pressure (BP) is an integral component of the pretest evaluation. Subsequent clinical decisions should be based on the average of two or more BP readings measured during each of two or more visits following an initial screening (4). Specific techniques for measuring BP are critical to accuracy and detection of high BP (Box 3-4). Optimal BP with respect to cardiovascular risk is systolic BP < 120 mm Hg and diastolic BP < 80 mm Hg (4). In addition to high BP readings, unusually low readings should also be evaluated for clinical significance. Tables 3-1 and 3-2 and Box 3-5 provide guidelines for the classification of hypertension, as recommended by the Joint National Committee on Prevention, Detection, Evaluation, and Treatment of High Blood Pressure (JNC VI) (4). Lifestyle modification including weight control, increased physical activity, alcohol moderation, restriction of dietary sodium, adequate intake of dietary calcium, potassium, and magnesium, stress management, smoking cessation, and possible discontinuation of certain medications known to elevate BP (birth control pills, antihistamines, corticosteroids, and others) for patients with elevated BP remains the cornerstone of all antihypertensive therapies (4).

Cholesterol and Lipoproteins

An increased blood cholesterol level, specifically a high concentration of low-density lipoprotein (LDL) cholesterol or a low concentration of high-density lipoprotein (HDL) cholesterol, increases the risk of CAD. Conversely, lowering total cholesterol and LDL cholesterol reduces the risk. The National Cholesterol Education Program (NCEP) Guidelines (5) can be used to classify individuals based on cholesterol and lipoprotein concentrations (Fig. 3-1), determine what type and when follow-up testing is desired (Figs. 3-1 and 3-2), and provide information on which treatment decisions

---

BOX 3-4. Procedures for Assessment of Resting Blood Pressure*

- Patients should be seated for at least 5 min in a chair with their back supported and their arms bared and supported at heart level. Patients should refrain from smoking cigarettes or ingesting caffeine during the 30 min preceding the measurement.
- Under special circumstances, measuring supine and standing positions may be indicated.
- Wrap cuff firmly around upper arm at heart level; align cuff with brachial artery.
- The appropriate cuff size must be used to ensure accurate measurement. The bladder within the cuff should encircle at least 80% of the upper arm. Many adults require a large adult cuff.
- Place stethoscope bell below the antecubital space over the brachial artery.
- Quickly inflate cuff pressure to 20 mm Hg above estimated systolic BP.
- Slowly release pressure at rate equal to 2 to 3 mm Hg/s, noting first Korotkoff sound.
- Continue releasing pressure, noting when sound becomes muffled (4th phase diastolic BP) and when sound disappears (5th phase diastolic BP). For classification purposes, the latter is used.

*Modified from Sixth Report of the Joint Committee on Prevention, Detection, Evaluation, and Treatment of High Blood Pressure (JNCVI), Public Health Service, National Institutes of Health, National Heart, Lung and Blood Institute, NIH Publication No. 98-4080, November 1997.

---

can be made (Table 3-3). The primary goal of lipid management is to lower LDL cholesterol below 100 mg/dL in persons with CAD or other atherosclerotic vascular disease; below 130 mg/dL in a primary prevention setting if two or more CAD risk factors are present; or below 160 mg/dL in a primary prevention setting if fewer than two CAD risk factors are present. For both primary and secondary prevention, secondary goals of lipid management are to lower triglycerides below 200 mg/dL and increase HDL cholesterol above 35 mg/dL (6,7).

The link between triglycerides and CAD is complex. Elevated serum triglycerides are positively correlated with CAD in univariant analysis. However, in multivariate analysis controlling for other risk factors (such as BP, physical inactivity, and obesity), the effect of triglycerides is diminished. Elevated triglyceride levels have also been positively linked to lower levels of HDL cholesterol as well as small dense LDL particle size (LDL subclass pattern B). Both of these conditions have been associated with a greater risk of atherosclerosis (8). Elevated serum triglycerides may indicate the need to evaluate the presence of alcohol abuse, diabetes, steroid use, dietary patterns, and obesity. The NCEP has provided a separate classification scheme for serum triglycerides (Table 3-4). Increased physical activity, coupled with other forms of nonpharmacological therapy (e.g., weight loss in obese patients, alcohol restriction), is recommended for all patients with elevated serum triglycerides. Drug treatment should be considered when nonpharmacologic approaches fail to lower serum triglycerides adequately in patients with CAD or a strong coronary risk profile. In patients with marked hypertriglyceridemia (>500 mg/dL), drug therapy may also be warranted to reduce the risk of pancreatitis (8).

Blood Profile Analyses

Multiple analysis blood profiles are commonly performed in clinical exercise programs. Such profiles may provide useful information about an individual's overall health status and ability to exercise and may help to explain ECG abnormalities. Because of varied methods of assaying blood samples, some caution is advised when comparing blood chemistries from different laboratories. Table 3-5 gives normal ranges for selected blood chemistries, derived from a variety of sources. For many patients with CAD, medications for dyslipidemia and hypertension are common. Many of these medications act in the liver to lower blood cholesterol and in the kidneys to lower blood

---

TABLE 3-1. Classification of Blood Pressure (BP) for Adults Aged 18 Years and Older[*,†,‡,§]

Category	Systolic BP (mm Hg)		Diastolic BP (mm Hg)
Optimal	<120	and	<80
Normal	120–129	and	80–84
High normal	130–139	or	85–89
Hypertension			
Stage 1	140–159	or	90–99
Stage 2	160–179	or	100–109
Stage 3	≥180	or	≥110

*Reprinted with permission from Sixth Report of the Joint Committee on Prevention, Detection, Evaluation, and Treatment of High Blood Pressure (JNCVI), Public Health Service, National Institutes of Health, National Heart, Lung and Blood Institute, NIH Publication No. 98-4080, November 1997.

†Not taking antihypertensive medication and not acutely ill. When systolic and diastolic BPs fall into different categories, the higher category should be selected to classify the individual's BP status. For example, 160/92 mm Hg should be classified as stage 2 hypertension and 174/120 mm Hg should be classified as stage 3 hypertension. Isolated systolic hypertension is defined as systolic BP ≥ 140 mm Hg and diastolic BP < 90 mm Hg and staged appropriately (e.g., 170/82 mm Hg is defined as stage 2 isolated systolic hypertension). In addition to classifying stages of hypertension on the basis of average BP levels, clinicians should specify presence or absence of target organ disease and additional risk factors. This specificity is important for risk classification and treatment (see Table 3-2).

‡Optimal BP with respect to cardiovascular risk is below 120/80 mm Hg. However, unusually low readings should be evaluated for clinical significance.

§Based on the average of two or more readings taken at each of two or more visits after an initial screening.

TABLE 3-2. Risk Stratification and Treatment*,†

Blood Pressure Stages (mm Hg)	Risk Group A (No Risk Factors; No TOD/CCD)‡	Risk Group B (At Least 1 Risk Factor Not Including Diabetes; No TOD/CCD)	Risk Group C (TOD/CCD and/or Diabetes, With or Without Other Risk Factors)
High-normal 130–139/85–89	Lifestyle modification	Lifestyle modification	Drug therapy§
Stage 1 140–159/90–99	Lifestyle modification (up to 12 months)	Lifestyle modification (up to 6 months)¶	Drug therapy
Stages 2 and 3 ≥160/≥100	Drug therapy	Drug therapy	Drug therapy

For example, a patient with diabetes and a blood pressure of 142/94 mm Hg plus left ventricular hypertrophy should be classified as having stage 1 hypertension with target organ disease (left ventricular hypertrophy) and with another major risk factor (diabetes). This patient would be categorized as stage 1, Risk Group C, and recommended for immediate initiation of pharmacologic treatment.

*Reprinted with permission from Sixth Report of the Joint Committee on Prevention, Detection, Evaluation, and Treatment of High Blood Pressure (JNCVI), Public Health Service, National Institutes of Health, National Heart, Lung and Blood Institute, NIH Publication No. 98-4080, November 1997.

†Lifestyle modification should be adjunctive therapy for all patients recommended for pharmacologic therapy.

‡Target organ disease (TOD)/clinical cardiovascular disease (CCD) (see Box 3-5).

¶ For patients with multiple risk factors, clinicians should consider drugs as initial therapy as well as lifestyle modification.

§For those with heart failure, renal insufficiency, or diabetes.

pressure. One should pay particular attention to liver function tests such as alanine transaminae (ALT), aspartate transaminase (AST), and bilirubin as well as to renal (kidney) function tests such as creatinine, blood urea nitrogen (BUN), and BUN/creatinine ratio in patients on such medications. Indication of volume depletion and excess potassium can be seen in the potassium and sodium measurements. These tests should be applied judiciously and not used as finite ranges of normal.

Many new and possibly important risk factors for CAD are currently being studied. Of these, elevated levels of serum homocysteine, lipoprotein

---

BOX 3-5. Components of Cardiovascular Risk Stratification in Patients With Hypertension*

Major Risk Factors[†]
- Smoking
- Dyslipidemia
- Diabetes mellitus
- Age older than 60 years
- Sex (men and postmenopausal women)
- Family history of cardiovascular disease: women under age 65 or men under age 55

Target Organ Damage/Clinical Cardiovascular Disease
- Heart diseases
    - Left ventricular hypertrophy
    - Angina/prior myocardial infarction
    - Prior coronary revascularization
    - Heart failure
- Stroke or transient ischemic attack
- Neuropathy
- Peripheral arterial disease
- Retinopathy

*Reprinted with permission from Sixth Report of the Joint Committee on Prevention, Detection, Evaluation, and Treatment of High Blood Pressure (JNC VI), Public Health Service, National Institutes of Health, National Heart, Lung and Blood Institute, NIH Publication No. 98-4080, November 1997.

†Note: Although not originally included in the JNC VI categorization, a sedentary lifestyle and obesity should be considered as major risk factors.

(a), fibrinogen, tissue-type plasminogen activator (tPA), and C-reactive protein appear to be associated in a variety of ways with increased susceptibility to atherosclerosis and/or thrombus formation (blood clotting).

Pulmonary Function

Pulmonary function assessment via routine spirometry is another test often used, particularly in patients who have a diagnosed pulmonary disease or who present with a medical history or physical examination that warrants assessment of basic lung function. While many spirometric tests are available, the most commonly used include forced vital capacity (FVC), forced expiratory volume in 1 second ($FEV_{1.0}$), $FEV_{1.0}/FVC$ ratio, and maximal voluntary ventilation (MVV). Normal values for lung function are based on age, gender, and height. As such, there are no "best" reference equations for predicting normal lung function, and considerable variability exists for commonly used prediction equations. Automated and computerized equipment often arbitrarily selects equations so that measured values may be compared with normal values. Table 3-6 provides a commonly used set of prediction equations (9,10). Even when properly performed, pulmonary

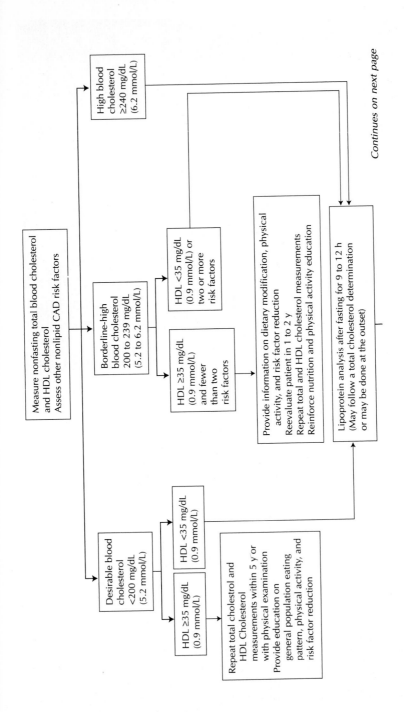

Measure nonfasting total blood cholesterol and HDL cholesterol
Assess other nonlipid CAD risk factors

Desirable blood cholesterol <200 mg/dL (5.2 mmol/L)

HDL ≥35 mg/dL (0.9 mmol/L)

HDL <35 mg/dL (0.9 mmol/L)

Repeat total cholestrol and HDL Cholesterol measurements within 5 y or with physical examination
Provide education on general population eating pattern, physical activity, and risk factor reduction

Borderline-high blood cholesterol 200 to 239 mg/dL (5.2 to 6.2 mmol/L)

HDL ≥35 mg/dL (0.9 mmol/L) and fewer than two risk factors

HDL <35 mg/dL (0.9 mmol/L) or two or more risk factors

Provide information on dietary modification, physical activity, and risk factor reduction
Reevaluate patient in 1 to 2 y
Repeat total and HDL cholesterol measurements
Reinforce nutrition and physical activity education

High blood cholesterol ≥240 mg/dL (6.2 mmol/L)

Lipoprotein analysis after fasting for 9 to 12 h (May follow a total cholesterol determination or may be done at the outset)

Continues on next page

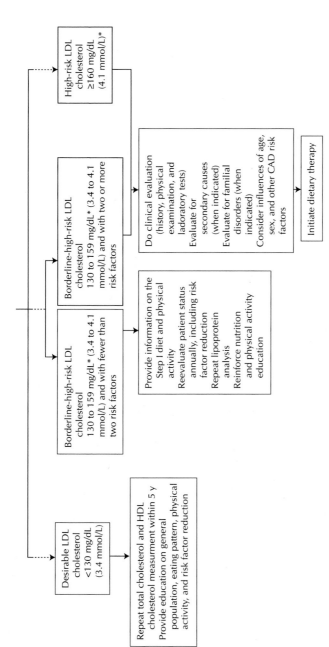

FIGURE 3-1. Lipoprotein analysis useful for identifying at-risk adults and determining appropriate follow-up regarding evaluation and therapy. *On the basis of the average of two determinations. If the first two LDL-cholesterol test results differ by more than 30 mg/dL (0.7 mmol/L), a third test result should be obtained within 1 to 8 weeks and the average of the three tests used. (Reprinted with permission from Expert Panel on Detection, Evaluation, and Treatment of High Blood Cholesterol in Adults. Summary of the Second Report of the National Cholesterol Education Program [NCEP] Expert Panel on Detection, Evaluation, and Treatment of High Blood Cholesterol in Adults [Adult Treatment Panel II]. JAMA 1993;269:3015–3023.)

The figure presents the following flow:

Desirable LDL cholesterol <130 mg/dL (3.4 mmol/L) → Repeat total cholesterol and HDL cholesterol measurement within 5 y Provide education on general population, eating pattern, physical activity, and risk factor reduction

Borderline-high-risk LDL cholesterol 130 to 159 mg/dL* (3.4 to 4.1 mmol/L) and with fewer than two risk factors → Provide information on the Step I diet and physical activity Reevaluate patient status annually, including risk factor reduction Repeat lipoprotein analysis Reinforce nutrition and physical activity education

Borderline-high-risk LDL cholesterol 130 to 159 mg/dL* (3.4 to 4.1 mmol/L) and with two or more risk factors → Do clinical evaluation (history, physical examination, and laboratory tests) Evaluate for secondary causes (when indicated) Evaluate for familial disorders (when indicated) Consider influences of age, sex, and other CAD risk factors

High-risk LDL cholesterol ≥160 mg/dL (4.1 mmol/L)*

Initiate dietary therapy

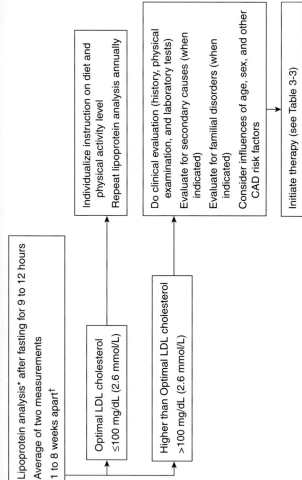

FIGURE 3-2. Lipoprotein analysis in adults with evidence of CAD or other atherosclerotic vascular disease. *Lipoprotein analysis should be performed when the patient is not in the recovery phase from an acute coronary or other medical event that would lower the usual low-density lipoprotein (LDL) cholesterol level. †If the first two LDL-cholesterol test results differ by more than 30 mg/dL (0.7 mmol/L), a third test result should be obtained within 1 to 8 weeks, and the average value of the three tests used. (Reprinted with permission from Expert Panel on Detection, Evaluation, and Treatment of High Blood Cholesterol in Adults. Summary of the Second Report of the National Cholesterol Education Program [NCEP] Expert Panel on Detection, Evaluation, and Treatment of High Blood Cholesterol in Adults [Adult Treatment Panel II]. JAMA 1993;269:3015–3023.)

TABLE 3-3. Treatment Decisions Based on LDL Cholesterol Level*

Patient Category	Initiation Level	LDL Goal
Dietary Therapy		
Without CAD and with <2 risk factors	≥160 mg/dL (4.1 mmol/L)	<160 mg/dL (4.1 mmol/L)
Without CAD and with ≥2 risk factors	≥130 mg/dL (3.4 mmol/L)	<130 mg/dL (3.4 mmol/L)
With CAD	>100 mg/dL (2.6 mmol/L)	≤100 mg/dL (2.6 mmol/L)
Drug Treatment		
Without CAD and with <2 risk factors	≥190 mg/dL (4.9 mmol/L)	<160 mg/dL (4.1 mmol/L)
Without CAD and with ≥2 risk factors	≥160 mg/dL (4.1 mmol/L)	<130 mg/dL (3.4 mmol/L)
With CAD	≥130 mg/dL (3.4 mmol/L)	≤100 mg/dL (2.6 mmol/L)

*Reprinted with permission from Expert Panel on Detection, Evaluation, and Treatment of High Blood Cholesterol in Adults. Summary of the Second Report of the National Cholesterol Education Program (NCEP) Expert Panel on Detection, Evaluation, and Treatment of High Blood Cholesterol in Adults (Adult Treatment Panel II). JAMA 1993;269:3015–3023.

CAD, coronary artery disease.

 TABLE 3-4. Classification of Fasting Serum Triglyceride Levels*

Serum Triglycerides	Classification	Comments
<200 mg/dL (<2.26 mmol/L)	Normal	
200–399 mg/dL (2.26–4.51 mmol/L)	Borderline high	Check for accompanying primary or secondary dyslipidemias
400–999 mg/dL (4.52–11.28 mmol/L)	High	Check for accompanying primary or secondary dyslipidemias
≥1000 mg/dL (≥11.29 mmol/L)	Very high	Increased risk for acute pancreatitis

*Adapted from Expert Panel on Detection, Evaluation, and Treatment of High Blood Cholesterol in Adults. Summary of the Second Report of the National Cholesterol Education Program (NCEP) Expert Panel on Detection, Evaluation, and Treatment of High Blood Cholesterol in Adults (Adult Treatment Panel II). JAMA 1993;269:3015–3023.

TABLE 3-5. Typical Ranges of Normal Values for Selected Blood Variables in Adults*

Variable	Men	Neutral	Women
Hemoglobin (g/dL)	13.5–17.5		11.5–15.5
Hematocrit (%)	40–52		36–48
Red cell count ($\times10^{12}$/L)	4.5–6.5		3.9–5.6
Mean cell hemoglobin concentration (MCHC)		30–35 (g/dL)	
White blood cell count		4–11 ($\times10^9$/L)	
Platelet count		150–450 ($\times10^9$/L)	
Fasting glucose		60–109 mg/dL	
Blood urea nitrogen (BUN)		4–24 mg/dL	
Creatinine		0.3–1.4 mg/dL	
BUN/Creatinine ratio		7–27	
Uric acid (mg/dL)	4.0–8.9		2.3–7.8
Sodium		135–150 mEq/L	
Potassium		3.5–5.5 mEq/L	
Chloride		98–110 mEq/L	
Osmolality		278–302 mOsm/kg	
Calcium		8.5–10.5 mg/dL	
Calcium, ion		4.0–5.2 mg/dL	
Phosphorus		2.5–4.5 mg/dL	
Protein, total		6.0–8.5 g/dL	
Albumin		3.0–5.5 g/dL	
Globulin		2.0–4.0 g/dL	
A/G ratio		1.0–2.2	
Iron, total (μg/dL)	40–190		35–180
Liver Function Tests			
Bilirubin		<1.5 mg/dL	
(SGOT) (AST)	8–46 μ/L		7–34 μ/L
(SGPT) (ALT)	7–46 μ/L		4–35 μ/L

*Certain variables must be interpreted in relation to the normal range of the issuing laboratory. SGOT, serum glutamic-oxaloacetic transaminase; AST, aspartate transaminase (formerly SGOT); SGPT, serum glutamic-pyruvic transaminase; ALT, alanine transaminase (formerly SGPT).

function tests must be interpreted with caution due to the degree of subject cooperation necessary to achieve peak values and the wide range of interindividual variability in "normal" responses. For this reason, Table 3-6 also gives the "lower limit of normal" for each variable. Subtracting this value from that calculated from the equation provides a better basis for determining whether a test result should be evaluated further.

Table 3-7 presents typical effects of obstructive or restrictive pulmonary disease on spirometric and airflow volume measurements (11). It should

TABLE 3-6. Pulmonary Function Prediction Equations With Corresponding Values Constituting the Lower Limits of Normal*

	Prediction Equation	Lower Limits of Normal[†]
Women		
FVC (L)	$= (0.0414 \times \text{Height, cm}) - (0.0232 \times \text{Age}) - 2.20$	-0.73
$FEV_{1.0}$ (L)	$= (0.0268 \times \text{Height, cm}) - (0.0251 \times \text{Age}) - 0.38$	-0.55
$FEV_{1.0}/FVC$ (%)	$= (-0.2145 \times \text{Height, cm}) - (0.1523 \times \text{Age}) + 124.5$	-11.1
MVV (L/min)	$= 40 \times FEV_{1.0}$ (L)	N/A
Men		
FVC (L)	$= (0.0774 \times \text{Height, cm}) - (0.0212 \times \text{Age}) - 7.75$	-0.84
$FEV_{1.0}$ (L)	$= (0.0566 \times \text{Height, cm}) - (0.0233 \times \text{Age}) - 4.91$	-0.68
$FEV_{1.0}/FVC$ (%)	$= (-0.1314 \times \text{Height, cm}) - (0.1490 \times \text{Age}) + 110.2$	-9.2
MVV (L/min)	$= 40 \times FEV_{1.0}$ (L)	N/A

*These equations are valid for white men and women ages 18 to 85.

†Subtracting this value from that calculated from the prediction equation provides the lower limit of normal. For African Americans and Asians, multiply the predicted FVC and $FEV_{1.0}$ values by 0.85. The lower limits of normal should likewise be multiplied by 0.85. FVC and FEV equations are from Miller A. Pulmonary function tests in clinical and occupational lung disease. Orlando: Grune & Stratton, 1986; the predicted MVV equation is from Wasserman K, Hansen JE, Sue DY, et al. Principles of Exercise Testing. Philadelphia: Lea & Febiger, 1987:79.

 TABLE 3-7. Typical Effect of Obstructive and Restrictive Pulmonary Disease on Spirometric Volume and Flow Measurements*

Measurement	Obstructive[†]	Restrictive[†]
Tidal volume (TV)	N or ↑	N or ↓
Inspiratory capacity (IC)	N or ↓	N or ↓
Expiratory reserve volume (ERV)	N or ↓	N or ↓
Vital capacity (VC)	N or ↓	↓
Forced vital capacity (FVC)	N or ↓	↓
Residual volume (RV)	↑	N or ↓
Functional residual volume (FRV)	↑	N or ↓
Total lung capacity (TLC)	↑	↓
Forced expiratory volume in 1 sec ($FEV_{1.0}$)	↓	N
$FEV_{1.0}/FVC$	↓	N or ↑
Forced expiratory flow rate between 25% and 75% FVC	↓	N or ↓
Maximal voluntary ventilation (MVV)	↓	N or ↓
Peak expiratory flow	↓	N or ↓

*Adapted from Sadowsky HS. Pulmonary diagnostic tests and procedures. In: Hillegass EA, Sadowsky HS, eds. Essentials of Cardiopulmonary Physical Therapy. 4th ed. Philadelphia: WB Saunders, 1994.

†N = normal; ↓ = decreased; ↑ = increased.

be emphasized, however, that pulmonary function test results provide information that is closely related to other clinical data and as such should not be interpreted in isolation.

CONTRAINDICATIONS TO EXERCISE TESTING

There are certain individuals for whom the risks of exercise testing outweigh the potential benefits. For these patients it is important to carefully assess risk versus benefit when deciding whether the exercise test should be performed. Box 3-6 outlines absolute and relative contraindications to exercise testing (12). Exercise tests should not be performed by patients with absolute

---

BOX 3-6. Contraindications to Exercise Testing*

Absolute
- A recent significant change in the resting ECG suggesting significant ischemia, recent myocardial infarction (within 2 days) or other acute cardiac event
- Unstable angina
- Uncontrolled cardiac arrhythmias causing symptoms or hemodynamic compromise
- Severe symptomatic aortic stenosis
- Uncontrolled symptomatic heart failure
- Acute pulmonary embolus or pulmonary infarction
- Acute myocarditis or pericarditis
- Suspected or known dissecting aneurysm
- Acute infections

Relative†
- Left main coronary stenosis
- Moderate stenotic valvular heart disease
- Electrolyte abnormalities (e.g., hypokalemia, hypomagnesemia)
- Severe arterial hypertension (i.e., systolic BP of >200 mm Hg and/or a diastolic BP of >110 mm Hg) at rest
- Tachyarrhythmias or bradyarrhythmias
- Hypertrophic cardiomyopathy and other forms of outflow tract obstruction
- Neuromuscular, musculoskeletal, or rheumatoid disorders that are exacerbated by exercise
- High-degree atrioventricular block
- Ventricular aneurysm
- Uncontrolled metabolic disease (e.g., diabetes, thyrotoxicosis, or myxedema)
- Chronic infectious disease (e.g., mononucleosis, hepatitis, AIDS)

*Modified from Gibbons RA, Balady GJ, Beasely JW, et al. ACC/AHA guidelines for exercise testing. J Am Coll Cardiol 1997;30:260–315.

†Relative contraindications can be superseded if benefits outweigh risks of exercise. In some instances, these individuals can be exercised with caution and/or using low-level end points, especially if they are asymptomatic at rest.

TABLE 3-8. Serum Enzymes (Myocardial Tissue Damage or Necrosis)

Enzyme	Normal Value*	Time Course of Change (When Abnormally Elevated)
CK myocardial band (CK-MB)	<5% of total CK	Appears at 4–6 hours; peaks 12–24 hours; returns to normal within 72 hours
Creatine phosphokinase (CPK or CK)	Females 10–70 U/L Males 25–90 U/L	Appears within hours and peaks at about 24 hours without reperfusion; returns to normal within 2–4 days
Troponin I	<0.5 ng/mL	Appears about 4–6 hours; peaks at 24 hours, remains elevated 5–10 days

*Normal values vary depending on the laboratory and the method used. The SGOT and LDH enzymes are no longer used as "cardiac enzymes" and have been replaced by the others.

contraindications until those conditions are stabilized or adequately treated. Patients with relative contraindications may be tested only after careful evaluation of the risk/benefit ratio. It should be emphasized, however, that contraindications might not apply in certain specific clinical situations, such as soon after acute myocardial infarction, revascularization procedure, or bypass surgery or to determine the need for, or benefit of, drug therapy. Finally, conditions exist that preclude reliable diagnostic ECG information from exercise testing (e.g., left bundle-branch block, digitalis therapy). The test may still provide useful information on exercise capacity, arrhythmias, and hemodynamic responses to exercise. In these conditions, additional evaluative techniques such as echocardiography or nuclear imaging can be added to the exercise test to improve sensitivity, specificity, and diagnostic capabilities.

Immediate exercise testing of selected low-risk patients presenting to the emergency department with chest pain (i.e., within 4 to 8 hours) is being increasingly employed to "rule out myocardial infarction" (13). Generally, these patients include those who are no longer symptomatic and who have unremarkable ECGs and serial cardiac enzymes. Table 3-8 is a quick reference source for serum concentrations of enzymes commonly used as indices of myocardial damage or necrosis.

INFORMED CONSENT

Obtaining adequate informed consent from participants prior to exercise testing and participation in a supervised exercise program is an important ethical and legal consideration (see Chapter 13). Although the content and extent of consent forms may vary, enough information must be present in the informed consent process to ensure that the participant knows and understands the purposes and risks associated with the test or exercise program. The consent form should include a statement indicating that the patient has been given an opportunity to ask questions about the procedure and has sufficient information to give informed consent. If the subject to be tested is a minor, a legal guardian or parent must sign the consent form. It is advisable to check with authoritative bodies (hospital risk management, institutional review boards, legal counsel) to determine what is appropriate for an acceptable informed consent process. Sample consent forms for exercise testing and rehabilitation are provided in Figs. 3-3 and 3-4. No sample form should be adopted for a specific program unless approved by local legal counsel.

When the test is for purposes other than diagnosis or prescription, i.e., for experimental purposes, this should be indicated on the Informed Consent Form, and applicable policies for the testing of human subjects must be implemented. A copy of the Policy on Human Subjects for Research is available from the ACSM on request.

Because most consent forms include a statement that emergency equipment is available, the program must ensure that available personnel are legally authorized to carry out emergency procedures that use such equipment. This is of particular importance when defibrillators are present because use of defibrillators is limited to medical practitioners or others specifically authorized by law.

Patient Instructions

Explicit instructions for patients prior to exercise testing increase test validity and data accuracy. Whenever possible, written instructions along with a description of the evaluation should be provided well in advance of the appointment so the patient can prepare adequately. The following points should be considered for inclusion in such preliminary instructions; however, specific instructions vary with test type and purpose:

- Patients should refrain from ingesting food, alcohol, or caffeine or using tobacco products within 3 hours of testing.
- Patients should be rested for the assessment, avoiding significant exertion or exercise on the day of the assessment.
- Clothing should permit freedom of movement and include walking or running shoes. Women should bring a loose-fitting, short-sleeved blouse that buttons down the front and should avoid restrictive undergarments.
- If the evaluation is on an outpatient basis, patients should be made aware that the evaluation may be fatiguing and that they may wish to have someone accompany them to the assessment to drive home afterward.

continues on page 56

Informed Consent for an Exercise Test

1. Purpose and Explanation of the Test

   You will perform an exercise test on a cycle ergometer or a motor-driven treadmill. The exercise intensity will begin at a low level and will be advanced in stages depending on your fitness level. We may stop the test at any time because of signs of fatigue or changes in your heart rate, electrocardiogram (ECG), or blood pressure, or symptoms you may experience. It is important for you to realize that you may stop when you wish because of feelings of fatigue or any other discomfort.

2. Attendant Risks and Discomforts

   There exists the possibility of certain changes occurring during the test. These include abnormal blood pressure, fainting, irregular, fast or slow heart rhythm, and in rare instances, heart attack, stroke, or death. Every effort will be made to minimize these risks by evaluation of preliminary information relating to your health and fitness and by careful observations during testing. Emergency equipment and trained personnel are available to deal with unusual situations that may arise.

3. Responsibilities of the Participant

   Information you possess about your health status or previous experiences of heart-related symptoms (such as shortness of breath with low-level activity, pain, pressure, tightness, heaviness in the chest, neck, jaw, back and/or arms) with physical effort may affect the safety of your exercise test. Your prompt reporting of these and any other unusual feelings with effort during the exercise test itself is of great importance. You are responsible for fully disclosing your medical history, as well as symptoms that may occur during the test. You are also expected to report all medications (including non-prescription) taken recently and, in particular, those taken today, to the testing staff.

4. Benefits to be Expected

   The results obtained from the exercise test may assist in the diagnosis of your illness, in evaluating the effect of your medications or in evaluating what type of physical activities you might do with low risk.

5. Inquiries

   Any questions about the procedures used in the exercise test or the results of your test are encouraged. If you have any concerns or questions, please ask us for further explanations.

6. Use of Medical Records

   The information that is obtained during exercise testing will be treated as privileged and confidential. It is not to be released or revealed to any person except your referring physician without your written consent. The information obtained, however, may be used for statistical analysis or scientific purposes with your right to privacy retained.

7. Freedom of Consent

   I hereby consent to voluntarily engage in an exercise test to determine my exercise capacity and state of cardiovascular health. My permission to perform this exercise test is given voluntarily. I understand that I am free to stop the test at any point, if I so desire.

I have read this form, and I understand the test procedures that I will perform and the attendant risks and discomforts. Knowing these risks and discomforts, and having had an opportunity to ask questions that have been answered to my satisfaction. I consent to participate in this test.

_____   _____
Date   Signature of Patient

_____   _____
Date   Signature of Witness

_____   _____
Date   Signature of Physician or Authorized Delegate

FIGURE 3-3. Sample of informed consent form for an exercise test.

Informed Consent for an Outpatient Cardiac Rehabilitation Program

1. Explanation of Outpatient Cardiac Rehabilitation Program

   You will be placed in a rehabilitation program that will include physical exercises, educational activities, and other health-related services. The levels of exercise which you will undertake will be based on your cardiovascular response to an exercise test and other clinical information. You will be given clear instructions regarding the amount and kind of regular exercise you should do. Your exercise sessions may be adjusted by the program staff and physician, depending on your progress. At your physician's discretion, you may be given the opportunity for re-evaluation with a graded exercise test ____ months after the initiation of the rehabilitation program, and ____ months thereafter. Other tests may be recommended as needed.

2. Monitoring

   Your blood pressure will be monitored as required. You agree to learn how to count your own pulse rate and record it before, during, and after each exercise session, as instructed by program staff members. You agree to report to the rehabilitation staff any unusual, new or worsened symptoms associated with your exercise program. These include but are not limited to unusual shortness of breath with low level activity, pain, pressure, tightness, heaviness in the chest, neck, jaw, back and/or arms, unusual fatigue with exercise, unusually fast, slow or irregular heart rate, faintness or dizziness.

3. Attendant Risks and Discomforts

   There exists the possibility of certain changes occurring during exercise sessions. These include abnormal blood pressure, fainting, irregular, fast, or slow heart rhythm, and in rare instances, heart attack, stroke, or death. Every effort will be made to minimize those risks by provision of appropriate supervision during exercise. Emergency equipment and trained personnel are available to deal with unusual situations that may arise.

4. Benefits to be Expected

   Participation in the rehabilitation program may help to evaluate which activities you may safely engage in during your daily life. No assurance can be given that the rehabilitation program will increase your exercise tolerance, although considerable evidence indicates improvement is usually achieved.

5. Responsibility of the Participant

   To promote your safety and gain benefit, you must give priority to regular attendance and adherence to the prescribed intensity, duration, frequency, progression, and type of activity. To achieve the best possible care:

   DO *NOT*

   - Withhold any information pertinent to symptoms from any staff member.
   - Exceed your target heart rate.
   - Exercise when you do not feel well.
   - Exercise within 2 hours after eating or using tobacco products or alcohol.
   - Use extremely hot water during showering after exercise (avoid sauna, steam bath, and similar extreme temperatures).

FIGURE 3-4. Sample of informed consent for an outpatient cardiac rehabilitation program.

Informed Consent for an Outpatient Cardiac Rehabilitation Program
(*continued*)

DO
- Report any unusual symptoms that you experience before, during, or after exercise. (You may help assure the safety and well-being of others in the program if you would also report any unusual symptoms you notice in others.)
- Check in with the staff after showering/dressing before leaving the site.
- Follow, without exception, all recommendations made by staff concerning the limits on any exercise, weight control, or health-related activities which you may be encouraged to do and document by recordings.

6. Use of Medical Records
   The information that is obtained while you are a participant in the Cardiac Rehabilitation Program will be treated as privileged and confidential. It is not to be released or revealed to any person except your referring physician without your written consent. The information obtained, however, may be used for statistical analysis or scientific purposes with your right to privacy retained.

7. Inquiries
   Any questions about the rehabilitation program are welcome. If you have any doubts or questions, please ask us for further explanation.

8. Freedom of Consent
   I agree to voluntarily participate in the Cardiac Rehabilitation Program. I understand that I am free to deny any consent if I so desire, both now and at any point in the program.

I acknowledge that I have read this form in its entirety or it has been read to me, and I understand my responsibility in the Rehabilitation Program in which I will be engaged. I accept the risks, rules, and regulations set forth. Knowing these, and having had an opportunity to ask questions which have been answered to my satisfaction, I consent to participate in this Rehabilitation Program.

_____   _____
Date   Signature of Patient

_____   _____
Date   Signature of Witness

_____   _____
Date   Signature of Physician or Authorized Delegate

FIGURE 3-4. (*continued*)

- If the test is for diagnostic purposes, it may be helpful for patients to discontinue prescribed cardiovascular medications, but only with physician approval. Currently prescribed antianginal agents alter the hemodynamic response to exercise and significantly reduce the sensitivity of ECG changes for ischemia. Patients taking intermediate- or high-dose β-blocking agents may be asked to taper their medication over a 2- to 4-day period to minimize hyperadrenergic withdrawal responses.
- If the test is for functional purposes, *patients should continue their medication regimen* on their usual schedule so that the exercise responses will be consistent with responses expected during exercise training.
- Patients should bring a list of their medications, including dosage and frequency of administration, to the assessment and should report the last actual dose taken. As an alternative, patients may wish to bring their medications with them for the clinician to record.

References

1. Fuster V, Pearson TA. 27th Bethesda Conference: Matching the intensity of risk factor management with the hazard for coronary disease events. September 14–15, 1995. J Am Coll Cardiol 1996;27:957–1047.
2. Berra K, Froelicher E. Exercise testing. In: Cardiac Nursing. 3rd ed. Philadelphia: JB Lippincott, 1995:135–154.
3. Ritchie JL, Batemen TM, Bonow RO, et al. Guidelines for clinical use of cardiac radionuclide imaging. Report of the American College of Cardiology/American Heart Association Task Force on Assessment of Diagnostic and Therapeutic Cardiovascular Procedures (Subcommittee on Coronary Artery Bypass Graft Surgery). J Am Coll Cardiol 1991;17:543–589.
4. Sixth Report of the Joint Committee on Prevention, Detection, Evaluation, and Treatment of High Blood Pressure (JNCVI), Public Health Service, National Institutes of Health, National Heart, Lung and Blood Institute, NIH Publication No. 98-4080, November 1997.
5. Expert Panel on Detection, Evaluation, and Treatment of High Blood Cholesterol in Adults. Summary of the Second Report of the National Cholesterol Education Program (NCEP) Expert Panel on Detection, Evaluation, and Treatment of High Blood Cholesterol in Adults (Adult Treatment Panel II). JAMA 1993;269:3015–3023.
6. American Heart Association Science Advisory. Guide to primary prevention of cardiovascular diseases. A statement for healthcare professionals from the task force on risk reduction. Circulation 1997;95:2329–2331.
7. American Heart Association Medical/Scientific Statement. Preventing heart attack and death in patients with coronary disease. Circulation 1995;92:2–4.
8. NIH Consensus Development Panel on Triglyceride, High-Density Lipoprotein, and Coronary Heart Disease. Triglyceride, high-density lipoprotein, and coronary heart disease. JAMA 1993;269:505–510.
9. Miller A. Pulmonary function tests in clinical and occupational lung disease. Orlando: Grune & Stratton, 1986.
10. Wasserman K, Hansen JE, Sue DY, et al. Principles of Exercise Testing. Philadelphia: Lea & Febiger, 1987:79.
11. Sadowsky HS. Pulmonary diagnostic tests and procedures. In: Hillegass EA, Sadowsky HS, eds. Essentials of Cardiopulmonary Physical Therapy. 4th ed. Philadelphia: WB Saunders, 1994.
12. Gibbons RA, Balady GJ, Beasely JW, et al. ACC/AHA guidelines for exercise testing. J Am Coll Cardiol 1997;30:260–315.
13. Lewis WR, Amsterdam EA. Evaluation of the patient with 'rule out myocardial infarction'. Arch Intern Med 1996;156:41–45.

⑥ Chapter 4
Physical Fitness Testing and Interpretation

The term "physical fitness" has been defined in many ways. Most definitions of physical fitness refer strictly to the capacity for movement, and the following definition is typical in this regard: *A set of attributes that people have or achieve that relates to the ability to perform physical activity* (1). Such definitions are, by nature, broad and can be interpreted as encompassing an array of fitness components, some of which relate to athletic performance but not to health. Accordingly, the term "health-related physical fitness" has been used to denote fitness as it pertains to disease prevention and health promotion. One definition of health-related physical fitness is: *A state characterized by (a) an ability to perform daily activities with vigor, and (b) a demonstration of traits and capacities that are associated with low risk of premature development of the hypokinetic diseases (i.e., those associated with physical inactivity)* (2).

Although many different literal definitions of physical fitness exist, there is relative uniformity in the *operational* definition of physical fitness. It has almost always been viewed as a multifactorial construct that includes several components. Each component is a movement-related trait or capacity that is considered to be largely independent of the others. *Health-related physical fitness* typically includes cardiorespiratory endurance, body composition, muscular strength and endurance, and flexibility. The concept that underlies health-related physical fitness is that better status in each of the components is associated with lower risk for development of disease and/or functional disability. Note that informed consent procedures similar to those described in Chapter 3 must be followed when fitness tests are performed.

Purposes of Fitness Testing

Measurement of physical fitness is a common and appropriate practice in preventive and rehabilitative exercise programs. The purposes of fitness testing in such programs include the following:

- Educating participants about their present fitness status relative to health-related standards and age- and gender-matched norms.
- Providing data that are helpful in development of exercise prescriptions to address all fitness components.
- Collecting baseline and follow-up data that allow evaluation of progress by exercise program participants.
- Motivating participants by establishing reasonable and attainable fitness goals.
- Stratifying risk.

A fundamental goal of preventive and rehabilitative exercise programs is promotion of health. Therefore, such programs should focus on enhancement of the health-related components of physical fitness. This chapter provides guidelines for the measurement and evaluation of health-related physical fitness in presumably healthy adults.

BASIC PRINCIPLES AND GUIDELINES

The information obtained from physical fitness testing, in combination with the individual's health and medical information, can be used by the health/fitness professional to help an individual achieve specific fitness goals. A sound, well-conducted physical fitness test measures what it purports to measure (i.e., is valid), is reliable, and is relatively inexpensive and easy to administer. Additionally, the test should yield results that can be directly and appropriately compared to normative data.

Pretest Instructions

Before administering a physical fitness test, certain measures should be taken to ensure client safety and comfort. A minimal recommendation is that individuals complete a questionnaire such as the PAR-Q (see Chapter 2) before coming to the testing facility. Individuals should also be given precise instructions regarding the fitness tests before coming to the testing facility. In general, individuals should be instructed to do the following:

- Wear comfortable, loose-fitting clothing consistent with testing.
- Drink plenty of fluids over the 24-hour period preceding the test to ensure normal hydration prior to the testing.
- Avoid food, tobacco, alcohol, and caffeine for at least 3 hours before testing.
- Avoid exercise or strenuous physical activity the day of the test.
- Get an adequate amount of sleep (6 to 8 hours) the night before the test.

Test Order

Prior to the participant's arrival at the test site, the following should be accomplished:

- Have all forms, score sheets, tables, graphs, and other paper work for the test's administration.
- Calibrate all equipment to be used: metronome, cycle ergometer, calipers, and so on.
- Organize equipment so that tests can follow in sequence.
- Set room temperature to 70 to 74°F (21 to 23°C).

When multiple tests are to be administered, the organization of the testing session can be very important, depending on what physical fitness components are to be evaluated. Resting measurements such as heart rate, blood pressure, height, weight, and body composition should be obtained first. When all fitness components are assessed in a single session, resting measurements should be followed (in order) by tests of cardiorespiratory endurance, muscular fitness, and flexibility. Testing cardiorespiratory endurance after assessing muscular fitness (which elevates heart rate) can produce inaccurate results regarding an individual's cardiorespiratory endurance status—particularly when submaximal tests are used. Likewise, dehydration resulting from cardiorespiratory endurance tests might influence body composition values if measured by bioelectrical impedance analysis (BIA).

Test Environment

The test environment is important for test validity and reliability. Test anxiety, emotional problems, food in the stomach, bladder distention, and room temperature and ventilation should be controlled as much as possible. To minimize anxiety, the test procedures should be explained adequately, and the test environment should be quiet and private. The room should be equipped with a comfortable seat and/or examination table to be used for resting blood pressure and heart rate and/or electrocardiographic (ECG) recordings, in addition to the standard testing equipment required. The demeanor of personnel should be one of relaxed confidence to put the subject at ease. Testing procedures should not be rushed, and all procedures must be explained clearly prior to initiating the process. These seemingly minor tasks are easily accomplished and are important in achieving valid and reliable test results.

Body Composition

It is well established that excess body fat is associated with hypertension, type 2 diabetes, and hyperlipidemia (3). The prevalence of overweight U.S.

adults was found to be 33% in 1988–1991, with some populations (Mexican-American and non-Hispanic black women) approaching 50% (4). This represented an 8% increase in prevalence over a 10-year time span. An increase in the prevalence of overweight children was also observed over a similar time period, but the increase was primarily attributed to the heaviest children being heavier (5). Unfortunately, the heaviest children are more at risk of carrying the problem of overweight into adulthood. Consequently, measurement of body composition as it relates to health is a concern throughout the life span.

Body composition refers to the relative percentage of body weight that is fat and fat-free tissue. Body composition can be estimated with both laboratory and field techniques which vary in terms of complexity, cost, and accuracy. Different assessment techniques are briefly reviewed in this section; however, the detail associated with obtaining measurements and calculating estimates of body fat for all of these techniques is beyond the scope of this text. A more detailed description is provided in Heyward and Stolarczyk's *Applied Body Composition Assessment* (6), and Roche, Heymsfield, and Lohman's *Human Body Composition* (7). Prior to collecting data for body composition assessment, the technician must be trained, routinely practiced in the techniques, and have already demonstrated reliability in his or her measurements, independent of the technique being used.

Densitometry

Body composition can be estimated from a measurement of whole-body density, using the ratio of body mass to body volume. In this technique, which has been used as a reference or criterion standard for assessing body composition, the body is divided into two components: the fat mass (FM) and the fat-free mass (FFM). The limiting factor in the measurement of body density is the accuracy of the body volume measurement because body mass is measured simply as body weight. Body volume can be measured by hydrostatic (underwater) weighing and by plethysmography.

HYDROSTATIC (UNDERWATER) WEIGHING

This technique of measuring body composition is based on Archimedes' principle, which states that when a body is immersed in water, it is buoyed by a counterforce equal to the weight of the water displaced. This loss of weight in water, corrected for the density of water, allows calculation of body volume. However, the volume of air in the lungs at the time of measurement (usually residual volume) must be accounted for, as shown in the following formula:

$$\text{Body density} = \frac{\text{Weight in air}}{\left[\dfrac{(\text{Weight in air} - \text{Weight in water})}{\text{Density of water}} - \text{Residual volume}\right]}$$

Bone and muscle tissue are more dense than water, whereas fat tissue is less dense. Therefore, a person with more FFM for the same total body mass weighs more in water and has a higher body density and lower percentage of body fat. Although hydrostatic weighing is a standard method for measuring body volume, several sources of error are inherent in the procedure (8):

- The common formulas used to convert body density to percent fat assume a density of 0.900 g/mL for the fat mass and 1.100 g/mL for the density of the fat-free mass (see below). However, it has become clear that the density of the FFM is not constant, but varies with growth, maturation, aging, gender, and ethnicity. Use of a single equation to convert body density to percent body fat for all populations can result in systematic errors. In addition, within any group of the same gender, age, and ethnicity, the density of the FFM will vary from individual to individual, resulting in an error of estimate of about ±2% body fat, even when the measurement technique is carried out flawlessly. Techniques that divide body mass into three (fat, water, and solids; or fat, mineral, and lean soft tissue) or four (fat, water, mineral, and protein) components allow for accurate estimates of the density of the FFM. This, in turn, results in more accurate equations to estimate body fatness from body density.
- Measurement of lung residual volume (RV) is needed for accurate calculation of body density. The most accurate way is to measure RV at the time underwater weight is measured, but RV measured prior to the test (with subject in testing posture) is also considered acceptable. Regression equations using age and height to predict RV, or formulas using a fraction of vital capacity to predict RV, introduce large errors into the calculation of body density.
- Underwater weight is more accurately measured using a force-transducer system than using a spring-loaded autopsy scale.
- Finally, hydrostatic weighing requires expensive, special equipment, and the procedure is somewhat complicated and time-consuming. For some individuals, submersion of the head underwater might be difficult or anxiety-provoking.

PLETHYSMOGRAPHY

Body volume can also be measured by air displacement rather than water displacement. One commercial system uses a dual-chamber plethysmograph that measures body volume by changes in pressure in a closed chamber. This new technology shows great promise and can more easily accommodate individuals who cannot perform the procedures associated with underwater weighing (9,10).

Once body density has been determined, percent body fat can be calculated. Two of the most common prediction equations used to convert body density to percent body fat are derived from the two-component model of body composition (11,12):

$$\% \, fat = \frac{457}{Body \, Density} - 414.2$$

$$\% \, fat = \frac{495}{Body \, Density} - 450$$

However, as mentioned earlier, based on research using the three- and four-component models of body composition, a variety of new equations have been developed to increase the accuracy of the estimate of percent fat when applied to different populations. These equations (Table 4-1) are likely to improve over time as additional studies are done on larger samples within each population group (6).

Anthropometric Methods

Measurements of height, weight, circumferences, and skinfolds are used to estimate body composition. Although the skinfold method might be the

TABLE 4-1. Population-Specific Formulas for Conversion of Body Density (Db) to Percent Body Fat*

Population	Age	Gender	% Body Fat[†]
Race			
American Indian	18–60	Female	(4.81/Db)–4.34
Black	18–32	Male	(4.37/Db)–3.93
	24–79	Female	(4.85/Db)–4.39
Hispanic	20–40	Female	(4.87/Db)–4.41
Japanese Native	18–48	Male	(4.97/Db)–4.52
		Female	(4.76/Db)–4.28
	61–78	Male	(4.87/Db)–4.41
		Female	(4.95/Db)–4.50
White	7–12	Male	(5.30/Db)–4.89
		Female	(5.35/Db)–4.95
	13–16	Male	(5.07/Db)–4.64
		Female	(5.10/Db)–4.66
	17–19	Male	(4.99/Db)–4.55
		Female	(5.05/Db)–4.62
	20–80	Male	(4.95/Db)–4.50
		Female	(5.01/Db)–4.57
Levels of Body Fatness			
Anorexia	15–30	Female	(5.26/Db)–4.83
Obese	17–62	Male	(5.00/Db)–4.56

*Adapted from Heyward VH, Stolarczyk LM. Applied Body Composition Assessment. Champaign, IL: Human Kinetics, 1996.

†Percent body fat is obtained by multiplying the value calculated from the equation by 100.

most difficult, it provides better estimations of body fatness than those based only on height, weight, and circumferences (10).

BODY MASS INDEX

The body mass index (BMI), or Quetelet index, is used to assess weight relative to height and is calculated by dividing body weight in kilograms by height in meters squared (kg/m^2). Obesity-related health problems increase beyond a BMI of 25 for most people, and the Expert Panel on the Identification, Evaluation, and Treatment of Overweight and Obesity in Adults (13) lists a BMI of 25.0 to 29.9 kg/m^2 for overweight and a BMI of greater than or equal to 30.0 kg/m^2 for obesity. However, due to the relatively large standard error of estimating percent fat from BMI ($\pm5\%$ fat), it should not be used to determine an individual's body fatness during a fitness assessment (10).

WAIST-TO-HIP CIRCUMFERENCE

The pattern of body fat distribution is recognized as an important predictor of the health risks of obesity (14). Individuals with more fat on the trunk, especially abdominal fat, are at increased risk of hypertension, type 2 diabetes, hyperlipidemia, coronary artery disease, and premature death compared with individuals who are equally fat, but have more of their fat on the extremities. Traditionally, the waist-to-hip ratio (WHR—the circumference of the waist divided by the circumference of the hips) has been used as a simple method for determining body fat pattern (15). Waist is measured at the narrowest part of the torso (above the umbilicus and below the xiphoid process); hip, at the maximal circumference of the hips or buttocks region, whichever is larger (above the gluteal fold). Health risk increases with WHR, and standards for risk vary with age and gender. For example, health risk is *very high* for young men when WHR is more than 0.94 and for young women when WHR is more than 0.82. For ages 60 to 69 years, the WHR values are greater than 1.03 for men and greater than 0.90 for women for the same risk classification (6,15). More recently, the focus has shifted from WHR to waist circumference alone (13).

The waist circumference can be used alone as an indicator of health risk because abdominal obesity is the issue. The expert panel on obesity and health risk, mentioned earlier in the BMI section, provided a classification of disease risk based on both BMI and waist circumference (13) as shown in Table 4-2.

SKINFOLD MEASUREMENTS

Body composition determined from skinfold measurements correlates well ($r = 0.70$–0.90) with body composition determined by hydrostatic weighing. The principle behind this technique is that the amount of subcutaneous fat is proportional to the total amount of body fat. However, the exact proportion of subcutaneous-to-total fat varies with gender, age, and ethnicity (16). Therefore, regression equations used to convert sum of skinfolds to percent fat must consider these variables for greatest accuracy. Box 4-1 presents a standardized description of skinfold sites and procedures. To improve the accuracy of the measurement, it is recommended that one train with a skilled technician, use videotapes that demonstrate proper technique, and attend workshops for that purpose. The accuracy of pre-

TABLE 4-2. Classification of Disease Risk Based on Body Mass Index (BMI) and Waist Circumference*

| | BMI, kg/m² | Disease Risk[†] Relative to Normal Weight and Waist Circumference[‡] | |
		Men, ≤102 cm; Women, ≤88 cm	Men, >102 cm; Women, >88 cm
Underweight	<18.5	. . .	. . .
Normal[§]	18.5–24.9	. . .	. . .
Overweight	25.0–29.9	Increased	High
Obesity, class			
I	30.0–34.9	High	Very high
II	35.0–39.9	Very high	Very high
III	≥40	Extremely high	Extremely high

*Modified from Expert Panel. Executive summary of the clinical guidelines on the identification, evaluation, and treatment of overweight and obesity in adults. Arch Intern Med 1998;158:1855–1867.

†Disease risk for type 2 diabetes, hypertension, and cardiovascular disease. Ellipses indicate that no additional risk at these levels of BMI was assigned.

‡A gender neutral value for waist circumference (>100 cm) has also been suggested as an index of obesity (see Table 2-1).

§Increased waist circumference can also be a marker for increased risk even in persons of normal weight.

dicting percent fat from skinfolds is ±3.5% assuming that appropriate techniques and equations have been used (6).

Various regression equations have been developed to predict body density or percent fat from skinfold measurements. For example, Box 4-2 lists generalized equations that allow calculation of percent fat or density without a loss in prediction accuracy for a wide range of individuals (17,18). However, if a population-specific equation is needed, Heyward and Stolarczyk provide a quick reference guide to match the client to the correct equation based on gender, age, ethnicity, fatness, and sport (6).

Other Techniques

The following body composition techniques include one popular field technique, a new methodology used primarily in a research or clinical setting, and finally, one for which more research is needed before it can be recommended generally.

BIOELECTRICAL IMPEDANCE ANALYSIS

Bioelectrical impedance analysis (BIA) is an easy-to-administer, noninvasive, and safe method of assessing body composition in a fitness setting.

BOX 4-1. Standardized Description of Skinfold Sites and Procedures

Skinfold Site

- Abdominal — Vertical fold; 2 cm to the right side of the umbilicus
- Triceps — Vertical fold; on the posterior midline of the upper arm, halfway between the acromion and olecranon processes, with the arm held freely to the side of the body
- Biceps — Vertical fold; on the anterior aspect of the arm over the belly of the biceps muscle, 1 cm above the level used to mark the triceps site
- Chest/Pectoral — Diagonal fold; one-half the distance between the anterior axillary line and the nipple (men) or one-third of the distance between the anterior axillary line and the nipple (women)
- Medial Calf — Vertical fold; at the maximum circumference of the calf on the midline of its medial border
- Midaxillary — Vertical fold; on the midaxillary line at the level of the xiphoid process of the sternum (An alternate method is a horizontal fold taken at the level of the xiphoid/sternal border in the midaxillary line.)
- Subscapular — Diagonal fold (at a 45° angle); 1 to 2 cm below the inferior angle of the scapula
- Suprailiac — Diagonal fold; in line with the natural angle of the iliac crest taken in the anterior axillary line immediately superior to the iliac crest
- Thigh — Vertical fold; on the anterior midline of the thigh, midway between the proximal border of the patella and the inguinal crease (hip)

Procedures

- All measurements should be made on the right side of the body
- Caliper should be placed 1 cm away from the thumb and finger, perpendicular to the skinfold, and halfway between the crest and the base of the fold
- Pinch should be maintained while reading the caliper
- Wait 1 to 2 s (and not longer) before reading caliper
- Take duplicate measures at each site and retest if duplicate measurements are not within 1 to 2 mm
- Rotate through measurement sites or allow time for skin to regain normal texture and thickness

---

BOX 4-2. Generalized Skinfold Equations*

Men

- **7-Site Formula** (chest, midaxillary, triceps, subscapular, abdomen, suprailiac, thigh)
  Body Density = 1.112 − 0.00043499 (Sum of 7 Skinfolds) + 0.00000055 (Sum of 7 Skinfolds)^2 − 0.00028826 (Age)
- **3-Site Formula** (chest, abdomen, thigh)
  Body Density = 1.10938 − 0.0008267 (Sum of 3 Skinfolds) + 0.0000016 (Sum of 3 Skinfolds)^2 − 0.0002574 (Age)
- **3-Site Formula** (chest, triceps, subscapular)
  Body Density = 1.1125025 − 0.0013125 (Sum of 3 Skinfolds) + 0.0000055 (Sum of 3 Skinfolds)^2 − 0.000244 (Age)

Women

- **7-Site Formula** (chest, midaxillary, triceps, subscapular, abdomen, suprailiac, thigh)
  Body Density = 1.097 − 0.00046971 (Sum of 7 Skinfolds) + 0.00000056 (Sum of 7 Skinfolds)^2 − 0.00012828 (Age)
- **3-Site Formula** (triceps, suprailiac, thigh)
  Body Density = 1.099421 − 0.0009929 (Sum of 3 Skinfolds) + 0.0000023 (Sum of 3 Skinfolds)^2 − 0.0001392 (Age)
- **3-Site Formula** (triceps, suprailiac, abdominal)
  Body Density = 1.089733 − 0.0009245 (Sum of 3 Skinfolds) + 0.0000025 (Sum of 3 Skinfolds)^2 − 0.0000979 (Age)

*Adapted from Jackson AS, Pollock ML. Practical assessment of body composition. Physician Sport Med 1985;13:76–90.

BIA involves passing a small electric current through the body and measuring the impedance or opposition to current flow (6). Fat-free tissue (body water) is a good conductor of electrical current, whereas fat is not. The resistance to current flow is thus inversely related to FFM and total body water, both of which can be predicted by this technique. In general, the prediction of percent fat from BIA measurements is similar to that of skinfolds, *as long as the recommended protocol is followed.* The subject must do the following:

- Abstain from eating or drinking within 4 hours of the assessment.
- Avoid moderate or vigorous physical activity within 12 hours of the assessment.
- Void completely before the assessment.
- Abstain from alcohol consumption within 48 hours of the assessment.
- Ingest no diuretic agents, including caffeine, prior to the assessment unless prescribed by a physician.

Failure to follow these guidelines increases the error in measurement. In addition, one must determine if the equations programmed into the analyzer's computer are valid and accurate for the populations being measured (6).

DUAL ENERGY X-RAY ABSORPTIOMETRY

Dual energy x-ray absorptiometry (DXA; sometimes abbreviated DEXA) is a new technology that can be used to assess total bone mineral as well as regional estimates of bone, fat, and lean tissues. It uses a three-component model to predict body fatness and offers advantages over the densitometry technique described earlier (19). DXA is typically found in a clinical setting and can be used to measure body composition across the life span.

NEAR-INFRARED INTERACTANCE

Near-infrared interactance (NIR) is based on the principles of light absorption and reflection using near-infrared spectroscopy to provide information about the chemical composition of the body. Further research is needed to develop and cross-validate gender-specific equations for infrared interactance, and to determine whether this technique is an accurate method for assessing body composition (6).

Tables 4-3 and 4-4 provide percentile values for percent body fat in men and women, respectively (10). These values are based on a selected population; exact percent body fatness values associated with an increased health risk have yet to be defined.

TABLE 4-3. Body Composition (% Body Fat) for Men*

Percentile	Age				
	20–29	30–39	40–49	50–59	60+
90	7.1	11.3	13.6	15.3	15.3
80	9.4	13.9	16.3	17.9	18.4
70	11.8	15.9	18.1	19.8	20.3
60	14.1	17.5	19.6	21.3	22.0
50	15.9	19.0	21.1	22.7	23.5
40	17.4	20.5	22.5	24.1	25.0
30	19.5	22.3	24.1	25.7	26.7
20	22.4	24.2	26.1	27.5	28.5
10	25.9	27.3	28.9	30.3	31.2

*Data provided by the Institute of Aerobics Research, Dallas, TX (1994). Study population for the data set was predominately white and college educated. The following may be used as descriptors for the percentile rankings: well above average (90), above average (70), average (50), below average (30), and well below average (10).

TABLE 4-4. Body Composition (% Body Fat) for Women*					
	Age				
Percentile	**20–29**	**30–39**	**40–49**	**50–59**	**60+**
90	14.5	15.5	18.5	21.6	21.1
80	17.1	18.0	21.3	25.0	25.1
70	19.0	20.0	23.5	26.6	27.5
60	20.6	21.6	24.9	28.5	29.3
50	22.1	23.1	26.4	30.1	30.9
40	23.7	24.9	28.1	31.6	32.5
30	25.4	27.0	30.1	33.5	34.3
20	27.7	29.3	32.1	35.6	36.6
10	32.1	32.8	35.0	37.9	39.3

*Data provided by the Institute for Aerobics Research, Dallas, TX (1994). Study population for the data set was predominately white and college educated. The following may be used as descriptors for the percentile rankings: well above average (90), above average (70), average (50), below average (30), and well below average (10).

CARDIORESPIRATORY FITNESS

Cardiorespiratory fitness is related to the ability to perform large muscle, dynamic, moderate-to-high intensity exercise for prolonged periods. Performance of such exercise depends on the functional state of the respiratory, cardiovascular, and skeletal muscle systems. Cardiorespiratory fitness is considered health-related because (a) low levels of cardiorespiratory fitness have been associated with a markedly increased risk of premature death from all causes and specifically from cardiovascular disease, (b) increases in cardiorespiratory fitness are associated with a reduction in death from all causes, and (c) high levels of cardiorespiratory fitness are associated with higher levels of habitual physical activity, which are, in turn, associated with many health benefits (20–22).

The Concept of Maximal Oxygen Uptake

Maximal oxygen uptake ($\dot{V}O_{2max}$) is accepted as the criterion measure of cardiorespiratory fitness. Maximal oxygen uptake is the product of the maximal cardiac output (L/min) and arterial-venous oxygen difference (mL O_2/L). The two- to three-fold difference in $\dot{V}O_{2max}$ (L/min) that exists across populations is due primarily to differences in maximal cardiac output; therefore, $\dot{V}O_{2max}$ is related to the functional capacity of the heart.

Open-circuit spirometry is used to measure $\dot{V}O_{2max}$. In this procedure, the subject breathes through a low-resistance valve (with nose occluded) while pulmonary ventilation and expired fractions of O_2 and CO_2 are measured. Measurement procedures have been considerably simplified since the days of collecting expired gas in Douglas bags and using chemical gas analyzers to determine the O_2 and CO_2 content. Modern automated systems provide ease of use and a detailed printout of test results that save time and effort (23). However, attention to detail relative to calibration is still essential to obtain accurate results. Because of the costs associated with equipment, space, and personnel needed to carry out these tests, direct measurement of $\dot{V}O_{2max}$ is generally reserved for research or clinical settings.

When direct measurement of $\dot{V}O_{2max}$ is not feasible or desirable, a variety of submaximal and maximal exercise tests can be used to estimate $\dot{V}O_{2max}$. These tests have been validated by examining (a) the correlation between directly measured $\dot{V}O_{2max}$ and the $\dot{V}O_{2max}$ estimated from physiologic responses to submaximal exercise (e.g., heart rate at a specified power output); or (b) the correlation between directly measured $\dot{V}O_{2max}$ and test performance (e.g., time to run 1 or 1.5 miles, or time to volitional fatigue using a standard graded exercise test protocol).

Maximal versus Submaximal Exercise Testing

The decision to use a maximal or submaximal exercise test depends largely on the reasons for the test, the type of subject to be tested, and the availability of appropriate equipment and personnel. $\dot{V}O_{2max}$ can be estimated with reasonable accuracy during conventional exercise test protocols, by considering test duration at a given grade and speed on a treadmill or power output on a cycle ergometer, using the prediction equations found in Appendix D. Maximal tests have the disadvantage of requiring participants to exercise to the point of volitional fatigue and might require physician supervision (see Chapter 2) and emergency equipment. Maximal exercise testing, however, offers increased sensitivity in the diagnosis of coronary artery disease in asymptomatic individuals (see Chapter 5).

Because maximal exercise testing is not a feasible method of assessing cardiorespiratory endurance for the vast majority of health/fitness practitioners, submaximal exercise tests are commonly used. The basic aim of submaximal exercise testing is to determine the heart rate (HR) response to one or more submaximal work rates and use the results to predict $\dot{V}O_{2max}$ (24).

Submaximal exercise tests make several assumptions:

- A steady-state heart rate is obtained for each exercise work rate.
- A linear relationship exists between heart rate and work rate.
- The maximal heart rate for a given age is uniform.
- Mechanical efficiency (i.e., $\dot{V}O_2$ at a given work rate) is the same for everyone.

Some of these assumptions are easily met (i.e., steady-state heart rate can be verified), while others (e.g., estimated maximal heart rate) introduce unknown errors into the prediction of $\dot{V}O_{2max}$. Although submaximal exercise testing is not as precise as maximal exercise testing, it provides a reasonably accurate reflection of an individual's fitness at a lower cost and reduced risk, and requires less time and effort on the part of the subject. When an individual is given repeated submaximal exercise tests over a period of weeks or months and the heart rate response to a fixed work rate decreases over time, it is likely that the individual's cardiorespiratory fitness has improved, independent of the accuracy of the $\dot{V}O_{2max}$ prediction. The details for various submaximal protocols are presented later in this chapter.

Modes of Testing

Field tests requiring an all-out effort, and submaximal treadmill, cycle ergometer, and step tests can be used as modes of testing to predict $\dot{V}O_{2max}$. There are advantages and disadvantages of each mode:

- *Field tests* consist of walking or running a certain distance in a given time; i.e., 12-minute run test, the 1-mile walk test, the 1.5-mile run test for time. The advantages of field tests are that large numbers of individuals can be tested at one time and little equipment (e.g., a stopwatch) is needed. The disadvantages are that they are all presumably maximal tests, and by their nature, are unmonitored. However, $\dot{V}O_{2max}$ can be estimated from test results.
- *Motor driven treadmills* can be used for submaximal and maximal testing and are often used for diagnostic testing. They provide a common form of physiologic stress (i.e., walking) and can accommodate the least to the most fit individuals across the continuum of walking to running speeds. Nevertheless, a practice session might be necessary in some cases to permit habituation and reduce anxiety. On the other hand, treadmills are usually expensive, not easily transportable, and make some measurements (blood pressure) difficult.
- *Mechanically braked cycle ergometers* are excellent test modalities for submaximal and maximal testing. They are relatively inexpensive, easily transportable, and allow blood pressure and the electrocardiogram (if appropriate) to be easily measured. The main disadvantage is that cycling is an unfamiliar method of exercise for many Americans, often resulting in limiting localized muscle fatigue. Cycle ergometers provide a non–weight-bearing test modality in which work rates are easily adjusted in small work-rate increments, and subjects tend to be least anxious using this device (25). The cycle ergometer must be calibrated and the subject must maintain the proper pedal rate because most tests require that heart rate be measured at specific work rates. Electronic cycle ergometers can deliver the same work rate across a range of pedal rates, but calibration might require special equipment not available in most laboratories.

- *Step testing* is an excellent modality for predicting cardiorespiratory fitness by measuring the heart rate response to one or more step rates (or step heights), or by measuring postexercise recovery heart rates. Step tests require little or no equipment; steps are easily transportable; stepping skill requires no practice; the test is usually of short duration; and stepping is excellent for mass testing (25,26). Postexercise (recovery) heart rates decrease with improved cardiorespiratory fitness and test results are easy to explain to participants (26). Special precautions might be needed for those who have balance problems or are extremely deconditioned.

FIELD TESTS

Two of the most widely used running tests for assessing cardiorespiratory fitness are the Cooper 12-minute test and the 1.5-mile test for time. The objective in the 12-minute test is to cover the greatest distance in the allotted time period, and for the 1.5-mile test it is to run the distance in the shortest period of time. $\dot{V}O_{2max}$ can be estimated from the equations in Appendix D. Although field tests are easy to administer, an individual's level of motivation and pacing ability can have a profound impact on test results. Of greater potential importance is the risk that exists during such testing because individuals are encouraged to put forth a maximal effort. These all-out run tests might be inappropriate for sedentary individuals at increased risk for cardiovascular and musculoskeletal complications.

The Rockport One-Mile Fitness Walking Test has gained wide popularity as an effective means for estimating cardiorespiratory fitness. In this test, an individual walks 1 mile as fast as possible, preferably on a track or a level surface, and heart rate is measured in the final minute, during the last one-quarter mile. An alternative is to measure a 10-second heart rate immediately on completion of the 1-mile walk, but this may overestimate the $\dot{V}O_{2max}$ compared to when heart rate is measured during the walk. $\dot{V}O_{2max}$ is estimated from a regression equation (found in Appendix D) based on weight, age, gender, walk time, and heart rate (27).

SUBMAXIMAL EXERCISE TESTS

Both single-stage and multi-stage submaximal exercise tests are available to estimate $\dot{V}O_{2max}$ from simple heart rate measurements. It is recommended that an electrocardiograph, heart rate monitor, or a stethoscope be used to determine heart rate. The submaximal heart rate response is easily altered by a number of environmental (heat and/or humidity), dietary (time since last meal), and behavioral (smoking, previous activity) factors. These variables must be controlled to have a valid and reliable estimate that can be used as a reference point in a person's fitness program. In addition, the test mode (cycle, treadmill, or step) should be consistent with the primary activity used by the participant to address specificity of training issues. Standardized procedures for submaximal testing are presented in Box 4-3; pretest instructions were presented at the beginning of this chapter.

> ## BOX 4-3. General Procedures for Submaximal Testing of Cardiorespiratory Endurance Using a Cycle Ergometer
>
> 1. The exercise test should begin with a 2- to 3-min warm-up to acquaint the client with the cycle ergometer and prepare him or her for the exercise intensity in the first stage of the test.
> 2. The specific protocol consists of 3-min stages with appropriate increments in work rate.
> 3. The client should be properly positioned on the cycle ergometer (i.e., upright posture, 5° bend in the knee at maximal leg extension, hands in proper position on handlebars).
> 4. Heart rate should be monitored at least 2 times during each stage, near the end of the second and third minutes of each stage. If heart rate > 110 beats·min^{-1}, steady-state heart rate (i.e., 2 heart rates within 6 beats·min^{-1}) should be reached before the work rate is increased.
> 5. Blood pressure should be monitored in the later portion of each stage and repeated (verified) in the event of a hypotensive or hypertensive response.
> 6. Perceived exertion should be monitored near the end of each stage using either the 6–20 or the 0–10 scale (Table 4-6).
> 7. Client appearance and symptoms should be monitored regularly.
> 8. The test should be terminated when the subject reaches 85% of age-predicted maximal heart rate (70% of heart rate reserve), fails to conform to the exercise test protocol, experiences adverse signs or symptoms, requests to stop, or experiences an emergency situation.
> 9. An appropriate cool-down/recovery period should be initiated consisting of either:
>   a. continued pedaling at a work rate equivalent to that of the first stage of the exercise test protocol or lower; or,
>   b. a passive cool-down if the subject experiences signs of discomfort or an emergency situation occurs.
> 10. All physiologic observations (e.g., heart rate, blood pressure, signs and symptoms) should be continued for at least 4 min of recovery unless abnormal responses occur, which would warrant a longer posttest surveillance period.

Cycle Ergometer Tests The Åstrand-Ryhming cycle ergometer test is a single-stage test lasting 6 minutes (28). For the population studied, these researchers observed that at 50% of $\dot{V}O_{2max}$, average heart rate was 128 beats·min^{-1} for males, and for females, 138 beats·min^{-1}. If a female was working at a $\dot{V}O_2$ of 1.5 L·min^{-1} and her HR was 138 beats·min^{-1}, then her $\dot{V}O_{2max}$ was estimated to be 3.0 L·min^{-1}. The suggested work rate is based on gender and an individual's fitness status as follows:

males—unconditioned: 300 or 600 kg·m·min^{-1} (50 or 100 watts)
males—conditioned: 600 or 900 kg·m·min^{-1} (100 or 150 watts)
females—unconditioned: 300 or 450 kg·m·min^{-1} (50 or 75 watts)
females—conditioned: 450 or 600 kg·m·min^{-1} (75 or 100 watts)

The pedal rate is set at 50 rpm. The goal is to obtain HR values between 125 and 170 beats·min^{-1}, and HR is measured during the fifth and sixth minute of work. The average of the two heart rates is then used to estimate $\dot{V}O_{2max}$ from a nomogram (Fig. 4-1). This value must then be adjusted

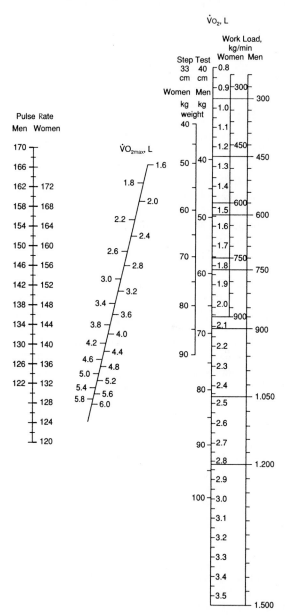

FIGURE 4-1. Modified Åstrand-Ryhming nomogram. (Reprinted with permission from Åstrand P-O, Ryhming I. A nomogram for calculation of aerobic capacity [physical fitness] from pulse rate during submaximal work. J Appl Physiol 1954;7:218–221.)

for age (because maximal HR decreases with age) by multiplying the $\dot{V}O_{2max}$ value by the following correction factors (29):

Age	Correction Factor
15	1.10
25	1.00
35	0.87
40	0.83
45	0.78
50	0.75
55	0.71
60	0.68
65	0.65

In contrast to the single-stage test, Maritz et al. (30) measured HR at a series of submaximal work rates and extrapolated the response to the subject's age-predicted maximal heart rate. This has become one of the most popular assessment techniques to estimate $\dot{V}O_{2max}$, and the YMCA test is a good example (18). The YMCA protocol uses two to four, 3-minute stages of continuous exercise (Fig. 4-2). The test is designed to raise the steady-state HR of the subject to between 110 beats·min^{-1} and 85% of the age-predicted maximal HR for at least two consecutive stages. An important point to remember is that two consecutive HR measurements must be obtained within this HR range to predict $\dot{V}O_{2max}$. In the YMCA protocol, each work rate is performed for 3 minutes, and heart rates are recorded during the final 15 to 30 seconds of the second and third minutes. If these heart rates are not within 6 beats·min^{-1} of each other, then that work rate is maintained for an additional minute. The heart rate measured during the last minute of each stage is plotted against work rate. The line generated from the plotted points is then extrapolated to the age-predicted maximal heart rate (e.g., 220 − age), and a perpendicular line is dropped to the x-axis to estimate the work rate that would have been achieved if the person had worked to maximum (Fig. 4-3). $\dot{V}O_{2max}$ can be estimated from the work rate using the formula in Appendix D. The two lines noted as ±1 SD in Figure 4-3 show what the estimated $\dot{V}O_{2max}$ would be if the subject's true maximal HR were 168 or 192 beats·min^{-1}, rather than 180 beats·min^{-1}. Part of the error involved in estimating $\dot{V}O_{2max}$ from submaximal HR responses occurs because the formula (220 − age) can provide only an estimate of maximal HR.

Treadmill Tests   The primary exercise modality for submaximal exercise testing has traditionally been the cycle ergometer, although in many settings, treadmills have been used. The same end point (85% of age-predicted maximal HR) is used, and the stages of the test should be 3 minutes or longer to ensure a steady-state HR response at each stage. The HR values are extrapolated to age-predicted maximal HR, and $\dot{V}O_{2max}$ is estimated using

	1st Stage	150 kgm/min (0.5 kg)

	HR < 80	HR 80–89	HR 90–100	HR > 100
2nd Stage	750 kgm/min (2.5 kg)*	600 kgm/min (2.0 kg)	450 kgm/min (1.5 kg)	300 kgm/min (1.0 kg)
3rd Stage	900 kgm/min (3.0 kg)	750 kgm/min (2.5 kg)	600 kgm/min (2.0 kg)	450 kgm/min (1.5 kg)
4th Stage	1050 kgm/min (3.5 kg)	900 kgm/min (3.0 kg)	750 kgm/min (2.5 kg)	600 kgm/min (2.0 kg)

Directions
1. Set the first work rate at 150 kgm/min (0.5 kg at 50 rpm)
2. If the HR in the third minute of the stage is:
   less than (<) 80, set the second stage at 750 kgm/min (2.5 kg at 50 rpm)
   80–89, set the second stage at 600 kgm/min (2.0 kg at 50 rpm)
   90–100, set the second stage at 450 kgm/min (1.5 kg at 50 rpm)
   greater than (>) 100, set the second stage at 300 kgm/min (1.0 kg at 50 rpm)
3. Set the third and fourth (if required) stages according to the work rates in the columns below the second loads.

FIGURE 4-2. YMCA cycle ergometry protocol. *Resistance settings shown here are appropriate for an ergometer with a flywheel of 6 m/rev.

the formula in Appendix D from the highest grade and/or speed that would have been achieved if the person had worked to maximum. Most common treadmill protocols (see Chapter 5) can be used, but the duration of each stage should be at least 3 minutes.

Step Tests Step tests have also been used to estimate $\dot{V}O_{2max}$. Åstrand and Ryhming (28) used a single-step height of 33 cm for women and 40 cm for men at a rate of 22.5 steps·min^{-1}. These tests require oxygen uptakes of about 25.8 and 29.5 mL·kg^{-1}·min^{-1}, respectively. Heart rate is measured as described above for the cycle test, and $\dot{V}O_{2max}$ is estimated from the nomogram (see Fig. 4-1). In contrast, Maritz et al. (30) used a single-step height (30.5 cm) and four-step rates to systematically increase the work rate. A steady-state HR was measured for each step rate and a line formed from these HR values was extrapolated to age-predicted maximal HR; the maximal work rate was determined as described above for the YMCA cycle test.

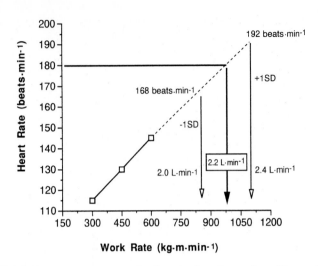

FIGURE 4-3. Heart rate responses to 3 submaximal work rates for a 40-year old, sedentary female weighing 64 kg. $\dot{V}O_{2max}$ was estimated by extrapolating the heart rate (HR) response to the age-predicted maximal HR of 180 beats·min^{-1} (based on 220 − age). The work rate that would have been achieved at that HR was determined by dropping a line from that HR value to the x-axis. $\dot{V}O_{2max}$, estimated using the formula in Appendix D and expressed in L·min^{-1}, was 2.2 L·min^{-1}. The other 2 lines estimate what the $\dot{V}O_{2max}$ would have been if the subject's true maximal HR was ±1 SD from the 180 beats·min^{-1} value.

$\dot{V}O_{2max}$ can be estimated from the formula for stepping in Appendix D. Such step tests should be modified to suit the population being tested. The Canadian Home Fitness Test has demonstrated that such testing can be used on a large scale and at low cost (26,31).

Instead of estimating $\dot{V}O_{2max}$ from HR responses to several submaximal work rates, a wide variety of step tests have been developed to categorize cardiovascular fitness on the basis of a person's recovery HR following a standardized step test. The 3-Minute YMCA Step Test is a good example of such a test. This test uses a 12-inch (30.5 cm) bench, with a stepping rate of 24 steps·min^{-1} (estimated oxygen cost of 25.8 mL·kg^{-1}·min^{-1}). After exercise is completed, the subject immediately sits down, and heart rate is counted for 1 minute. Counting must start within 5 seconds of the end of exercise. Heart rate values are used to obtain a qualitative rating of fitness from published normative tables (18).

Table 4-5 provides normative values for $\dot{V}O_{2max}$ (mL·kg^{-1}·min^{-1}), with specific reference to age and gender. Research suggests that a $\dot{V}O_{2max}$ below the 20th percentile for age and gender is associated with an increased risk of death from all causes (20). However, caution should be exercised when using these data to determine the fitness status for any given individual. One must consider whether the data set was based on a representative population, used the same test (mode; maximal versus submaximal; stage duration; etc.), and whether $\dot{V}O_{2max}$ was estimated or measured directly. Perhaps a more useful approach is to use the baseline test as a reference point to chart progress in cardiorespiratory fitness over time.

TABLE 4-5. Percentile Values for Maximal Aerobic Power (mL·kg⁻¹·min⁻¹)*

Percentile	Age				
	20–29	**30–39**	**40–49**	**50–59**	**60+**
Men					
90	51.4	50.4	48.2	45.3	42.5
80	48.2	46.8	44.1	41.0	38.1
70	46.8	44.6	41.8	38.5	35.3
60	44.2	42.4	39.9	36.7	33.6
50	42.5	41.0	38.1	35.2	31.8
40	41.0	38.9	36.7	33.8	30.2
30	39.5	37.4	35.1	32.3	28.7
20	37.1	35.4	33.0	30.2	26.5
10	34.5	32.5	30.9	28.0	23.1
Women					
90	44.2	41.0	39.5	35.2	35.2
80	41.0	38.6	36.3	32.3	31.2
70	38.1	36.7	33.8	30.9	29.4
60	36.7	34.6	32.3	29.4	27.2
50	35.2	33.8	30.9	28.2	25.8
40	33.8	32.3	29.5	26.9	24.5
30	32.3	30.5	28.3	25.5	23.8
20	30.6	28.7	26.5	24.3	22.8
10	28.4	26.5	25.1	22.3	20.8

*Data provided by Institute for Aerobics Research, Dallas, TX (1994). Study population for the data set was predominately white and college educated. A modified Balke treadmill test was used with $\dot{V}O_{2max}$ estimated from the last grade/speed achieved. The following may be used as descriptors for the percentile rankings: well above average (90), above average (70), average (50), below average (30), and well below average (10).

Cardiorespiratory Test Sequence and Measures

Typically, HR, blood pressure, and rating of perceived exertion (RPE) are measured during exercise tests. After the initial screening process, selected baseline measurements should be obtained prior to the start of the exercise test. Taking a resting ECG prior to exercise testing assumes that trained personnel are available to interpret the ECG and provide medical guidance. When diagnostic testing is not being done, and when apparently healthy individuals are being tested with submaximal tests, an ECG is not necessary. At a minimum, resting HR and blood pressure measurements should be obtained immediately prior to exercise, during each stage of the exercise testing protocol (typically every 2 or 3 minutes), and at 1- or 2-minute intervals during the recovery period. The recovery period should consist of at least 4 minutes of low-intensity exercise (e.g., walking at 2 to 3 mph [54 to 80 m·min⁻¹] or low-load cycling [75 to 150 kg·m·min⁻¹]). This period of low-intensity exercise should continue until HR and blood pressure stabilize, but not necessarily until they reach preexercise levels.

Heart rate can be determined using several techniques, including radial or carotid pulse palpation, auscultation with a stethoscope, or the use of pulse monitors. The pulse palpation technique involves "feeling" the pulse by placing the first and second fingers over an artery (usually the radial artery located near the thumbside of the wrist or the carotid artery located in the neck near the larynx). The pulse is typically counted for either 10 or 15 seconds, and then multiplied by 6 or 4, respectively, to determine the per-minute HR. Although the carotid pulse might be easier to obtain, one should not press too hard with the palpating fingers because this could produce a marked bradycardia in the presence of a hypersensitive carotid sinus reflex. For the auscultation method, the bell of the stethoscope should be placed to the left of the sternum just above the level of the nipple. This method is most accurate when the heart sounds are clearly audible and the subject's torso is relatively stable. Over the years, several automated heart rate monitors have been developed. Heart rate monitors ("watches") have proven to be accurate and reliable, provided there is no outside electrical interference (e.g., emissions from the display consoles of computerized exercise equipment).

Blood pressure should be measured with the subject's arm relaxed and not grasping a handrail (treadmill) or handlebar (cycle ergometer). To help ensure accurate readings, the use of an appropriate-sized blood pressure cuff is important. The rubber bladder of the blood pressure cuff should encircle at least two-thirds of the subject's upper arm. If the subject's arm is large, a normal-size adult cuff will be too small, making the readings higher than they actually are (the converse is also true). Blood pressure measurements should be taken with a mercury sphygmomanometer adjusted to eye level or a recently calibrated aneroid manometer. Systolic and diastolic blood pressure measurements can be used as indicators for stopping an exercise test (see next section).

Rating of perceived exertion (RPE) is a valuable and reliable indicator in monitoring an individual's exercise tolerance. Often used while conducting graded exercise tests, perceived exertion ratings correlate highly with exercise heart rates and work rates. Borg's RPE scale was developed to allow the exerciser to subjectively rate his or her feelings during exercise, taking into account personal fitness level, environmental conditions, and general fatigue levels (32). Currently, two RPE scales are widely used: the original or category scale, which rates exercise intensity on a scale of 6 to 20, and the revised or category-ratio scale of 0 to 10. This category-ratio scale uses terminology better understood by the subject, thereby providing the tester with more valid information by which to further direct the test.

The greatest value of the RPE scale is that it provides exercisers of all fitness levels with easily understood guidelines regarding exercise intensity. It has been found that a cardiorespiratory training effect and the threshold for blood lactate accumulation are achieved at a rating of "somewhat hard" to "hard," which approximates a rating of 12 to 16 on the category scale or 4 to 5 on the category-ratio scale. Both RPE scales are shown in Table 4-6.

During exercise testing, the RPE can be used as an indication of impending fatigue. Most subjects reach their subjective limit of fatigue at an RPE of 18 to 19 (very, very hard) on the category Borg scale of 9 to 10 (very, very strong) on the category-ratio scale; therefore, RPE can effectively be used to monitor progress toward maximal exertion during exercise testing. Clinical and practical experience indicate, however, that approximately 5 to 10% of individuals tend to underestimate RPE during the early and middle stages of an exercise test. It is important to use standardized instructions to reduce problems of misinterpretation of RPE. The following are recommended instructions for using the RPE scale during exercise testing (33):

"During the exercise test we want you to pay close attention to how hard you feel the exercise work rate is. This feeling should reflect your total amount of exertion and fatigue, combining all sensations and feelings of physical stress, effort, and fatigue. Don't concern yourself with any one factor such as leg pain, shortness of breath or exercise intensity, but try to concentrate on your total, inner feeling of exertion. Try not to underestimate or overestimate your feelings of exertion; be as accurate as you can."

TABLE 4-6. Category and Category-Ratio Scales for Ratings of Perceived Exertion (RPE)*

Category Scale		Category-Ratio Scale	
6	0	Nothing at all	"No I"
7 Very, very light	0.3		
8	0.5	Extremely weak	Just noticeable
9 Very light	0.7		
10	1	Very weak	
11 Fairly light	1.5		
12	2	Weak	Light
13 Somewhat hard	2.5		
14	3	Moderate	
15 Hard	4		
16	5	Strong	Heavy
17 Very hard	6		
18	7	Very strong	
19 Very, very hard	8		
20	9		
	10	Extremely strong	"Strongest I"
	11		
	•	Absolute maximum	Highest possible

*Copyright Gunnar Borg. Reproduced with permission.

Note: On the Category-Ratio Scale, "I" represents intensity.

For correct usage of the Borg scales, it is necessary to follow the administration and instructions given in Borg G. Borg's Perceived Exertion and Pain Scales. Champaign, IL: Human Kinetics, 1998.

> ## BOX 4-4. General Indications for Stopping an Exercise Test in Low-Risk Adults*
>
> - Onset of angina or angina-like symptoms.
> - Significant drop (20 mm Hg) in systolic blood pressure or a failure of the systolic blood pressure to rise with an increase in exercise intensity.
> - Excessive rise in blood pressure: systolic pressure > 260 mm Hg or diastolic pressure > 115 mm Hg.
> - Signs of poor perfusion: light-headedness, confusion, ataxia, pallor, cyanosis, nausea, or cold and clammy skin.
> - Failure of heart rate to increase with increased exercise intensity.
> - Noticeable change in heart rhythm.
> - Subject requests to stop.
> - Physical or verbal manifestations of severe fatigue.
> - Failure of the testing equipment.

*Assumes that testing is nondiagnostic and is being performed without direct physician involvement or electrocardiographic monitoring. For clinical testing, Box 5-3 provides more definitive and specific termination criteria.

Test Termination Criteria

Graded exercise testing, whether maximal or submaximal, is a safe procedure when subject screening and testing guidelines (see Chapter 2) are adhered to. Occasionally, for safety reasons, the test may have to be terminated prior to the subject reaching a measured $\dot{V}O_{2max}$, volitional fatigue, or a predetermined end point (i.e., 85% age-predicted maximal HR). General indications—those that do not rely on physician involvement or ECG monitoring—for stopping an exercise test are outlined in Box 4-4. More specific termination criteria for clinical or diagnostic testing are provided in Chapter 5.

MUSCULAR FITNESS

Muscular fitness is a health-related fitness component because it improves or maintains the following:

> - The fat-free mass and resting metabolic rate, which is related to weight gain
> - Bone mass, which is related to osteoporosis
> - Glucose tolerance, which is related to type 2 diabetes
> - Musculotendinous integrity, which is related to a lower risk of injury, including low-back pain
> - The ability to carry out the activities of daily living, which is related to self-esteem

Accordingly, the ACSM has included muscular fitness in its recent position stand on the quantity and quality of exercise to achieve and maintain fitness (34). The term "muscular fitness" has been used to describe the integrated status of muscular strength (maximal force a muscle can generate at a given velocity) and muscular endurance (ability of a muscle to make repeated contractions or to resist muscular fatigue) (35,36). The assessment of muscular strength and endurance represents a continuum with "muscular strength" at one end of the assessment scale and "muscular endurance" at the other. Tests allowing few repetitions of a task are measuring strength, while those in which great numbers of repetitions can be done are measuring endurance. Before common tests to measure muscular fitness are described, there are some points worth noting (35,36):

- Muscular strength and muscular endurance are specific to the muscle or muscle group, the type of muscular contraction (static or dynamic; concentric or eccentric), the speed of muscular contraction (slow or fast), and the joint angle being tested (static contraction). Accordingly, the results of any one test are specific to the procedures used, and no single test exists for evaluating total body muscular strength or muscular endurance.
- Individuals should be put through familiarization/practice sessions with the equipment and protocol to be used in order to obtain a reliable score that can be used to track true physiological adaptations over time.
- Safety measures related to the equipment to be used and the use of spotters (when necessary) should be reviewed.
- Improvements in an individual's muscular fitness over time can use the absolute strength values (e.g., kilograms lifted), but when comparisons are made between individuals, the values should be expressed per kilogram of body weight (kg/kg). However, for the latter comparisons, caution must be used in the interpretation of the scores because the norms may not be representative of the individual being measured or the exact test (free weight versus machine weight) being used.

MUSCULAR STRENGTH

Muscular strength refers to the maximal force (properly expressed in Newtons, although kg is commonly used as well) that can be generated by a specific muscle or muscle group. Static or isometric strength can be measured conveniently using a variety of devices, including cable tensiometers and handgrip dynamometers. Unfortunately, measures of static strength are specific to both the muscle group and joint angle involved in testing and, therefore, their utility in describing overall muscular strength is limited. Peak force development in such tests is commonly referred to as the maximum voluntary contraction.

When testing involves movement of the body (e.g., a push-up) or an external load, then dynamic strength is being evaluated. The "gold standard" of dynamic strength testing is the 1-repetition maximum (1-RM), the heaviest weight that can be lifted only once using good form. The following represents the basic steps in 1-RM testing following familiarization/practice sessions (35):

1. The subject performs a light warm-up of 5 to 10 repetitions at 40 to 60% of perceived maximum.
2. Following a 1-minute rest with light stretching, the subject does 3 to 5 repetitions at 60% to 80% of perceived maximum.
3. The subject should be close to a perceived 1-RM in Step 2. A small amount of weight is added, and a 1-RM lift is attempted. If the lift is successful, a rest period of 3 to 5 minutes is provided. The goal is to find the 1-RM within 3 to 5 maximal efforts. The process of titrating the increase in weight up to a true 1-RM can be improved by prior familiarization sessions that allow approximation of the 1-RM. Clear communication with the subject is needed to facilitate determination of the 1-RM. This process continues until a failed attempt occurs.
4. The 1-RM is reported as the weight of the last successfully completed lift.

TABLE 4-7. Upper Body Strength*,†

| | Age | | | | |
Percentile	20–29	30–39	40–49	50–59	60+
Men					
90	1.48	1.24	1.10	.97	.89
80	1.32	1.12	1.00	.90	.82
70	1.22	1.04	.93	.84	.77
60	1.14	.98	.88	.79	.72
50	1.06	.93	.84	.75	.68
40	.99	.88	.80	.71	.66
30	.93	.83	.76	.68	.63
20	.88	.78	.72	.63	.57
10	.80	.71	.65	.57	.53
Women					
90	.90	.76	.71	.61	.64
80	.80	.70	.62	.55	.54
70	.74	.63	.57	.52	.51
60	.70	.60	.54	.48	.47
50	.65	.57	.52	.46	.45
40	.59	.53	.50	.44	.43
30	.56	.51	.47	.42	.40
20	.51	.47	43	.39	.38
10	.48	.42	38	.37	.33

*One repetition maximum bench press, with bench press weight ratio = weight pushed/body weight.

†Data provided by the Institute for Aerobics Research, Dallas, TX (1994). Adapted from ACSM's Guidelines for Exercise Testing and Prescription. 5th ed. Study population for the data set was predominately white and college educated. A Universal dynamic variable resistance (DVR) machine was used to measure the 1-RM. The following may be used as descriptors for the percentile rankings: well above average (90), above average (70), average (50), below average (30), and well below average (10).

One can use a 6-RM or 10-RM as a measure of muscular fitness, but estimating a 1-RM from such tests is problematic. This is due to the marked variation in the number of repetitions one can perform at a fixed percent of a 1-RM for different muscle groups (e.g., leg press versus bench press) (37,38). At the very least, the 6-RM or 10-RM can be used to simplify the testing procedures outlined above to measure a 1-RM. In addition, if the participant is following a 10- to 12-RM weight training program, improvement in muscular fitness can be tracked over time independent of the true 1-RM. However, for research purposes the true 1-RM should be measured (35). Valid measures of general upper body strength include the 1-RM values for bench press or military press. Corresponding indices of lower body strength include 1-RM values for leg press or leg extension. Norms for the bench press and leg press are provided in Tables 4-7 and 4-8, respectively.

Isokinetic testing involves the assessment of maximal muscle tension throughout a range of joint motion set at a constant angular velocity (e.g., 60° per second). Equipment that allows control of the speed of joint rotation

TABLE 4-8. Leg Strength*,†

| | Age | | | | |
Percentile	20–29	30–39	40–49	50–59	60+
Men					
90	2.27	2.07	1.92	1.80	1.73
80	2.13	1.93	1.82	1.71	1.62
70	2.05	1.85	1.74	1.64	1.56
60	1.97	1.77	1.68	1.58	1.49
50	1.91	1.71	1.62	1.52	1.43
40	1.83	1.65	1.57	1.46	1.38
30	1.74	1.59	1.51	1.39	1.30
20	1.63	1.52	1.44	1.32	1.25
10	1.51	1.43	1.35	1.22	1.16
Women					
90	1.82	1.61	1.48	1.37	1.32
80	1.68	1.47	1.37	1.25	1.18
70	1.58	1.39	1.29	1.17	1.13
60	1.50	1.33	1.23	1.10	1.04
50	1.44	1.27	1.18	1.05	.99
40	1.37	1.21	1.13	.99	.93
30	1.27	1.15	1.08	.95	.88
20	1.22	1.09	1.02	.88	.85
10	1.14	1.00	.94	.78	.72

*One repetition maximum leg press with leg press weight ratio = weight pushed/body weight.

†Data provided by the Institute for Aerobics Research, Dallas, TX (1994). Adapted from ACSM's Guidelines for Exercise Testing and Prescription. 5th ed. Study population for the data set was predominately white and college educated. A Universal dynamic variable resistance (DVR) machine was used to measure the 1-RM. The following may be used as descriptors for the percentile rankings: well above average (90), above average (70), average (50), below average (30), and well below average (10).

(degrees/sec) as well as the ability to test movement around various joints (e.g., knee, hip, shoulder, elbow) is available from several commercial sources. Such devices measure peak rotational force or torque, but an important drawback is that this equipment is extremely expensive compared to other strength-testing modalities (35,36).

MUSCULAR ENDURANCE

Muscular endurance is the ability of a muscle group to execute repeated contractions over a period of time sufficient to cause muscular fatigue, or to maintain a specific percentage of the maximum voluntary contraction for a prolonged period of time. Simple field tests such as a curl-up (crunch) test (39,40) or the maximum number of push-ups that can be performed without rest (41) may be used to evaluate the endurance of the abdominal

---

BOX 4-5. Push-up and Curl-up (Crunch) Test Procedures for Measurement of Muscular Endurance

Push-up
1. The push-up test is administered with male subjects in the standard "up" position (hands shoulder width apart, back straight, head up, using the toes as the pivotal point) and female subjects in the modified "knee push-up" position (legs together, lower leg in contact with mat with ankles plantar-flexed, back straight, hands shoulder width apart, head up).
2. The subject must lower the body until the chin touches the mat. The stomach should not touch the mat (41).
3. For both men and women, the subject's back must be straight at all times and the subject must push up to a straight arm position.
4. The maximal number of push-ups performed consecutively without rest is counted as the score.

Curl-up (Crunch)
1. Individual assumes a supine position on a mat with the knees at 90°. The arms are at the side, with fingers touching a piece of masking tape. A second piece of masking tape is placed 8 cm (for those who are ≥45 y) or 12 cm (for those who are <45 y) beyond the first (40).*
2. A metronome is set to 40 beats·min⁻¹ (50 beats·min⁻¹ for the Canadian standardized test) and the individual does slow, controlled curl-ups to lift the shoulder blades off the mat (trunk makes a 30° angle with the mat) in time with the metronome (20 curl-ups/min). The low back should be flattened before curling up.
3. Individual performs as many curl-ups as possible without pausing, up to a maximum of 75.†

*Alternatives include (a) having the hands held across the chest, with the head activating a counter when the trunk reaches a 30° position (39) and placing the hands on the thighs and curling up until the hands reach the knee caps (40). Elevation of the trunk to 30° is the important aspect of the movement.

†An alternative includes doing as many curl-ups as possible in 1 minute (39).

TABLE 4-9. Percentiles by Age Groups and Gender for Push-ups*

Percentile	Age									
	20–29		30–39		40–49		50–59		60–69	
Gender	M	F	M	F	M	F	M	F	M	F
90	41	32	32	31	25	28	24	23	24	25
80	34	26	27	24	21	22	17	17	16	15
70	30	22	24	21	19	18	14	13	11	12
60	27	20	21	17	16	14	11	10	10	10
50	24	16	19	14	13	12	10	9	9	6
40	21	14	16	12	12	10	9	5	7	4
30	18	11	14	10	10	7	7	3	6	2
20	16	9	11	7	8	4	5	1	4	—
10	11	5	8	4	5	2	4	—	2	—

*Based on data from the Canada Fitness Survey, 1981. (Reprinted from Canadian Standardized Test of Fitness (CSTF) Operations Manual. 3rd ed. With permission of Fitness Canada, Fitness and Amateur Sport Canada, Ottawa, 1986.) The following may be used as descriptors for the percentile rankings: well above average (90), above average (70), average (50), below average (30), and well below average (10).

muscle groups and upper body muscles, respectively. Although scientific data to support this hypothesis are lacking, poor abdominal strength/endurance is commonly thought to contribute to muscular low back pain (42). Procedures for conducting the push-up and curl-up (crunch) muscular endurance tests are given in Box 4-5, and norms and percentiles are provided in Tables 4-9 and 4-10, respectively.

Resistance training equipment can also be adapted to measure muscular endurance by selecting an appropriate submaximal level of resistance and measuring the number of repetitions or the duration of static contraction before fatigue. For example, the YMCA bench press test involves performing standardized repetitions at a rate of 30 lifts/min. Men are tested using an 80-pound barbell and women using a 35-pound barbell. Subjects are scored by the number of successful repetitions (18).

FLEXIBILITY

Flexibility is the ability to move a joint through its complete range of motion. It is important in athletic performance (e.g., ballet, gymnastics) and in the ability to carry out the activities of daily living. Consequently, maintaining flexibility of all joints facilitates movement; in contrast, when an activity moves the structures of a joint beyond a joint's shortened range of motion, tissue damage can occur.

Flexibility depends on a number of specific variables, including distensibility of the joint capsule, adequate warm-up, and muscle viscosity. Addi-

TABLE 4-10. Percentiles by Age Groups and Gender for Partial Curl-up*

Percentile	Age									
	20–29		30–39		40–49		50–59		60–69	
Gender	M	F	M	F	M	F	M	F	M	F
90	75	70	75	55	75	50	74	48	53	50
80	56	45	69	43	75	42	60	30	33	30
70	41	37	46	34	67	33	45	23	26	24
60	31	32	36	28	51	28	35	16	19	19
50	27	27	31	21	39	25	27	9	16	13
40	24	21	26	15	31	20	23	2	9	9
30	20	17	19	12	26	14	19	0	6	3
20	13	12	13	0	21	5	13	0	0	0
10	4	5	0	0	13	0	0	0	0	0

*Based on data from Canadian Standardized Test of Fitness Operations Manual. 3rd ed. Ottawa: Canadian Society for Exercise Physiology in cooperation with Fitness Canada, Government of Canada, 1986. See reference 40. The following may be used as descriptors for the percentile rankings: well above average (90), above average (70), average (50), below average (30), and well below average (10).

tionally, compliance ("tightness") of various other tissues such as ligaments and tendons affects the range of motion. Just as muscular strength is specific to the muscles involved, flexibility is joint specific. Therefore, no single flexibility test can be used to evaluate total body flexibility. Laboratory tests usually quantify flexibility in terms of range of motion, expressed in degrees. Common devices for this purpose include various goniometers, electrogoniometers, the Leighton flexometer, inclinometers, and tape measures. Visual estimates of range of motion can be useful in fitness screening, but are inaccurate relative to directly measured range of motion. These estimates can include neck and trunk flexibility, hip flexibility, lower extremity flexibility, shoulder flexibility, and postural assessment (43).

The sit-and-reach test has been commonly used to assess low back and hip-joint flexibility; however, it is not a good measure of low-back function when the distance reached is the only measure. To improve its use as a test of low back and hip-joint flexibility, the following steps are suggested (44):

- The test administrator should examine the quality of the movement including the angle of the sacrum (near 90° or more) and the "smoothness" of the spinal curve.
- Only one leg should be measured at a time to evaluate symmetry.
- If a sit-and-reach box is used, consider modifying it to allow plantar flexion because it has a significant effect on performance.

Poor lower back and hip flexibility may, in conjunction with poor abdominal strength/endurance or other causative factors, contribute to development of muscular low back pain. This hypothesis, however, remains to be substantiated from a scientific perspective. Methods for administering this test, including steps to correct for proportional differences in arm and leg lengths (45), are presented in Box 4-6. Percentile data on two sit-and-reach tests are presented in Tables 4-11 and 4-12.

BOX 4-6. Trunk Flexion (Sit-and-Reach) Test Procedures*

Pretest: Participant should perform a short warm-up prior to this test and include some stretches (e.g., modified hurdler's stretch). It is also recommended that the participant refrain from fast, jerky movements, which may increase the possibility of an injury. The participant's shoes should be removed.

1. For the YMCA sit-and-reach test, a yardstick is placed on the floor and tape is placed across it at a right angle to the 15-inch mark. The participant sits with the yardstick between the legs, with legs extended at right angles to the taped line on the floor. Heels of the feet should touch the edge of the taped line and be about 10 to 12 inches apart. If a standard sit-and-reach box is available, heels should be placed against the edge of the box.

2. The participant should slowly reach forward with both hands as far as possible, holding this position momentarily. Be sure that the participant keeps the hands parallel and does not lead with one hand. Fingertips can be overlapped and should be in contact with the yardstick or measuring portion of the sit-and-reach box.

3. The score is the most distant point (in inches or centimeters) reached with the fingertips. The best of three trials should be recorded. To assist with the best attempt, the participant should exhale and drop the head between the arms when reaching. Testers should ensure that the knees of the participant stay extended; however, the participant's knees should not be pressed down. The participant should breathe normally during the test and should not hold his or her breath at any time. Norms for the YMCA test are presented in Table 4-11.

4. The sit-and-reach test is also done using a sit-and-reach box. The participant sits with the legs fully extended with the soles of the feet against the box. The other directions are as described above. Norms for a sit-and-reach box test are provided in Table 4-12. Note that these norms use a sit-and-reach box in which the "zero" point is set at the 26 cm mark (41). If you are using a box in which the zero point is set at 23 cm (e.g., Fitnessgram), subtract 3 cm from each value in this table.

*Diagrams of these procedures are available elsewhere (18,41).

TABLE 4-11. Percentiles by Age Groups and Gender for YMCA Sit-and-Reach Test (Inches)*

	Age										
Percentile	**18–25**		**26–35**		**36–45**		**46–55**		**56–65**		**>65**	
Gender	**M**	**F**	**M**	**F**	**M**	**F**	**M**	**F**	**M**	**F**	**M**	**F**
90	22	24	21	23	21	22	19	21	17	20	17	20
80	20	22	19	21	19	21	17	20	15	19	15	18
70	19	21	17	20	17	19	15	18	13	17	13	17
60	18	20	17	20	16	18	14	17	13	16	12	17
50	17	19	15	19	15	17	13	16	11	15	10	15
40	15	18	14	17	13	16	11	14	9	14	9	14
30	14	17	13	16	13	15	10	14	9	13	8	13
20	13	16	11	15	11	14	9	12	7	11	7	11
10	11	14	9	13	7	12	6	10	5	9	4	9

*Based on data from YMCA of the USA (reference 18). The following may be used as descriptors for the percentile rankings: well above average (90), above average (70), average (50), below average (30), and well below average (10).

TABLE 4-12. Percentiles by Age Groups for Trunk Forward Flexion Using a Sit-and-Reach Box (cm)*

	Age									
Percentile	**20–29**		**30–39**		**40–49**		**50–59**		**60–69**	
Gender	**M**	**F**	**M**	**F**	**M**	**F**	**M**	**F**	**M**	**F**
90	42	43	40	42	37	40	38	40	35	37
80	38	40	37	39	34	37	32	37	30	34
70	36	38	34	37	30	35	29	35	26	31
60	33	36	32	35	28	33	27	32	24	30
50	31	34	29	33	25	31	25	30	22	28
40	29	32	27	31	23	29	22	29	18	26
30	26	29	24	28	20	26	18	26	16	24
20	23	26	21	25	16	24	15	23	14	23
10	18	22	17	21	12	19	12	19	11	18

*Based on data from the Canada Fitness Survey, 1981. Reprinted from Canadian Standardized Test of Fitness (CSTF) Operations Manual. 3rd ed. With permission of Fitness Canada, Fitness and Amateur Sport Canada, Ottawa, 1986. The following may be used as descriptors for the percentile rankings: well above average (90), above average (70), average (50), below average (30), and well below average (10).

Note: These norms are based on a sit-and-reach box in which the "zero" point is set at 26 cm. When using a box in which the "zero" point is set at 23 cm, subtract 3 cm from each value in this table.

References

1. Casperson CJ, Powell KE, Christenson GM. Physical activity, exercise and physical fitness: Definitions and distinctions for health-related research. Public Health Rep 1985;100:126–131.
2. Pate RR. The evolving definition of physical fitness. Quest 1988;40:174–179.
3. National Institutes of Health. Health implications of obesity: National Institutes of Health consensus development statement. Ann Intern Med 1985;103:1073–1077.
4. Kuczmarski RJ, Flegal KM, Campbell SM, et al. Increasing prevalence of overweight among US adults. JAMA 1994;272:205–211.
5. Troiano RP, Flegal KM. Overweight children and adolescents: description, epidemiology, and demographics. Pediatrics 1998;101:497–504.
6. Heyward VH, Stolarczyk LM. Applied Body Composition Assessment. Champaign, IL: Human Kinetics, 1996.
7. Roche AF, Heymsfield SB, Lohman TG, eds. Human Body Composition. Champaign, IL: Human Kinetics, 1996.
8. Going BS. Densitometry. In: Roche AF, Heymsfield SB, Lohman TG, eds. Human Body Composition. Champaign, IL: Human Kinetics, 1996:3–23.
9. Dempster P, Aitkens S. A new air displacement method for the determination of human body composition. Med Sci Sports Exerc 1995;27:1692–1697.
10. Lohman TG, Houtkooper L, Going SB. Body fat measurement goes high-tech. ACSM's Health Fitness J 1997;1:30–35.
11. Brozek J, Grande F, Anderson J, et al. Densitometric analysis of body composition: revision of some quantitative assumptions. Ann NY Acad Sci 1963;110:113–140.
12. Siri WE. Body composition from fluid spaces and density. Univ Calif Donner Lab Med Phys Rep, March 1956.
13. Expert Panel. Executive summary of the clinical guidelines on the identification, evaluation, and treatment of overweight and obesity in adults. Arch Intern Med 1998;158:1855–1867.
14. Van Itallie TB. Topography of body fat: relationship to risk of cardiovascular and other diseases. In: Lohman TG, Roche AF, Martorell R, eds. Anthropometric Standardization Reference Manual. Champaign, IL: Human Kinetics, 1988.
15. Bray GA, Gray DS. Obesity. Part 1-Pathogenesis. West J Med 1988;149:429–441.
16. Roche AF. Anthropometry and ultrasound. In: Roche AF, Heymsfield SB, Lohman TG, eds. Human Body Composition. Champaign, IL: Human Kinetics, 1996:167–189.
17. Jackson AS, Pollock ML. Practical assessment of body composition. Physician Sport Med 1985;13:76–90.
18. Golding LA, Myers CR, Sinning WE, eds. Y's Way to Physical Fitness. 3rd ed. Champaign, IL: Human Kinetics, 1989.
19. Lohman TG. Dual energy x-ray absorptiometry. In: Roche AF, Heymsfield SB, Lohman TG, eds. Human Body Composition. Champaign, IL: Human Kinetics, 1996:63–78.
20. Blair SN, Kohl HW III, Paffenbarger RS Jr, et al. Physical fitness and all-cause mortality: a prospective study of healthy men and women. JAMA 1989;262:2395–2401.
21. Blair SN, Kohl HW III, Barlow CE, et al. Changes in physical fitness and all-cause mortality. A prospective study of healthy and unhealthy men. JAMA 1995;273:1093–1098.
22. Paffenbarger RS Jr, Hyde RT, Wing AL, et al. The association of changes in physical-activity level and other lifestyle characteristics with mortality among men. N Engl J Med 1993;328:538–545.
23. Davis JA. Direct determination of aerobic power. In: Maud PJ, Foster C, eds. Physiological Assessment of Human Fitness. Champaign, IL: Human Kinetics, 1995:9–17.
24. McConnell TR. Cardiorespiratory assessment of apparently healthy populations. In: Roitman JL, ed. ACSM's Resource Manual for Guidelines for Exercise Testing and Prescription. 3rd ed. Baltimore: Williams & Wilkins, 1998:347–353.
25. Shephard RJ, Allen C, Benade AJS, et al. Standardization of submaximal exercise tests. Bull World Health Organ 1968;38:765–775.
26. Jetté M, Campbell J, Mongeon J, et al. The Canadian home fitness test as a predictor of aerobic capacity. Can Med Assoc J 1976;114:680–682.
27. Kline GM, Porcari JP, Hintermeister R, et al. Estimation of $\dot{V}O_{2max}$ from a one-mile track walk, gender, age, and body weight. Med Sci Sports Exerc 1987;19:253–259.
28. Åstrand P-O, Ryhming I. A nomogram for calculation of aerobic capacity (physical fitness) from pulse rate during submaximal work. J Appl Physiol 1954;7:218–221.
29. Åstrand I. Aerobic work capacity in men and women with special reference to age. Acta Physiol Scand 1960;49(suppl 169):45–60.
30. Maritz JS, Morrison JF, Peter J, et al. A practical method of estimating an individual's maximal oxygen uptake. Ergonomics 1961;4:97–122.
31. Shephard RJ, Thomas S, Weller I. The Canadian home fitness test: 1991 update. Sports Med 1991;11:358–366.

32. Noble BJ, Borg GAV, Jacobs I, et al. A category-ratio perceived exertion scale: relationship to blood and muscle lactates and heart rate. Med Sci Sports Exerc 1983;15:523–528.
33. Morgan W, Borg G. Perception of effort in the prescription of physical activity. In: Nelson T, ed. Mental health and emotional aspects of sports. Chicago: American Medical Association, 1976:126–129.
34. American College of Sports Medicine Position Stand. The recommended quantity and quality of exercise for developing and maintaining cardiorespiratory and muscular fitness, and flexibility in healthy adults. Med Sci Sports Exerc 1998;30:975–991.
35. Kramer WJ, Fry AC. Strength testing: development and evaluation of methodology. In: Maud PJ, Foster C, eds. Physiological Assessment of Human Fitness. Champaign, IL: Human Kinetics, 1995:115–138.
36. Graves JE, Pollock ML, Bryant CX. Assessment of muscular strength and endurance. In: Roitman JL, ed. ACSM's Resource Manual for Guidelines for Exercise Testing and Prescription. 3rd ed. Baltimore: Williams & Wilkins, 1998:363–367.
37. Hoeger WWK, Barette SL, Hale DR, et al. Relationship between repetitions and selected percentages of one repetition maximum. J Appl Sport Sci Res 1987;1:11–13.
38. Hoeger WWK, Hopkins DR, Barette SL, et al. Relationship between repetitions and selected percentages of one repetition maximum: a comparison between untrained and trained males and females. J Appl Sport Sci Res 1990;4:47–54.
39. Diener MH, Golding LA, Diener D. Validity and reliability of a one-minute half sit-up test of abdominal muscle strength and endurance. Sports Med Training Rehab 1995;6:105–119.
40. Faulkner RA, Springings ES, McQuarrie A, et al. A partial curl-up protocol for adults based on an analysis of two procedures. Can J Sport Sci 1989;14:135–141.
41. Canadian Standardized Test of Fitness Operations Manual. 3rd ed. Ottawa: Fitness and Amateur Sport Canada, 1986.
42. Jackson AW, Morrow JR, Brill PA, et al. Relations of sit-up and sit-and-reach to low back pain in adults. J Orthop Sports Phys Ther 1998;27:22–26.
43. Protas EJ. Flexibility and range of motion. In: Roitman JL, ed. ACSM's Resource Manual for Guidelines for Exercise Testing and Prescription. 3rd ed. Baltimore: Williams & Wilkins, 1998:368–377.
44. Liemohn WP. Flexibility and low-back function. In: Howley ET, Franks BD, eds. Health Fitness Instructor's Handbook. Champaign, IL: Human Kinetics, 1997:247–262.
45. Hoeger WWK, Hoeger SA. Lifetime Physical Fitness and Wellness. Englewood, CO: Morton Publishing, 1998:124.

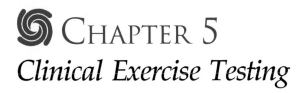 CHAPTER 5
Clinical Exercise Testing

Standard graded exercise tests are used in clinical applications to assess the patient's ability to tolerate increasing intensities of exercise while electrocardiographic (ECG), hemodynamic, and symptomatic responses are monitored for manifestations of myocardial ischemia, electrical instability, or other exertion-related abnormalities.

INDICATIONS AND APPLICATIONS

The exercise test may be used for diagnostic, prognostic, and therapeutic applications, especially in regard to exercise prescription (see Chapter 8).

Diagnostic Exercise Testing

Diagnostic exercise testing is best used in patients with an intermediate probability of angiographically significant coronary artery disease (CAD) as determined by age, gender, and symptoms (Table 5-1). Asymptomatic individuals generally represent those with a low likelihood (i.e., <10%) of significant CAD. Diagnostic exercise testing in asymptomatic individuals is generally not indicated. However, exercise testing may be useful in asymptomatic persons when multiple risk factors are present (1), indicating at least a moderate risk of experiencing a serious cardiovascular event within 5 years (2). It may also be indicated in those who are about to start a vigorous exercise program (see Chapter 2), or those involved in occupations in which cardiovascular events may affect public safety. In general, patients with a high probability of disease (i.e., typical angina, prior coronary revascularization or myocardial infarction [MI]) are tested to assess residual myocardial ischemia and prognosis rather than for diagnostic purposes. Although exercise electrocardiography for diagnostic purposes is less accurate in women, test sensitivity is not affected; thus, a standard exercise test remains the initial diagnostic evaluation of choice.

TABLE 5-1. Pretest Likelihood of Coronary Artery Disease*†

Age	Gender	Typical Definite Angina Pectoris	Atypical/Probable Angina Pectoris	Nonanginal Chest Pain	Asymptomatic
30–39	Men	Intermediate	Intermediate	Low	Very low
	Women	Intermediate	Very low	Very low	Very low
40–49	Men	High	Intermediate	Intermediate	Low
	Women	Intermediate	Low	Very low	Very low
50–59	Men	High	Intermediate	Intermediate	Low
	Women	Intermediate	Intermediate	Low	Very low
60–69	Men	High	Intermediate	Intermediate	Low
	Women	High	Intermediate	Intermediate	Low

*No data exist for patients who are <30 or >69 years, but it can be assumed that prevalence of CAD increases with age. In a few cases, patients with ages at the extremes of the decades listed may have probabilities slightly outside the high or low range. High indicates >90%; intermediate, 10–90%; low, <10%; and very low, <5%.

†Reprinted with permission from Gibbons RA, Balady GJ, Beasely JW, et al. ACC/AHA guidelines for exercise testing. J Am Coll Cardiol 1997;30:260–315.

Exercise Testing for Disease Severity and Prognosis

Exercise testing is useful in the evaluation of persons with known or suspected CAD. Data derived from the exercise test are most useful when considered in context with other clinical data. Data regarding symptoms, functional capacity, and myocardial ischemia during the exercise test must be considered together. The magnitude of ischemia caused by a coronary lesion is generally proportional to the degree of ST-segment depression, the number of electrocardiographic (ECG) leads involved, and the duration of ST-segment depression in recovery. It is inversely proportional to the ST slope, the double product at which the ST-segment depression occurs, and the maximal heart rate, systolic blood pressure, and metabolic equivalent (MET) level achieved. Several numerical indices of prognosis have been published (3,4) including the Duke treadmill exercise score (3) (Fig. 5-1), which has been validated on a population of inpatients referred for cardiac catheterization and outpatients (men and women) referred for noninvasive evaluation of CAD, but without recent MI or coronary revascularization. This nomogram is considered by many to be the major advance in exercise testing over the past decade, as is demonstrated by its inclusion in all of the major guidelines.

Exercise Testing After Myocardial Infarction

Exercise testing after MI can be performed before or soon after hospital discharge (as early as 4 days after MI) for prognostic assessment, activity prescription, and evaluation of medical therapy. Submaximal tests may be used prior to hospital discharge at 4 to 6 days after acute MI. Low-level exercise testing provides sufficient data to make recommendations about the patient's ability to safely perform activities of daily living and serves as a guide for early ambulatory exercise therapy. Symptom-limited tests are usually performed at more than 14 days after MI (1). As contemporary therapies have led to dramatic reductions in mortality after MI, the use of exercise testing in the evaluation of prognosis has changed. Patients who have not undergone coronary revascularization and are unable to undergo exercise testing appear to have the worst prognosis. Other indicators of adverse prognosis in the post-MI patient include: ischemic ST-segment depression at a low level of exercise (particularly if accompanied by reduced left ventricular systolic function); functional capacity of less than 5 METs; and a hypotensive blood pressure response to exercise.

Functional Exercise Testing

Exercise testing is useful to determine functional capacity. This information can be valuable for activity counseling, exercise prescription, or disability assessment. Aerobic capacity may be reported as the percentage of expected

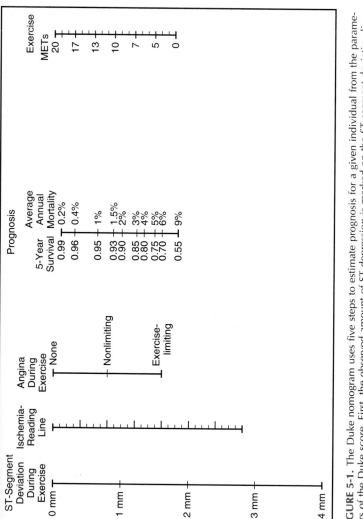

FIGURE 5-1. The Duke nomogram uses five steps to estimate prognosis for a given individual from the parameters of the Duke score. First, the observed amount of ST-depression is marked on the ST-segment deviation line. Second, the observed degree of angina is marked on the line for angina, and these two points are connected. Third, the point where this line intersects the ischemia reading line is noted. Fourth, the observed exercise tolerance is marked on the line for capacity exercise. Finally, the mark on the ischemia reading line is connected to the mark on the exercise capacity line, and the estimated 5-year survival or average annual mortality rate is read from the point at which this line intersects the prognosis scale.

METs for age using a nomogram (Fig. 5-2), with 100% being normal (separate nomograms are provided for referred men with suspected CAD and in healthy men) (5). Similar nomograms in women are not currently available.

EXERCISE TEST MODALITIES

The treadmill and cycle ergometer are the most commonly used devices in clinical exercise testing. Treadmill testing provides a more common form of physiologic stress (i.e., walking) in which subjects are more likely to attain a slightly higher oxygen consumption ($\dot{V}O_2$) and peak heart rate than

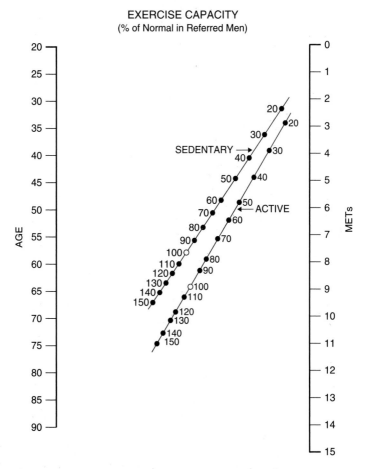

FIGURE 5-2. Nomograms of percent normal exercise capacity in men with suspected CAD who were referred for clinical exercise testing (this page) and in healthy men (page 96).

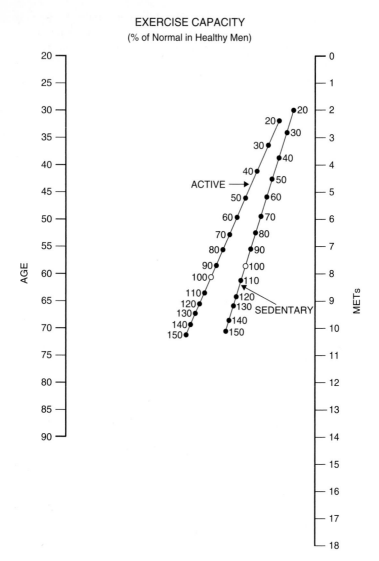

FIGURE 5-2. (continued)

during cycle ergometer testing (6,7). The treadmill should have a front rail and at least one side rail for patients to steady themselves. The patient should be told that he or she can hold on to the rails initially, but then should only use the rails for balance. An emergency stop button should be readily available.

Cycle ergometers are less expensive, require less space, and make less noise. Electronically braked cycle ergometers maintain the workload over a wide range of pedal rates. Because there is less movement of the patient's arms and thorax during cycling it is easier to obtain better quality ECG recordings and blood pressure measurements. However, stationary cycling is an unfamiliar method of exercise for many Americans and depends highly on patient motivation. Thus, the test may end prematurely (i.e., due to localized leg fatigue) before a cardiopulmonary end point has been achieved. Lower values for $\dot{V}O_{2max}$ during cycle ergometer testing (versus treadmill testing) can range from 5 to 25%, depending on the participant's conditioning and leg strength (8).

Arm ergometry is an alternative method of exercise testing for patients who cannot perform leg exercise. Because a smaller muscle mass is used during arm ergometry, $\dot{V}O_{2max}$ during arm exercise is generally 20 to 30% lower than that obtained during treadmill testing (9). Although this test has diagnostic utility (10), it has been largely replaced by the nonexercise pharmacologic stress techniques that are described below. Arm ergometer tests can be used for activity counseling and exercise prescription for individuals who perform primarily dynamic upper body work during occupational or leisure-time activities.

EXERCISE PROTOCOLS

The protocol employed for an exercise test should consider the purpose of the test, the specific outcomes desired, and the individual being tested. The most common exercise protocols and the predicted $\dot{V}O_2$ for each stage are illustrated in Figure 5-3. The Bruce treadmill test remains the most commonly used protocol; however, it employs relatively large increments (i.e., METs per stage) every 3 minutes. Consequently, patients often fail to attain a leveling off or plateauing of physiologic responses, and the exercise capacity may be markedly overestimated when it is predicted from exercise time or workload. Protocols with larger increments (e.g., Bruce, Ellestad) are better suited for screening younger and/or physically active individuals, whereas protocols with smaller increments (e.g., Naughton, Balke-Ware, USAFSAM), that is, 1 MET per stage or lower, are best for older or deconditioned individuals and patients with cardiovascular or respiratory disease.

Submaximal testing is an appropriate choice for predischarge, post-MI evaluations, and for patients who may be at high risk for threatening arrhythmias, abnormal blood pressure responses, or other adverse signs or symptoms. Submaximal tests can be useful for making activity recommendations, adjusting the medical regimen, and identifying the need for further interventions. These tests are frequently stopped at a predetermined level, such as a heart rate of 120 beats·min^{-1} or a MET level of 5, but this varies based on the patient and clinical judgment. When performed in this manner, submaximal tests have been useful in risk stratifying post-MI patients.

An alternative approach to incremental exercise testing that has gained popularity in recent years is the ramp protocol, in which work rate increases at a constant and continuous manner (11,12). Although ramp testing using a cycle ergometer has been available for many years, many of the major treadmill manufacturers have recently developed controllers that ramp speed and grade. Both individualized (11) and standardized ramp tests,

FUNCTIONAL CLASS	CLINICAL STATUS	O₂ COST mL·kg⁻¹·min⁻¹	METS	BICYCLE ERGOMETER (1 WATT = 6 KPM/MIN; FOR 70 KG BODY WEIGHT KPM/MIN)	BRUCE 3 MIN STAGES (MPH / GR)	KATTUS (MPH / GR)	BALKE-WARE (GRADE AT 3.3 MPH, 1-MIN STAGES)	ELLESTAD 3/2/3 MIN STAGES (MPH / GR)	USAFSAM (MPH / GR)	"SLOW" USAFSAM (MPH / GR)	McHENRY (MPH / GR)	STANFORD GRADE AT 3 MPH	STANFORD GRADE AT 2 MPH	METS
NORMAL AND I (HEALTHY, DEPENDENT ON AGE, ACTIVITY)		56.0	16		5.5 / 20		26	6 / 15						16
		52.5	15		5.0 / 18	4 / 22	25	5 / 15	3.3 / 25		3.3 / 21			15
		49.0	14				24							14
		45.5	13	1500	4.2 / 16	4 / 18	23		3.3 / 20		3.3 / 18			13
		42.0	12	1350		4 / 14	22				3.3 / 15	22.5		12
		38.5	11	1200			21	5 / 10	3.3 / 15	2 / 25		20.0		11
		35.0	10	1050	3.4 / 14	4 / 10	20					17.5		10
		31.5	9	900		3 / 10	19	4 / 10	3.3 / 10	2 / 20	3.3 / 12	15.0		9
	(SEDENTARY HEALTHY)	28.0	8	750		2 / 10	18			2 / 15	3.3 / 9	12.5		8
		24.5	7	600	2.5 / 12		17	3 / 10	3.3 / 5		3.3 / 6	10.0	17.5	7
		21.0	6	450			16			2 / 10		7.5	14	6
II (LIMITED)		17.5	5	300	1.7 / 10		15	1.7 / 10	3.3 / 0	2 / 5		5.0	10.5	5
		14.0	4	150	1.7 / 5		13				2.0 / 3	2.5	7	4
III (SYMPTOMATIC)		10.5	3		1.7 / 0					2 / 0		0.0	3.5	3
		7.0	2						2.0 / 0					2
IV		3.5	1											1

FIGURE 5-3. Common exercise protocols. Stage I of the conventional Bruce treadmill protocol starts at 1.7 mph, 10% grade. The "modified" Bruce protocol may start at 1.7 mph, 0% grade, or at 1.7 mph, 5% grade, as shown here.

such as the Bruce ramp (12), have been used. The former test individualizes the rate of increase in intensity based on the subject, and the latter matches work rates to equivalent time periods on the commonly used Bruce protocol, but increases in ramp fashion. Advantages of the ramp approach include the following:

- Avoidance of large and unequal increments in workload
- More accurate estimates of exercise capacity
- Facilitates individualizing the test (individualized ramp rate)
- Targeted test duration

Whichever exercise protocol is chosen, it should be individualized; for example, treadmill speed and increments in grade should be established based on the individual's capabilities. Ideally, increments in work rate should be chosen so that the total test time ranges between 8 and 12 minutes (11). For example, increments of 10 to 15 watts (1 W = 6.12 kg·m·min^{-1}) per min can be used on the cycle ergometer for elderly persons, deconditioned individuals, and patients with cardiovascular or pulmonary disease. Increases in grade of 1 to 3% per minute can be used for treadmill tests for these same populations.

Upper Body Exercise Testing

The arm cycle ergometer is the prototype of arm testing equipment. An arm cycle ergometer can be purchased as such, or modified from an existing stationary cycle ergometer by replacing the pedals with handles and mounting the unit on a table at shoulder height. Similar to leg cycle ergometers, these can be braked either mechanically or electrically. Work rates are adjusted by altering the cranking rates and/or resistance against the flywheel. Work rate increments of 10 W every 2 to 3 minutes, at a cranking rate of 60 revolutions per minute, have been applied to a broad spectrum of patients (13). Arm ergometry is best performed in the seated position with the fulcrum of the handle adjusted to shoulder height. Electrocardiographic leads should be placed to minimize muscle artifact from upper body movement. Blood pressure can be measured with the individual dropping one arm and continuing to arm crank with the other, or during brief rest periods between stages. However, systolic blood pressures taken by the standard cuff method immediately after arm crank ergometry are likely to underestimate "true" physiologic responses (14).

TESTING FOR RETURN TO WORK

The decision to return to work after a cardiac event is a complex one, with about 15 to 20% of patients failing to resume work (15). Both medical and nonmedical factors contribute to this loss of employment.

Work assessment and counseling are useful in optimizing return-to-work decisions. Early discussion of work-related issues with patients, preferably prior to hospital discharge, may help establish reasonable return-to-work expectations. Discussion with the patient could include a job analysis to 1) ascertain job demands and concerns; 2) establish tentative time lines for work evaluation and return; 3) individualize rehabilitation according to job demands; and 4) determine special work-related needs or job contacts (15). The appropriate time to return to work varies with type of cardiac event or interventional procedure, associated complications, and prognosis, but most uncomplicated patients can resume work within 8 weeks after the event.

The value of a symptom-limited treadmill or cycle ergometer graded exercise test (GXT) in evaluating and counseling patients on return-to-work status is well established (15). First, the patient's responses can help assess his or her prognosis. Secondly, measured or estimated peak MET capacity can be compared to the estimated aerobic requirements of the patient's job to assess expected relative energy demands (16). For most patients, physical demands are considered appropriate if the 8-hour energy expenditure requirement averages less than or equal to 50% peak METs and peak job demands (e.g., 5 to 45 minutes) are within guidelines prescribed for a home exercise program (e.g., 80% peak METs or lower). Most job tasks require less than 5 METs (15).

The GXT is the only type of exercise test needed to provide realistic advice on return-to-work status for the majority of cardiac patients. Some patients may benefit from further work testing if job demands differ substantially from that evaluated with GXT, especially patients with borderline physical work capacity in relationship to the anticipated job demands, those with concomitant left ventricular dysfunction, and/or those concerned about resuming a physically demanding job. Job tasks that produce disproportionate myocardial demands compared with a GXT include those requiring static muscular contraction, work combined with temperature stress, and intermittent heavy work (15). Typical physiologic responses include a greater pressor response to work involving a static muscular contraction, a progressive rise in heart rate and decrease in stroke volume over time for work in a hot environment, and a sudden increase in myocardial oxygen demands with intermittent heavy work. Whenever sufficient information is not available to determine a patient's ability to resume work within a reasonable degree of safety, tests simulating the task(s) in question can be administered. For patients in whom concerns exist regarding potential for serious arrhythmias or ischemia on the job, ambulatory ECG monitoring may be considered. Specialized work simulators (e.g., Baltimore Therapeutic and Valpar work simulators) are also available (17), although simple, inexpensive tests can be set up easily to evaluate types of work not evaluated with a GXT (15). Examples of the latter include weight carrying and repetitive lifting test protocols, which can be easily modified to meet specific job demands.

Weight Carrying Test

PURPOSE
The weight carrying test evaluates tolerance for light to heavy static work combined with light dynamic work.

GENERALIZED PROTOCOL

Comfortable treadmill walking speed (e.g., 2 mi·h^{-1}), 1- to 3-minute weight carrying stages, 1- to 3-minute rest periods interspersed between each stage, 10-pound increments/stage, weight (e.g., dumbbells) carried in one or both hands, blood pressure determined during (not after) weight carrying, ECG monitored.

EXAMPLE PROTOCOL

Stage	Duration (min)	Load (lb)	Speed (mi·h^{-1})	Predicted METs
1	3	0	2	2.4
2	3	20	2	3.0
3	3	30	2	4.2
4	3	40	2	5.0
5	2	50	2	4.8*

*Note: The slightly lower MET level listed for 50 pounds (4.8) versus 40 pounds (5.0) likely stems from the shorter walking time for the former (2 versus 3 minutes) and inability to achieve steady-state conditions.

Repetitive Lifting Test

PURPOSE

This test evaluates responses to intermittent static effort combined with light to moderate dynamic work.

GENERALIZED PROTOCOL

Repetitively lift weighted objects (e.g., boxes) from floor/pallet to work bench, 6-minute stages, 1- to 3-minute rest periods interspersed between each work stage, 10-pound stage increments, blood pressure determined while momentarily holding a weight load, ECG monitored.

EXAMPLE PROTOCOL

Stage	Load (lb)	Lift Rate	Predicted METs (8 lifts/min)
1	30	Self-paced	3.8
2	40	Self-paced	4.2
3	50	Self-paced	4.5
4	30,40,50	Self-paced	4.2

MEASUREMENTS

Common variables assessed during clinical exercise
rate and blood pressure, expired gases, ECG changes, an

Heart Rate and Blood Pressure

Heart rate and blood pressure should be measured before, during, and after the graded exercise test. Box 5-1 indicates the recommended frequency and sequence of these measures. A standardized procedure should be adopted for each laboratory so that baseline measures can be assessed more accurately when repeat testing is performed.

Although numerous devices have been developed to automate blood pressure measurement during exercise, none can be recommended unequivocally at the present time. Mercury manometers are favored over aneroid manometers, which require frequent and more difficult calibration. Boxes 3-4 and 5-2 suggest methods for blood pressure assessment at rest and potential sources of error during exercise, respectively. If systolic blood pressure appears to be decreasing with increasing exercise intensity, it should be taken again immediately (18). If a drop in systolic blood pressure of 10 mm Hg or more occurs with an increase in workload, or if it drops below the value obtained in the standing position prior to testing, the

---

BOX 5-1. Sequence of Measures for Heart Rate, Blood Pressure, Rating of Perceived Exertion (RPE), and Electrocardiogram (ECG) During Exercise Testing

Pretest
1. 12-lead ECG in supine and exercise postures
2. Blood pressure measurements in the supine position and exercise posture

Exercise*
1. 12-lead ECG recorded during last 15 seconds of every stage and at peak exercise (3-lead ECG observed/recorded every minute on monitor)
2. Blood pressure measurements should be obtained during the last minute of each stage[†]
3. Rating scales: RPE at the end of each stage, other scales if applicable

Posttest
1. 12-lead ECG immediately after exercise, then every 1 to 2 minutes for at least 5 minutes to allow any exercise-induced changes to return to baseline
2. Blood pressure measurements should be obtained immediately after exercise, then every 1 to 2 minutes until stabilized near baseline level
3. Symptomatic ratings should be obtained using appropriate scales as long as symptoms persist after exercise

these referenced variables should be assessed and recorded whenever adverse symp-
mal ECG changes occur.

anged or decreasing systolic blood pressure with increasing workloads should be
ied immediately).

> ## BOX 5-2. Potential Sources of Error in Blood Pressure Assessment
>
> Inaccurate sphygmomanometer
> Improper cuff size
> Auditory acuity of technician
> Rate of inflation or deflation of cuff pressure
> Experience of technician
> Reaction time of technician
> Improper stethoscope placement or pressure
> Background noise
> Allowing patient to hold treadmill handrails
> Certain physiologic abnormalities, e.g., damaged brachial artery, subclavian steal syndrome, atrioventricular fistula

test should be stopped, particularly if accompanied by adverse signs or symptoms (see Box 5-3 for test termination criteria).

Expired Gases

Because of the inaccuracies associated with estimating oxygen consumption and METs from work rate (i.e., treadmill speed and grade), many laboratories directly measure expired gases. The direct measurement of $\dot{V}O_2$ has been shown to be more reliable than estimated values from treadmill or cycle ergometer work rate. Peak $\dot{V}O_2$ is the most accurate measurement of functional capacity and is a useful index of overall cardiopulmonary health. Measurement of expired gases is not necessary for all clinical exercise testing, but the additional information can provide useful physiologic data. Heart and lung diseases may manifest as gas exchange abnormalities during exercise, and the information obtained is increasingly employed in clinical trials to objectively assess the response to specific interventions. Situations in which gas exchange measurements are appropriate include the following:

- When a precise cardiopulmonary response to a specific therapeutic intervention is required
- When a research question is being addressed
- When the etiology of exercise limitation or dyspnea is uncertain
- Evaluation of exercise capacity in patients with heart failure to assist in the estimation of prognosis and assess the need for transplantation
- When assisting in the development of an appropriate exercise prescription for cardiac rehabilitation

---

BOX 5-3. Indications for Terminating Exercise Testing*

Absolute Indications
- Drop in systolic blood pressure of ≥10 mm Hg from baseline blood pressure despite an increase in workload, when accompanied by other evidence of ischemia
- Moderate to severe angina
- Increasing nervous system symptoms (e.g., ataxia, dizziness, or near syncope)
- Signs of poor perfusion (cyanosis or pallor)
- Technical difficulties monitoring the ECG or systolic blood pressure
- Subject's desire to stop
- Sustained ventricular tachycardia
- ST elevation (≥1.0 mm) in leads without diagnostic Q-waves (other than V_1 or aVR)

Relative Indications
- Drop in systolic blood pressure of ≥10 mm Hg from baseline blood pressure despite an increase in workload, in the absence of other evidence of ischemia
- ST or QRS changes such as excessive ST depression (>2 mm horizontal or downsloping ST-segment depression) or marked axis shift
- Arrhythmias other than sustained ventricular tachycardia, including multifocal PVCs, triplets of PVCs, supraventricular tachycardia, heart block, or bradyarrhythmias
- Fatigue, shortness of breath, wheezing, leg cramps, or claudication
- Development of bundle-branch block or intraventricular conduction delay that cannot be distinguished from ventricular tachycardia
- Increasing chest pain
- Hypertensive response[†]

*Reprinted with permission from Gibbons RA, Balady GJ, Beasely JW, et al. ACC/AHA guidelines for exercise testing. J Am Coll Cardiol 1997;30:260–315.

†Systolic blood pressure of more than 250 mm Hg and/or a diastolic blood pressure of more than 115 mm Hg.

One commonly used component of the information obtained from expired gases is the ventilatory threshold (VT). Historically, this variable has described a breakpoint in ventilation during exercise, thought to be associated with lactate accumulation and muscle anaerobiosis. In truth, the VT probably reflects simply a balance between lactate production and removal in the blood (19). Because exercise beyond the VT is associated with metabolic acidosis, hyperventilation, and a reduced capacity to perform work, it has evolved into a useful physiologic measurement when evaluating interventions in patients with heart disease as well as studying limits of performance in healthy individuals.

Electrocardiographic Monitoring

A high-quality ECG is of paramount importance in an exercise test. Proper skin preparation is essential for recording the electrocardiogram. It is important to lower the resistance at the skin-electrode interface and thereby improve the signal-to-noise ratio. The general areas for electrode placement should be shaved, if hair is present, and cleansed with an alcohol-saturated gauze pad. The next step is to remove the superficial layer of skin using light abrasion with fine-grain emery paper or gauze. The electrodes are placed using anatomic landmarks that are most easily located with the patient supine (see Appendix C).

Bipolar systems have been used historically because of the relatively short time required for lead placement, the relative freedom from motion artifact, and the ease with which noise problems can be located. Clinically, bipolar leads have been replaced by the routine monitoring of 12 leads. Because electrodes placed on wrists and ankles obstruct exercise, these electrodes are affixed to the torso at the base of the limbs for exercise testing (20). Because torso leads may give a slightly different ECG configuration when compared with standard 12-lead resting ECG, use of torso leads should be noted on the ECG.

Signal processing techniques have made it possible to average ECG waveforms and to remove noise, but caution is urged because signal averaging can actually distort the signal (21). Moreover, most manufacturers do not specify how such procedures modify the ECG. It is therefore important to consider the "real time" ECG data first, using filtered data to aid in the interpretation if no distortion is obvious.

Subjective Ratings

The measurement of perceptual responses during exercise testing can provide useful clinical information. Somatic ratings of perceived exertion (RPE) and/or specific symptomatic complaints (degree of chest pain, burning, discomfort, dyspnea, or leg discomfort/pain) should be assessed routinely during clinical exercise tests. The patient is asked to provide subjective estimates during the last 15 seconds of each exercise intensity either verbally or manually. For example, the individual can provide a number verbally or point to a number if a mouthpiece or face mask is being used. The exercise technician should state the number out loud to confirm the correct rating.

Either the 6–20 category scale or the 0–10 category-ratio scale (see Chapter 4) may be used to assess RPE during exercise testing. Prior to the start of the exercise test, the patient should be given clear and concise instructions for use of the selected scale. Generic instructions for explaining either scale are provided in Chapter 4. The following instructions are recommended when using the 0–10 category-ratio scale:

"This is a scale for rating perceived exertion. Perceived exertion is the overall effort or distress of your body during exercise. The number 0 represents no perceived exertion or leg discomfort and the number 10 repre-

sents the greatest amount of exertion that you have ever experienced. At various times during the exercise test you will be asked to point to a number, which indicates your rating of perceived exertion at the time. One of the technicians will say the number out loud in order to make sure that we understand your selection. Do you have any questions?"

The 6–20 category scale has a history of extensive use in clinical exercise testing. In 1982, this scale was revised into a 0–10 category scale with ratio properties based on descriptors positioned alongside specific numbers. Although the 0–10 scale has theoretic advantages over the 6–20 scale, either instrument can be used to obtain RPE ratings.

When subjects become symptomatic during exercise, use of alternative rating scales that are specific to subjective symptoms are recommended. A frequently used scale for assessment of angina is as follows:

1+ Light, barely noticeable
2+ Moderate, bothersome
3+ Moderately severe, very uncomfortable
4+ Most severe or intense pain ever experienced

In general, a rating of 3, or a degree of chest discomfort that would cause the patient to stop normal daily activities, take a sublingual nitroglycerin tablet, or both, should be the exercise test stopping point (22)

Postexercise Period

If maximal sensitivity is to be achieved with an exercise test, patients should be supine during the postexercise period (23), although it is advantageous to record about 10 seconds of ECG data while the patient is in the upright position immediately after exercise. Having the patient perform a cool-down walk after the test may decrease the risk of hypotension but can attenuate the magnitude of ST-segment depression. When the test is being performed for nondiagnostic purposes, an active cool-down is usually preferable; for example, slow walking (1.0 to 1.5 mi·h^{-1}) or continued cycling against minimal resistance. Monitoring should continue for at least 5 minutes after exercise or until ECG changes return to baseline. ST-segment changes that occur only during the postexercise period, once thought likely to be false positive responses, have now been shown to be an important diagnostic part of the test (23). In patients who are severely dyspneic, the supine posture may exacerbate the condition, and sitting may be a more appropriate posture.

Indications for Exercise Test Termination

The absolute and relative indications for termination of an exercise test are listed in Box 5-3. Absolute indications are clear-cut, whereas relative indications may sometimes be reevaluated when sound clinical judgment supersedes the stated criteria.

EXERCISE TESTING WITH IMAGING MODALITIES

Cardiac imaging modalities are indicated when ECG changes are nondiagnostic, when it is important to determine the extent and distribution of ischemic myocardium, or when a positive or negative exercise ECG needs to be excluded or confirmed.

Exercise Echocardiography

Imaging modalities, such as echocardiography, can be combined with exercise ECG in an attempt to increase the sensitivity and specificity of stress testing, as well as to determine the extent of myocardium at risk for ischemia. Echocardiographic images at rest are compared with those obtained during cycle ergometry or immediately after treadmill exercise. Images must be obtained within 1 to 2 minutes after exercise because abnormal wall motion begins to normalize after this point.

Rest and stress images are compared side-by-side in a cineloop display that is gated during systole from the QRS complex. Myocardial contractility normally increases with exercise, whereas ischemia causes hypokinesis, akinesis, or dyskinesis of the affected segments. A test is considered positive if wall motion abnormalities such as hypokinesis, akinesis, or dyskinesis develop or worsen during exercise (24). Advantages of exercise echocardiography over nuclear testing include a significantly lower cost, the absence of exposure to ionizing radiation and a shorter amount of time for testing. Limitations include dependence on the operator for obtaining adequate, timely images. In addition, approximately 5% of patients have inadequate echocardiographic windows secondary to body habitus or lung interference (24).

Exercise Nuclear Imaging

Exercise tests with nuclear imaging are performed with ECG monitoring. There are several different imaging protocols using only technetium (Tc)-99m sestamibi (Cardiolite, Dupont Medical, North Billerica, MA) or thallous (thallium) chloride-201 or both (dual tracer with thallium rest images and sestamibi stress images). A common protocol with sestamibi is to perform rest images 30 to 60 minutes after intravenous administration of sestamibi followed by exercise (or pharmacologic stress) 1 to 3 hours later. Stress images are obtained 30 to 60 minutes after injecting sestamibi approximately 1 minute prior to completion of peak exercise. Comparison of the rest and stress images permit differentiation of fixed versus transient perfusion abnormalities.

Technetium-99m sestamibi permits higher dosing with less radiation exposure than thallium and results in improved images that are sharper and have less artifact and attenuation. Consequently, sestamibi is the preferred imaging agent when performing tomographic images of the heart using single photon emission computed tomography (SPECT). SPECT images are obtained with a gamma camera, which rotates 180 degrees around the patient, stopping at preset angles to record the image. Cardiac images are then displayed in slices from three different axes to allow visualization of the heart in three dimensions. Thus, multiple myocardial segments can be viewed individually, without the overlap of segments that occurs with planar imaging (25). Perfusion defects that are present during exercise but not seen at rest suggest myocardial ischemia. Perfusion defects that are present during exercise and persist at rest suggest previous MI or scar. In this manner, the extent and distribution of ischemic myocardium can be identified.

The limitations of sestamibi SPECT imaging include the exposure to ionizing radiation. Furthermore, additional equipment and personnel are required for image acquisition and interpretation, including a nuclear technician to administer the radioactive isotope and acquire the images, and a physician trained in nuclear medicine to reconstruct and interpret the images.

Pharmacologic Stress Testing

Patients unable to undergo exercise stress testing for reasons such as deconditioning, peripheral vascular disease, orthopedic disabilities, neurologic disease, and concomitant illness can often benefit from pharmacologic stress testing. The two most commonly used tests are dobutamine stress echocardiography and sestamibi or thallium scintigraphy with dipyridamole or adenosine. Indications for these tests include establishing a diagnosis of CAD, determining myocardial viability prior to revascularization, assessing prognosis after MI or in chronic angina, and evaluating cardiac risk preoperatively.

Dobutamine is infused intravenously starting at 5 $\mu g \cdot kg^{-1} \cdot min^{-1}$ and, if tolerated, increased to 10 $\mu g \cdot kg^{-1} \cdot min^{-1}$. Every 3 minutes thereafter the dose is increased by 10 $\mu g \cdot kg^{-1} \cdot min^{-1}$ until a maximal dose of 40 to 50 $\mu g \cdot kg^{-1} \cdot min^{-1}$ is reached or an end point is achieved. End points may include new or worsening wall-motion abnormalities, an adequate heart rate response, serious arrhythmias, angina, significant ST depression, intolerable side effects, and a significant increase or decrease in blood pressure. Atropine may be given if an adequate heart rate is not achieved or other end points have not been reached at peak dobutamine dose. Heart rate, blood pressure, ECG, and echocardiographic images are obtained throughout the infusion. Echocardiographic images are obtained similar to exercise echocardiography. A new or worsening wall motion abnormality constitutes a positive test for ischemia (26).

Vasodilators such as dipyridamole and adenosine are commonly used to assess coronary perfusion in conjunction with a nuclear imaging agent, such as thallium or sestamibi. Dipyridamole and adenosine cause maximal coronary vasodilation in normal epicardial arteries, but not in stenotic segments. As a result, a coronary steal phenomenon occurs, with a relatively increased flow to normal arteries and a relatively decreased flow to stenotic arteries. Perfusion imaging using either planar thallium or SPECT sestamibi under resting conditions is then compared with imaging obtained after coronary vasodilation (25). Interpretation is similar to that of exercise nuclear testing.

CONSIDERATIONS FOR PULMONARY PATIENTS

The vast majority of patients with chronic respiratory disease (e.g., asthma, chronic obstructive pulmonary disease [COPD], interstitial lung disease, and pulmonary vascular disease) seek medical attention because of exertional dyspnea or breathlessness. The medical history should include questions about the onset, frequency, severity, descriptive qualities, and activities/triggers that provoke dyspnea. Although the pathophysiology of the respiratory disease may cause breathlessness, any one of many temporally related events (e.g., weight gain, deconditioning, respiratory infection) might contribute to difficulty breathing.

It is helpful to quantify the severity of dyspnea as part of the medical history. Two different scales or questionnaires have been used to measure dyspnea intensity. One instrument uses a combination of the Baseline (BDI) and Transition (TDI) Dyspnea Indexes (27), which incorporate three components (task, effort, and function) that influence breathing to derive an overall estimate of dyspnea. Scores for baseline and transition ratings of dyspnea are obtained through an interview by a professional experienced in obtaining a clinical history for pulmonary disease. For each category, the interviewer asks open-ended questions about the patient's experience of breathlessness while simultaneously focusing on specific criteria for evaluating the intensity of dyspnea. Based on the patient's responses, the interviewer can grade the degree of impairment related to dyspnea.

Another useful instrument is the dyspnea component of the Chronic Respiratory Questionnaire (CRQ) (28), which considers the five most common activities that cause breathlessness for the individual. A list of 26 activities is read to the patient who responds whether shortness of breath occurred during that activity. After determining the five most common dyspnea-causing activities, the patient grades the severity of breathlessness on a scale of 1 ("extremely short of breath") to 7 ("not at all short of breath"). These scores are added to obtain an overall CRQ score ranging from 5 to 35. Both the BDI/TDI and the dyspnea scale of the CRQ have been shown to be valid, reliable, and responsive instruments (29).

Lung Function

Detailed information on selection and interpretation of lung function tests is provided in Chapter 3. The measured maximal voluntary ventilation

(MVV) or $FEV_{1.0} \times 35$ (or 40) can be used as an estimate of the predicted maximal exercise ventilation ($\dot{V}_{Emax}$) (30).

Exercise Testing of Pulmonary Patients

Exercise testing can be helpful for differentiating exertional breathlessness secondary to lung or cardiac diseases. Indications for cardiopulmonary exercise testing in pulmonary patients include the following (31):

- Cause of breathlessness remains unclear despite results from pulmonary function tests
- Patient's severity of breathlessness is disproportionate to objective data
- To distinguish whether cardiac or respiratory disease limits exercise tolerance
- Deconditioning, psychological factors (e.g., anxiety), or obesity are suspected causes for exertional dyspnea
- To evaluate for exercise-induced oxygen desaturation
- To select an appropriate intensity for exercise training

Although COPD is diagnosed by history and pulmonary function tests, spirometry may be used to estimate a patient's ventilatory capacity (but not the ventilatory requirements for exertional activities). Furthermore, many patients with COPD have concomitant CAD, deconditioning, or anxiety/depression that might also reduce exercise performance. Exercise testing can provide important clinical data about these and other possible conditions that might cause dyspnea and/or limit exercise performance in patients with COPD.

Measurement of ventilation is essential in exercise testing of patients with pulmonary disease. It is preferable to measure $\dot{V}_E$ and its components, frequency of respiration and tidal volume, as well as expired gases, O_2 and CO_2.

It is also important to measure gas partial pressures in pulmonary patients because oxygen desaturation may occur during exertion. Although measurement of P_aO_2 and P_aCO_2 from arterial blood has been the standard in the past, the availability of oximetry has replaced the need to routinely draw arterial blood in most patients. In patients with pulmonary disease, measurements of oxygen saturation (S_aO_2) from oximetry at rest correlate reasonably well with S_aO_2 measured from arterial blood (95% confidence limits are ±3 to 5% saturation) (32). Carboxyhemoglobin (COHb) levels greater than 4% and black skin may adversely affect the accuracy of pulse oximeters (33,34), and most oximeters are inaccurate at an S_aO_2 of 85% or less. If clinically warranted, arterial blood gases may be obtained.

As previously described, it is useful to measure dyspnea and leg discomfort during exercise in patients with respiratory disease. The 0–10 scale (35) is commonly used to quantify these symptoms (27).

METHODOLOGIC CONSIDERATIONS

Testing procedures for pulmonary patients are similar to those described for cardiac patients. Preparing the pulmonary patient physically and emotionally for testing is critical. A brief physical examination is important for screening purposes. The exercise test should be progressive and incremental; a ramp protocol can be used. Smaller and more frequent work increments are preferable to larger and less frequent increases. The exercise protocol should be individualized rather than using the same protocol for every patient. The optimal test duration is from 8 to 12 minutes (36). For most pulmonary patients, an exercise workload of 10 to 15 W/min will achieve the desired test duration.

SUPERVISION OF EXERCISE STRESS TESTING

The use of maximal or sign/symptom-limited exercise testing has expanded greatly to help guide decisions regarding medical management and surgical therapy in a broad spectrum of patients. For example, immediate exercise testing of selected low-risk patients presenting to the emergency department with chest pain is now increasingly employed to "rule out myocardial infarction" (37). Generally, these patients include those who are no longer symptomatic, with unremarkable ECGs and serial cardiac enzyme assays (e.g., no appreciable rise in the level of CK-MB) (see Table 3-8).

Before 1980, exercise tests were directly supervised by physicians more than 90% of the time (38,39). However, over the past 20 years, cost containment issues and time constraints on physicians have encouraged the use of specially trained health care professionals (e.g., nurses, exercise physiologists, physician assistants, and physical therapists) to administer selected exercise tests, with a physician immediately available for consultation or emergencies that may arise.

Considerations Regarding Medical Supervision

Although exercise testing is generally considered a safe procedure, both acute MI and cardiac arrest have been reported and can be expected to occur at a combined rate of *up to* 1 per 2500 tests (1). Thus, the contentious issue of responsibility for exercise test supervision probably stems, at least in part, from the increased risk of cardiovascular events during the procedure. To circumvent these concerns, a physician experienced in handling cardiovascular emergencies should be in close proximity to the testing area and immediately available in case of an untoward event.

Current Guidelines and Practices

In 1979, the American Heart Association first endorsed the concept that exercise testing may, in some instances, be delegated to "experienced paramedical personnel" (40). The degree of supervision can range from a properly trained nonphysician monitoring the testing of healthy younger persons (age < 40 y), to having a physician present to directly monitor the patient's blood pressure and ECG responses during exercise and recovery. Current standards for exercise testing suggest that nonphysician supervision is appropriate only for apparently healthy adults and low to moderate risk coronary patients, where permitted (1,41–44). Moreover, these guidelines endorse continuous physician presence for the testing of patients who are at increased risk of exercise-related cardiovascular complications (e.g., patient with aortic stenosis, exertional angina, heart failure, or high-grade arrhythmias). Despite these recommendations, empiric experience suggests that many larger hospitals and medical centers currently use paramedical personnel in the direct supervision of exercise testing, with a physician immediately available in the vicinity of the exercise testing area (45).

Competency Considerations

There is disagreement as to whether direct physician supervision of exercise tests in persons with known cardiovascular disease is routinely needed. Critics argue that if physician staff are readily available to evaluate selected patients before testing, specially trained paramedical specialists can appropriately screen for contraindications from the medical history and resting ECG, make a timely and accurate interpretation of ancillary signs and symptoms, and terminate an exercise test at a diagnostic intensity level (46). Specially trained health care professionals adhere to published contraindications to and end points for exercise testing and do so with caution and a minimum of personal interpretation. This premise is supported by data showing that the incidence of cardiovascular complications during exercise testing is no higher with "experienced paramedical personnel" than with direct physician supervision (45,46) (see Chapter 1).

It has been suggested that expertise, rather than physician presence per se, is the primary prerequisite to perform exercise testing, interpret the results, and safeguard the patient from excessive risk (47). This editorial further acknowledged that most exercise tests could be safely conducted by nonphysicians, such as exercise physiologists, nurses and technicians, *if* the person was experienced in exercise testing, fully trained in cardiopulmonary resuscitation, and supervised by a physician skilled in exercise testing who later provided a final interpretation. Relative to acute emergency management, the ability of trained paramedics to resuscitate patients is well-documented, even outside the hospital setting (48).

Although exercise tests are often directly or indirectly supervised by a cardiologist, general internists and family practice physicians with adequate training and experience are also qualified to conduct these tests. Recent guidelines suggest that medical residents perform at least 50 exercise stress tests to qualify for diagnostic stress testing in private practice, and that physicians should perform at least 25 exercise tests per year to maintain clinical competency (44).

Implications for Cost-Effectiveness

Although the cost of paramedical supervisory personnel (e.g., nurse or exercise physiologist and a technician) depends largely on the efficiency of exercise test scheduling, such staffing could probably be provided at a considerably lower cost than that of direct physician supervision; in addition, the physician would generally expect technical assistance. In the era of managed care, the use of specialized health care professionals for supervision of clinical exercise testing may represent a safe and cost-effective alternative to many hospitals and medical centers (49). Nevertheless, no supervising physician should embrace this recommendation without a thorough evaluation of reimbursement requirements and the status of state law as it applies to the performance of exercise testing by allied health professionals (50).

References

1. Gibbons RA, Balady GJ, Beasely JW, et al. ACC/AHA guidelines for exercise testing. J Am Coll Cardiol 1997;30:260–315.
2. Wilson PWF, D'Agostino RB, Levy D, et al. Prediction of coronary heart disease using risk factor categories. Circulation 1998;97:1837–1847.
3. Mark DB, Shaw L, Harrell FE, et al. Prognostic value of a treadmill exercise score in outpatients with suspected coronary artery disease. N Engl J Med 1991;325:849–853.
4. Froelicher VF, Morrow K, Brown M, et al. Prediction of atherosclerotic cardiovascular death in men using a prognostic score. Am J Cardiol 1994;73:133–138.
5. Morris CK, Myers JN, Froelicher VF, et al. Nomogram based on metabolic equivalents and age for assessing aerobic exercise capacity in men. J Am Coll Cardiol 1993;22:175–182.
6. Foster C, Pollock ML, Rod JL, et al. Evaluation of functional capacity during exercise radionuclide angiography. Cardiology 1983;70:85–93.
7. Myers J, Buchanan N, Walsh D, et al. Comparison of the ramp vs. standard exercise protocols. J Am Coll Cardiol 1991;17:1334–1342.
8. Pollock ML, Wilmore JH, Fox SM III. Exercise in Health and Disease: Evaluation and Prescription for Prevention and Rehabilitation. Philadelphia: WB Saunders, 1984.
9. Franklin BA. Exercise testing, training and arm ergometry. Sports Med 1985;2:100–119.
10. Balady GJ, Weiner DA, McCabe CH, et al. Value of arm exercise testing in detecting coronary artery disease. Am J Cardiol 1985;55:37–39.
11. Myers J, Buchanan N, Smith D, et al. Individualized ramp treadmill: observations on a new protocol. Chest 1992;101:236S–241S.
12. Kaminsky LA, Whaley MH. Evaluation of a new standardized ramp protocol: the BSU/Bruce ramp protocol. J Cardiopulm Rehabil 1998;18:438–443.
13. Balady GJ, Weiner DA, Rose L, et al. Physiologic responses to arm ergometry exercise relative to age and gender. J Am Coll Cardiol 1990;16:130–135.
14. Hollingsworth V, Bendick P, Franklin B, et al. Validity of arm ergometer blood pressures immediately after exercise. Am J Cardiol 1990;65:1358–1360.
15. Sheldahl LM, Wilke NA, Tristani FE. Evaluation and training for resumption of occupational and leisure-time physical activities in patients after a major cardiac event. Med Exerc Nutr Health 1995;4:273–289.
16. Ainsworth BE, Haskell WL, Leon AS, et al. Compendium of physical activities: classification of energy costs of human physical activities. Med Sci Sports Exer 1993;25:71–80.
17. Wilke NA, Sheldahl LM, Dougherty SM, et al. Baltimore therapeutic equipment work simulator: energy expenditure of work activities in cardiac patients. Arch Phys Med 1993;74:419–424.
18. Dubach P, Froelicher VF, Klein J, et al. Exercise-induced hypotension in a male population. Criteria, causes, and prognosis. Circulation 1989;78:1380–1387.
19. Myers J, Ashley E. Dangerous curves: a perspective on exercise, lactate, and anaerobic threshold. Chest 1997;111:787–795.
20. Gamble P, McManus H, Jensen D, et al. A comparison of the standard 12-lead electrocardiogram to exercise electrode placements. Chest 1984;85:616–622.
21. Milliken JA, Abdollah H, Burgraf GW. False-positive treadmill exercise tests due to computer signal averaging. Am J Cardiol 1990;65:946–948.

22. Myers J. Perception of chest pain during exercise testing in patients with coronary artery disease. Med Sci Sports Exerc 1994;26:1082–1086.

23. Lachterman B, Lehmann KG, Abrahamson D, et al. "Recovery only" ST segment depression and the predictive accuracy of the exercise test. Ann Intern Med 1990;112:11–16.

24. Armstrong W, Marcovitz PA. In: Braunwald E, ed. Stress Echocardiography. Heart Disease Updates. Philadelphia: WB Saunders, 1993:1–10.

25. Ritchie JL, Bateman TM, Bonow RO, et al. Guidelines for clinical use of cardiac radionuclide imaging. Report of the American College of Cardiology/American Heart Association Task Force on Assessment of Diagnostic and Therapeutic Cardiovascular Procedures (Subcommittee on Coronary Artery Bypass Graft Surgery). J Am Coll Cardiol 1991;17:543–589.

26. Poldermans D, Fioretti PM, Forster T, et al. Dobutamine stress echocardiography for assessment of perioperative cardiac risk in patients undergoing major vascular surgery. Circulation 1993;87:1506–1512.

27. Mahler DA, Weinberg DH, Wells CK, et al. The measurement of dyspnea: contents, interobserver agreement, and physiologic correlates of two new clinical indexes. Chest 1984;85:751–758.

28. Guyatt GH, Berman LB, Townsend M, et al. A measure of quality of life for clinical trials in chronic lung disease. Thorax 1987;42:773–778.

29. Mahler DA, Guyatt GH, Jones PW. Clinical measurement of dyspnea. In: Mahler DA, ed. Dyspnea. Mt. Kisco, NY: Futura Publishing, 1990.

30. Wasserman K, Hansen JE, Sue DY, et al. Principles of exercise testing and interpretation. Philadelphia: Lea & Febiger, 1987.

31. Mahler DA, Franco MJ. Clinical applications of cardiopulmonary exercise testing. J Cardiopulm Rehabil 1996;16:357–365.

32. Ries AL, Farrow JT, Clausen JL. Accuracy of two ear oximeters at rest and during exercise in pulmonary patients. Am Rev Respir Dis 1985;132:685–689.

33. Zeballos RJ, Weisman IM. Reliability of noninvasive oximetry in black subjects during exercise and hypoxia. Am Rev Respir Dis 1991;144:1240–1244.

34. Orenstein DM, Curtis SE, Nixon PA, et al. Accuracy of three pulse oximeters during exercise and hypoxemia in patients with cystic fibrosis. Chest 1993;104:1187–1190.

35. Borg GAV. Psychophysical bases of perceived exertion. Med Sci Sports Exerc 1982;14:377–381.

36. Buchfuhrer MJ, Hansen JE, Robinson TE, et al. Optimizing the exercise protocol for cardiopulmonary assessment. J Appl Physiol 1983;55:1558–1564.

37. Lewis WR, Amsterdam EA. Evaluation of the patient with 'rule out myocardial infarction.' Arch Intern Med 1996;156:41–45.

38. Rochmis P, Blackburn H. Exercise tests: a survey of procedures, safety, and litigation experience in approximately 170,000 tests. JAMA 1971;217:1061–1066.

39. Stuart RJ Jr, Ellestad MH. National survey of exercise stress testing facilities. Chest 1980;77:94–97.

40. Ellestad MH, Blomqvist CG, Naughton JP. Standards for adult exercise testing laboratories. Circulation 1979;59:421A–430A.

41. American Association of Cardiovascular and Pulmonary Rehabilitation. Guidelines for Cardiac Rehabilitation and Secondary Prevention Programs. 3rd ed. Champaign, IL: Human Kinetics, 1999:60.

42. Pina IL, Balady GJ, Hanson P, et al. Guidelines for clinical exercise testing laboratories. Circulation 1995;91:912–921.

43. Fletcher GF, Balady G, Froelicher VF, et al. Exercise standards. Circulation 1995;91:580–615.

44. Schlant RC, Friesinger GC, Leonard JJ. Clinical competence in exercise testing: a statement for physicians from the ACP/ACC/AHA task force on clinical privileges in cardiology. Circulation 1990;82:1884–1888.

45. Franklin BA, Gordon S, Timmis GC, et al. Is direct physician supervision of exercise stress testing routinely necessary? Chest 1997;111:262–265.

46. Shephard RJ. Safety of exercise testing—the role of the paramedical exercise specialist. Clin J Sports Med 1991;1:8–11.

47. Ellestad MH. Who should do exercise testing? Newsletter of the California Chapter of the American College of Cardiology, Spring 1993.

48. Liberthson RR, Nagel EL, Hirschman JC, et al. Prehospital ventricular defibrillation. Prognosis and follow-up course. N Engl J Med 1974;291:317–321.

49. Knight JA, Laubach CA, Butcher RJ, et al. Supervision of clinical exercise testing by exercise physiologists. Am J Cardiol 1995;75:390–391.

50. Editorial comment. The Exercise Standards and Malpractice Reporter 1989;3:74.

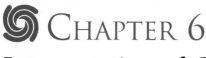 CHAPTER 6
Interpretation of Clinical Test Data

According to a World Health Organization Expert Committee on Rehabilitation, "the primary purpose of an exercise test is to determine the responses of the individual to efforts at given levels and from this information to estimate probable performance in specific life and occupational situations" (1). This chapter addresses the interpretation and clinical significance of exercise test results, with specific reference to screening for coronary artery disease (CAD), cardiovascular and electrocardiographic (ECG) responses, diagnostic value, and patients with pulmonary disorders.

EXERCISE TESTING AS A SCREENING TOOL FOR CORONARY ARTERY DISEASE

The probability of a patient having CAD cannot be estimated accurately from the exercise test result and the diagnostic characteristics of the test alone. It also depends on the likelihood of the patient having disease before the test is administered. Bayes theorem states that the posttest probability of a patient having disease is determined by the disease probability *before* the test and by the probability that the test will provide a true result. The probability of a patient having disease before the test is related, most importantly, to the patient's chest pain characteristics, but also to the patient's age, gender, and the presence of major risk factors for cardiovascular disease.

Clearly, exercise testing in individuals with known CAD (prior myocardial infarction, angiographically documented coronary stenoses, and/or prior coronary revascularization) is not used for diagnostic purposes (see Chapter 5). However, among individuals in whom the diagnosis is in question, the description of symptoms can be most helpful. Typical or definite angina (substernal chest discomfort that may radiate to the back, jaw, or arms; symptoms provoked by exertion or emotional stress and relieved by rest and/or nitroglycerin) makes the pretest probability so high that the test result does not dramatically change the probability of underlying CAD. Atypical angina (chest discomfort that lacks one of the above mentioned characteristics of typical angina) generally indicates an intermediate pretest likelihood of CAD in men older than 30 years and women older than 50 years (see Table 5-1).

The use of exercise testing in screening asymptomatic individuals is problematic in view of the low to very low pretest likelihood of CAD, even among symptom-free men and women older than 60 years (see Table 5-1). Exercise testing as a part of routine health screening in apparently healthy individuals is generally inappropriate (2). Such testing can have potential adverse consequences (psychologic, work and insurance status, costs for subsequent testing) by misclassifying a large percentage of those without CAD as having disease. As stated in Chapter 5, exercise testing in asymptomatic persons with multiple risk factors may provide some useful information, although this practice cannot be strongly recommended based on available data (2). It is likewise difficult to choose a chronological age beyond which exercise testing becomes valuable as a screening tool prior to beginning an exercise program because physiologic age often differs from chronological age. In general, if the exercise is more strenuous than vigorous walking, the guidelines in Table 2-2 are recommended. The potential ramifications resulting from mass screening must be considered and the results of such testing must be applied using the predictive model and Bayesian analyses. Test results should be considered as probability statements and not as absolutes.

Interpretation of Responses to Graded Exercise Testing

Before interpreting clinical test data, it is important to consider the purpose of the test (e.g., diagnostic or prognostic) and patient conditions that may influence the exercise test or its interpretation. Medical conditions influencing test interpretation include orthopedic limitations, pulmonary disease, obesity, neurologic disorders, and significant deconditioning. Medication effects (see Appendix A) and resting ECG abnormalities must also be considered, especially resting ST-segment changes secondary to conduction defects, left ventricular hypertrophy, and other factors that may contribute to spurious ST-segment depression.

Although somatic and myocardial oxygen consumption are directly related, this relationship can be altered by exercise training, drugs, and disease. For example, exercise-induced myocardial ischemia may cause left ventricular dysfunction, exercise impairment, and a hypotensive blood pressure response. Although the severity of symptomatic ischemia is inversely related to functional capacity, ejection fraction does not correlate well with exercise tolerance (3,4). Moreover, silent ischemia does not appear to adversely affect exercise capacity in patients with CAD (4).

The objective of exercise testing is to evaluate quantitatively and accurately the following variables: exercise tolerance or maximal aerobic power of the body ($\dot{V}O_{2max}$); hemodynamics, assessed by the heart rate (HR) and systolic/diastolic blood pressure (SBP/DBP) responses; associated changes in electrical functions of the heart (ECG waveforms), especially ST-segment displacement and supraventricular and ventricular arrhythmias; and limiting clinical signs or symptoms. Responses to exercise tests are useful in evaluating the need for and effectiveness of various types of therapeutic interventions.

Maximal Oxygen Uptake

Maximal oxygen uptake ($\dot{V}O_{2max}$), whether estimated from the work rate achieved or measured directly by gas analysis, provides important information about cardiovascular fitness and prognosis. In the absence of untoward signs or symptoms, patients should be encouraged to give their best effort so that maximal exercise tolerance can be determined. Population-specific nomograms (see Fig. 5-2) may be used when appropriate to compare the peak metabolic equivalents achieved on an exercise test with the expected $\dot{V}O_{2max}$ for a given age, gender, and activity status. Maximal oxygen uptake is not strongly related to ventricular function, and abnormal ventricular function does not always result in a low $\dot{V}O_{2max}$. Various objective and subjective indicators are useful to confirm that maximal effort has been elicited during graded exercise testing:

- Failure of HR to increase with further increases in exercise intensity.
- A plateau in oxygen uptake (or failure to increase oxygen uptake by 150 mL/min) with increased workload (5). This criterion has fallen into some disfavor because a plateau is inconsistently seen during continuous graded exercise tests and is confused by various definitions and how data are sampled during exercise.
- A respiratory exchange ratio greater than 1.15; however, there is considerable interindividual variability in this response.
- A postexercise venous lactic acid concentration of more than 8 mmol has also been used; however, there is great interindividual variability in this response.
- A rating of perceived exertion of more than 17 (6–20 scale).

Achievement of age-predicted maximal heart rate should not be used as an absolute test end point or as an indication that effort has been maximal, due to its high intersubject variability. The clinical indications for stopping an exercise test are presented in Box 5-3. Good judgment on the part of the physician and/or supervising staff remains the most important criteria for terminating exercise.

Heart Rate Response

Maximal heart rate (HR_{max}) may be predicted from age using any of several published equations (6). The relationship between age and HR_{max} for a large sample of subjects (i.e., the regression equation) is reproducible; however, interindividual variability is high (standard deviation is 10 to 12 beats·min^{-1}).

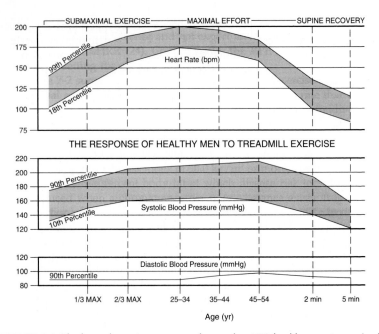

FIGURE 6-1. The hemodynamic responses of more than 700 healthy men to maximal treadmill exercise. Bands represent 80% of the population, with 10% having values exceeding the upper limit and 10% having lower values. (Reprinted with permission from Wolthius RA, Froelicher VF, Fischer J, et al. The response of healthy men to treadmill exercise. Circulation 1977;55:153–157.)

As a result, there is potential for considerable error in the use of methods that extrapolate submaximal test data to an age-predicted HR_{max}. Aerobic capacity, anthropometric measures such as height and weight, and body composition do not independently influence HR_{max}. The inability to appropriately increase heart rate during exercise (chronotropic incompetence) is associated with the presence of heart disease and a worse prognosis (7–9). A delayed decrease in the heart rate during the first minute of recovery (after exercise) is also a powerful predictor of overall mortality (10). Figure 6-1 presents the HR and SBP/DBP responses of more than 700 men to maximal treadmill exercise and provides percentile responses for comparative purposes (11).

Blood Pressure Response

The normal blood pressure response to dynamic upright exercise consists of a progressive increase in SBP, no change or a slight decrease in DBP, and a widening of the pulse pressure. The following are key points concerning interpretation of the blood pressure response to progressive dynamic exercise:

- A drop in SBP, or failure of SBP to increase with increased exercise intensity, is considered an abnormal test response. Exercise-induced decreases in SBP (exertional hypotension) may occur in patients with

CAD, valvular heart disease, cardiomyopathies, and serious arrhythmias. Occasionally, patients without clinically significant heart disease demonstrate exertional hypotension due to antihypertensive therapy, prolonged strenuous exercise, and vasovagal responses. However, exertional hypotension has been shown to correlate with myocardial ischemia, left ventricular dysfunction, and an increased risk of subsequent cardiac events (12,13). In some cases this response is improved after coronary bypass surgery (14).

- The normal postexercise response is a progressive decline in SBP. During passive recovery in an upright posture, SBP may decrease abruptly due to peripheral pooling (and usually normalizes upon resuming the supine position). SBP may remain below pretest resting values for several hours after the test. DBP may also drop during the postexercise period.
- The rate-pressure product or double product (SBP × HR) is an indicator of myocardial oxygen demand (15). Signs and symptoms of ischemia generally occur at a reproducible double product.
- Although an increase in DBP of more than 10 mm Hg during or after exercise may be associated with CAD (16), it more likely represents labile hypertension.
- In patients on vasodilators, calcium channel blockers, angiotensin-converting enzyme inhibitors, and α- and β-adrenergic blockers, the blood pressure response to exercise is variably attenuated and cannot be accurately predicted in the absence of clinical test data.

The normative data shown in Figure 6-1 are based on an exclusively male sample. Mean peak SBP and DBP by age and gender are provided in Table 6-1 (17). Although age-predicted maximal heart rates are comparable for men and women, men generally have higher systolic blood pressures (approximately 20 ± 5 mm Hg) during maximal treadmill testing. The gender difference, however, is no longer apparent after 70 years of age.

TABLE 6-1. Mean (±SD) Peak SBP and DBP (mm Hg) During Maximal Treadmill Exercise*

Age	Men SBP	Men DBP	Women SBP	Women DBP
18–29	182 ± 22	69 ± 13	155 ± 19	67 ± 12
30–39	182 ± 20	76 ± 12	158 ± 20	72 ± 12
40–49	186 ± 22	78 ± 12	165 ± 22	76 ± 12
50–59	192 ± 22	82 ± 12	175 ± 23	78 ± 11
60–69	195 ± 23	83 ± 12	181 ± 23	79 ± 11
70–79	191 ± 27	81 ± 13	196 ± 23	83 ± 11

*Reprinted with permission from Hiroyuki D, Allison TG, Squires RW, et al. Peak exercise blood pressure stratified by age and gender in apparently healthy subjects. Mayo Clin Proc 1996;71:445–452.

ECG Waveforms

Appendix C provides information to aid in the interpretation of resting and exercise electrocardiograms. Additional information is provided here with respect to common exercise-induced changes in ECG variables. The normal ECG response to exercise includes the following:

- Minor and insignificant changes in P wave morphology
- Superimposition of the P and T waves of successive beats
- Increases in septal Q wave amplitude
- Slight decreases in R wave amplitude
- Increases in T wave amplitude (although wide variability exists among subjects)
- Minimal shortening of the QRS duration
- Depression of the J point
- Rate-related shortening of the QT interval

However, some changes in ECG wave morphology may be indicative of underlying pathology. For example, while QRS duration tends to decrease slightly with exercise (and increasing HR) in normal subjects, it may increase in patients with either angina or left ventricular dysfunction. Exercise-induced P wave changes corresponding to P-pulmonale or P-mitrale are rarely seen and are of questionable significance. Many factors affect R-wave amplitude; consequently, such changes during exercise have no independent predictive power (18).

ST-SEGMENT DISPLACEMENT

ST-segment changes are widely accepted criteria for myocardial ischemia and injury. Interpretation of ST segments may be affected by the resting ECG configuration (e.g., bundle-branch blocks, left ventricular hypertrophy) and pharmacologic agents (e.g., digitalis therapy). There may be J-point depression and tall peaked T-waves at high exercise intensities and during recovery in normal subjects. Depression of the J point that leads to marked ST-segment upsloping is due to competition between normal repolarization and delayed terminal depolarization forces rather than to ischemia (19). Exercise-induced myocardial ischemia may be manifested by three different types of ST-segment changes on the ECG:

ST-segment elevation
- ST-segment elevation (early repolarization) may be seen in the normal resting ECG. Increasing HR may cause normally elevated ST segments to return to the isoelectric line.
- ST-segment elevation indicates myocardial injury (i.e., an acute transmural infarction) when followed by the evolution of significant Q-waves.

- Exercise-induced ST-segment elevation in leads displaying a previous Q wave infarction may be indicative of wall motion abnormalities or ventricular aneurysm (20,21); ST-segment elevation may also result from coronary spasm.
- Exercise-induced ST-segment elevation on an otherwise normal ECG (except in aVR or V_{1-2}) represents transmural ischemia, is very arrhythmogenic, and localizes the ischemia (22).

ST-segment depression
- ST-segment depression (depression of the J point and the slope over the following 80 msec) is the most common manifestation of exercise-induced myocardial ischemia.
- Horizontal or downsloping ST-segment depression is more indicative of subendocardial ischemia than is upsloping depression.
- Slowly upsloping ST-segment depression should be considered a borderline response, and added emphasis should be placed on other clinical and exercise variables.
- ST-segment depression does not localize the area of ischemia nor indicate which coronary artery is involved.
- The more leads with (apparent) ischemic ST-segment shifts, the more severe the disease.
- Significant ST-segment depression occurring only in recovery likely represents a true positive response, and should be considered an important diagnostic finding (23).

ST-segment normalization or absence of change
- Ischemia may be manifested by normalization of resting ST segments. ECG abnormalities at rest, including T-wave inversion and ST-segment depression, may return to normal during anginal symptoms and during exercise in some patients (4,24).

ST-segment depression can be quantitated manually or, more precisely, with the aid of a computer. Examples of the various criteria for ischemic ST-segment displacement, as well as some waveform changes previously discussed, are shown in Figure 6-2. Although several methods may be used to evaluate an abnormal ECG response, the ST-segment index (25), defined as the algebraic sum of the ST J-segment depression in millimeters and the ST slope in millivolts per second (mV/sec), has been correlated with angiographically documented CAD. A negative index (i.e., <0) is considered abnormal, assuming that the magnitude of ST-segment depression (from the baseline to the J point) is at least 1.0 mm. For example, slow upsloping ST-segment depression would be considered abnormal if the depression and slope were −2.0 mm and 1.0 mV/sec, respectively. The ST-segment index would be −1.0 in this case, suggesting an ischemic response (Fig. 6-3).

In patients with left bundle-branch block, ST-segment abnormalities that develop during exercise are uninterpretable with respect to evidence of myocardial ischemia (26). In rate-dependent left bundle-branch block, the HR at onset may be helpful in diagnosing CAD (27). In right bundle-branch block, exercise-induced ST-segment displacement in the anterior

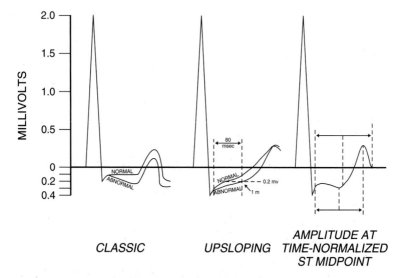

FIGURE 6-2. Standard visual and computer criteria for identifying ischemia. As shown, there are different ways of calculating ST-segment displacement. Some have suggested using the end of the T wave for measuring the midpoint of the ST segment, whereas others used the peak of the T wave. This change was made to have a more stable end point, since the former is more difficult to define than the latter. The ST integral requires delineation of the end of the QRS complex or J junction, and that the area measurement stops when the ST segment crossed the isoelectric line or as the T wave began. The ST integral used by most commercial systems initiates the area at a fixed period after the R wave and ends 80 msec thereafter. (*Continues at top of page 123.*)

precordial leads (V_1, V_2, and V_3) should not be used to diagnose ischemia; however, ST-segment changes in the lateral leads (V_4, V_5, and V_6) may be indicative of ischemia even in the presence of this anomaly (28).

ARRHYTHMIAS

Exercise-associated arrhythmias occur in healthy subjects as well as patients with cardiac disease. Increased sympathetic drive and changes in extracellular and intracellular electrolytes, pH, and oxygen tension contribute to disturbances in myocardial and conducting tissue automaticity and reentry, which are major mechanisms of arrhythmias.

Supraventricular Arrhythmias   Isolated premature atrial contractions are common and require no special precautions. Atrial flutter or atrial fibrillation may occur in organic heart disease or may reflect endocrine, metabolic, or drug effects (hyperthyroidism, alcoholic cardiomyopathy, alcohol consumption, and digoxin toxicity).

Sustained supraventricular tachycardia is occasionally induced by exercise and may require pharmacologic treatment or electroconversion if discontinuation of exercise or use of vagal reflex maneuvers fail to abolish the rhythm. Patients who experience paroxysmal atrial tachycardia may be evaluated by repeating the exercise test after appropriate treatment.

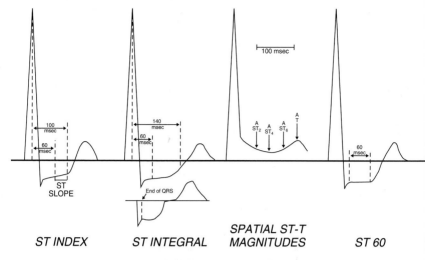

FIGURE 6-2. (*continued*)

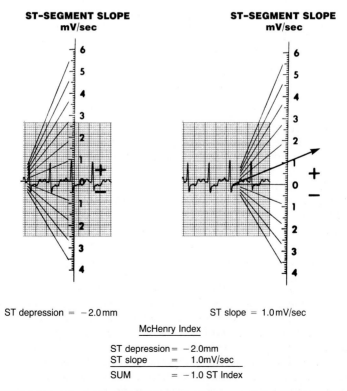

FIGURE 6-3. Example showing calculation of the ST-segment index (McHenry Index) by using a transparent overlay to determine the ST-segment slope and depression. An abnormal ECG response with upsloping ST-segment depression is shown.

Ventricular Arrhythmias Isolated premature ventricular complexes or contractions (PVCs) occur during exercise in 30 to 40% of healthy subjects and in 50 to 60% of patients with CAD. In some individuals, graded exercise induces PVCs whereas in others it reduces their occurrence. However, the suppression of resting ventricular arrhythmias during exercise *does not* exclude the presence of underlying CAD; conversely, PVCs that increase in frequency, complexity, or both do not necessarily signify underlying ischemic heart disease (29). Threatening forms of ventricular ectopy, including paired or multiform PVCs, salvos, and ventricular tachycardia, are likely to be associated with significant CAD and/or a poor prognosis if they occur in conjunction with signs and/or symptoms of myocardial ischemia (30,31), or in patients with a history of sudden cardiac death, cardiomyopathy, or valvular heart disease (32). Nonsustained exercise-induced ventricular tachycardia during routine treadmill testing is not associated with other complications during testing or with increased cardiovascular mortality (33). Moreover, the prevalence of exercise-induced ventricular tachycardia is low in most clinical laboratories and usually consists of three consecutive beats.

Criteria for terminating exercise tests based on ventricular ectopy include increasing frequency of PVCs, multiform appearance, and frequent coupling or any run of ventricular tachycardia (three or more PVCs in succession). The decision to terminate an exercise test should also be influenced by simultaneous evidence of myocardial ischemia or adverse signs or symptoms (see Box 5-3).

Symptoms

Although patients with exercise-induced ST-segment depression are often asymptomatic, when concomitant angina occurs, the likelihood that the ECG changes are due to CAD is significantly increased (34). In addition, angina pectoris *without* ischemic ECG changes may be as predictive of CAD as ST-segment changes alone (35). Both are currently considered independent variables that identify patients at increased risk for subsequent coronary events.

Diagnostic Value of Exercise Testing

The diagnostic value of conventional exercise testing for the detection of CAD is influenced by the principles of conditional probability (Box 6-1). The factors that determine the predictive outcome of exercise testing (and other diagnostic tests) are the sensitivity and specificity of the test procedure and the prevalence of CAD in the population tested. Sensitivity and specificity determine how effective the test is in making correct diagnoses in individuals with and without disease, respectively. Disease prevalence is an important determinant of the predictive value of the test. Moreover, non-ECG criteria, such as duration of exercise or maximal MET level, hemodynamic responses, symptoms of angina or dyspnea, and even the maximal blood

---

BOX 6-1. Sensitivity, Specificity, and Predictive Value of Diagnostic Graded Exercise Testing

Sensitivity = TP/(TP + FN) =
  the percentage of patients with CAD who will have an abnormal test
Specificity = TN/(TN + FP) =
  the percentage of patients without CAD who will have a negative test
Predictive Value (positive test) = TP/(TP + FP) =
  the percentage of patients with a positive test result who have CAD
Predictive Value (negative test) = TN/(TN + FN) =
  the percentage of patients with a negative test who do not have CAD

TP, true positive (positive exercise test and coronary artery disease [CAD]); FP, false positive (positive exercise test and no CAD); TN, true negative (negative exercise test and no CAD); FN, false negative (negative exercise test and CAD).

---

lactate level (36), if available, may be considered in the overall interpretation of exercise test results.

Sensitivity

Sensitivity refers to the percent of patients tested who have CAD and who demonstrate positive (abnormal) test results. Exercise ECG sensitivity for the detection of CAD usually is based on subsequent angiographically determined coronary artery stenosis of 70% or more in at least one vessel. A true positive exercise test (based on ST-segment depression of 1.0 mm or more) correctly identifies a patient with CAD. False negative test results show no or nondiagnostic ECG changes and fail to identify patients with underlying CAD.

Common factors that contribute to false negative exercise tests are summarized in Box 6-2. Test sensitivity is decreased by inadequate stress, drugs that attenuate cardiac demands to exercise or reduce myocardial ischemia (e.g., β-blockers, nitrates, and calcium channel blocking agents), and insufficient ECG lead monitoring. Accordingly, use of right precordial

---

BOX 6-2. Causes of False Negative Test Results

Failure to reach an ischemic threshold
Monitoring an insufficient number of leads to detect ECG changes
Failure to recognize non-ECG signs and symptoms that may be associated with underlying CAD (e.g., exertional hypotension)
Angiographically significant CAD compensated by collateral circulation
Musculoskeletal limitations to exercise preceding cardiac abnormalities
Technical or observer error

ECG, electrocardiogram; CAD, coronary artery disease.

leads along with the standard six left precordial leads during exercise electro-cardiography improves the sensitivity of exercise testing in the detection of CAD, similar to that of thallium-201 scintigraphy (37). Preexisting ECG changes, such as left ventricular hypertrophy, left bundle-branch block, or the preexcitation syndrome (Wolff-Parkinson-White), limit the ability to interpret exercise-induced ST-segment changes as ischemic ECG responses.

Specificity

The specificity of exercise tests refers to the percent of normal subjects (without CAD) who show a negative stress test. A true negative test correctly identifies a person without CAD. Many conditions may cause false positive exercise ECG responses (Box 6-3).

Reported values for the specificity and sensitivity of exercise ECG testing vary due to differences in patient selection, test protocols, ECG criteria for a positive test, and the angiographic definition of CAD. In studies that controlled for these variables, the pooled results show a sensitivity of 68% and a specificity of 77% (2).

Predictive Value

The predictive value of exercise testing is a measure of how accurately a test result (positive or negative) correctly identifies the presence or absence of CAD in patients tested. That is, the predictive value of an abnormal test is the percentage of those persons with an abnormal test who have the disease. Nevertheless, a test should not be classified as "negative" unless the patient has attained an adequate level of cardiovascular stress, generally

---

BOX 6-3. Causes of False Positive Test Results*

Resting repolarization abnormalities (e.g., left bundle-branch block)
Cardiac hypertrophy
Accelerated conduction defects (e.g., Wolff-Parkinson-White syndrome)
Digitalis
Nonischemic cardiomyopathy
Hypokalemia
Vasoregulatory abnormalities
Mitral valve prolapse
Pericardial disorders
Technical or observer error
Coronary spasm in the absence of significant CAD
Anemia
Female gender

*Selected variables may simply be associated with rather than causes of false positive test results.
CAD, coronary artery disease.

TABLE 6-2. Test Performance versus Predictive Value and Risk Ratio: A Model in a Population of 10,000

Disease Prevalence	Subjects	Number With Abnormal Test Results	Test Performance	Number With Normal Test Results
5%	500 diseased	450 (TP)	90% sensitivity	50 (FN)
		350 (TP)	70% sensitivity	150 (FN)
	9500 nondiseased	2850 (FP)	70% specificity	6650 (TN)
		950 (FP)	90% specificity	8550 (TN)
50%	5000 diseased	4500 (TP)	90% sensitivity	500 (FN)
		3500 (TP)	70% sensitivity	1500 (FN)
	5000 nondiseased	1500 (FP)	70% specificity	3500 (TN)
		500 (FP)	90% specificity	4500 (TN)

Disease Prevalence	Predictive Value of Abnormal Test		Risk Ratio*	
Sensitivity/Specificity	5%	50%	5%	50%
70%/90%	27%	88%	3	27
90%/70%	14%	75%	5	14
90%/90%	32%	90%	9	64
66%/84%	18%	80%	3	9

*Times that for normal subjects.

TP, true positive test result; FP, false positive test result; FN, false negative test result; TN, true negative test result.

defined as having achieved 85% or more of predicted maximal heart rate during the test. Predictive value cannot be estimated directly from a test's demonstrated specificity or sensitivity; it depends on the prevalence of disease in the population tested. Examples of this are shown in Table 6-2.

Comparison With Imaging Stress Tests

The overall sensitivity and specificity of exercise echocardiography ranges from 74 to 97% and 64 to 94%, respectively, with higher sensitivities in patients with multivessel disease (38). Patients with a normal exercise echocardiogram have a low risk of future cardiac events, including myocardial infarction and sudden cardiac death, as well as the need for coronary revascularization. Cardiac events are more likely to occur in patients with lower exercise capacities and in those unable to achieve 85% of predicted maximal heart rate (39). Exercise with concomitant technetium-Tc99m sestamibi

BOX 6-4. Electrocardiographic, Cardiorespiratory, and Hemodynamic Responses to Exercise Testing and Their Clinical Significance

Variable	Clinical Significance
ST-segment depression (ST ↓):	An abnormal ECG response is defined as ≥1.0 mm of horizontal or downsloping ST ↓ at 80 msec beyond the J point, suggesting myocardial ischemia.
ST-segment elevation (ST ↑):	ST ↑ in leads displaying a previous Q-wave MI almost always reflects an aneurysm or wall motion abnormality. In the absence of significant Q waves, exercise-induced ST ↑ is often associated with a fixed high-grade coronary stenosis.
Supraventricular arrthythmias:	Isolated atrial ectopic beats or short runs of SVT commonly occur during exercise testing and do not seem to have any diagnostic or prognostic significance for CAD.
Ventricular arrhythmias:	The suppression or progression of PVCs during exercise testing does not necessarily signify the absence or presence of ischemic CAD, respectively. Threatening forms of ventricular ectopy (e.g., frequent multiform PVCs, salvos, VT) are even more likely to be associated with CAD and a poor prognosis if they occur in the presence of significant ST ↓, ST ↑, angina pectoris, or combinations thereof.
Heart rate (HR):	The normal HR response to progressive exercise is a relatively linear increase, corresponding to 10 ± 2 beats/MET for inactive subjects. Chronotropic incompetence is signified by a peak exercise HR that is >2 SD (>20 beats·min^{-1}) below the age-predicted maximal HR for subjects who are limited by volitional fatigue and are not taking β-blockers.
Systolic blood pressure (SBP):	The normal response to exercise is a progressive increase in SBP, typically 10 ± 2 mm Hg/MET, with a possible plateau at peak exercise. Exercise testing should be discontinued with SBP values of >250 mm Hg. Exertional hypotension (SBP that fails to rise or falls [>10 mm Hg]) may signify myocardial ischemia and/or LV dysfunction. Maximal exercise SBP of <140 mm Hg suggests a poor prognosis.
Diastolic blood pressure (DBP):	The normal response to exercise is no change or a decrease in DBP. A DBP of >115 mm Hg is considered an end point for exercise testing. An increase of >15 mm Hg in DBP

	during treadmill testing may suggest severe CA even in the absence of ischemic ST ↓ .
Anginal symptoms:	Can be graded on a scale of 1 to 4, corresponding to perceptible but mild, moderate, moderate severe, and severe, respectively. Ratings of >2 (moderate) should generally be used as end poin for exercise testing.
Aerobic fitness:	Average values of $\dot{V}O_{2max}$, expressed as METs, expected in healthy sedentary men and women can be predicted from the following regressions: Men = (57.8 − .445 [age])/3.5; Women = (42.3 − .356 [age])/3.5. The FAI can be calculated as: % FAI = ([Predicted $\dot{V}O_{2max}$ − Observed $\dot{V}O_{2max}$]/Predicted $\dot{V}O_{2max}$) × 100.

ECG, electrocardiographic; ST ↓, ST-segment depression; ST ↑, ST-segment elevation; MI, myoca dial infarction; SVT, supraventricular tachycardia; PVCs, premature ventricular contractions; CAD coronary artery disease; VT, ventricular tachycardia; HR, heart rate; MET, metabolic equivalent; SD, standard deviation; LV, left ventricular; SBP, systolic blood pressure; DBP, diastolic blood pressure; $\dot{V}O_{2max}$, aerobic capacity; FAI, functional aerobic impairment.

(Cardiolite, Dupont Medical, North Billerica, MA) imaging has shown similar accuracy to exercise with thallous (thallium) chloride-201 imaging in the detection of myocardial ischemia. For planar imaging, the sensitivity and specificity of sestamibi have been measured at 84% and 83%, compared with 83% and 88% for thallium; for single photon emission computed tomography (SPECT) imaging they were 90% and 93%, compared with 89% and 76% for thallium. In addition, when normal, reversible, and nonreversible segments scanned with sestamibi and thallium are compared, there is 88% agreement with planar and 92% agreement with SPECT imaging (40,41).

Prognostic Applications of the Exercise Test

Risk or prognostic evaluation is a pivotal activity in medical practice on which many patient management decisions are based. In patients with CAD, several clinical factors contribute to patient outcome, including severity and stability of symptoms; left ventricular function; angiographic extent and severity of CAD; electrical stability of the myocardium; and the presence of other comorbid conditions. Unless cardiac catheterization and immediate coronary revascularization are indicated, an exercise test should be performed in persons with known or suspected CAD to assess risk of future cardiac events, and to assist in subsequent management decisions. As stated in Chapter 5, data derived from the exercise test are most useful when considered in the context of other clinical information. Important prognostic variables that can be derived from the exercise test are summarized in Box 6-4.

Use of the VA score (42) (validated for the male veteran population) and the Duke nomogram (43) (validated for the general population, including women) (see Fig. 5-1) can be helpful when applied appropriately. Patients who have recently suffered an acute myocardial infarction and received thrombolytic therapy and/or have undergone coronary revascularization generally have a low subsequent cardiac event rate. Exercise testing can still provide prognostic information in this population, as well as assist in activity counseling and exercise prescription.

Interpretation of Exercise Tests in Pulmonary Patients

The major abnormalities of cardiopulmonary exercise responses are ventilatory limitation and/or oxygen desaturation in patients with moderate to severe lung disease (asthma, chronic obstructive pulmonary disease [COPD], interstitial lung disease, and pulmonary vascular disease):

Ventilatory limitation
- Is assessed by calculating the $\dot{V}_{E\,max}$/maximal voluntary ventilation (MVV) ratio $\times$ 100% (approximately 50 to 70% in normal healthy individuals). In addition, the breathing reserve (BR), defined as 100% $-$ ($[\dot{V}_{E\,max}/MVV] \times 100\%$), is another method to consider ventilatory limitation (44).
- A $\dot{V}_{E\,max}$/MVV value of more than 70% or a low breathing reserve (<30%) is used to indicate a ventilatory limitation.

O_2 desaturation
- Gas exchange may be impaired during exercise in some patients with respiratory disease.
- A decrease in the percent saturation of arterial oxygen (S_aO_2) of 4% or more is considered abnormal.
- The resting (baseline) S_aO_2 and its position on the oxyhemoglobin curve is also important (e.g., a decrease in S_aO_2 from 91% at rest to 87% during exercise may lead to pulmonary vasoconstriction, cardiac dysfunction, or severe dyspnea, whereas a change from 97% at rest to 93% at peak exercise would not be expected to have important clinical consequences).
- Arterial blood gases may be measured in selected patients to provide more precise information about oxygenation as well as the partial pressure of carbon dioxide (P_aCO_2) and pH. In addition, the alveolar-arterial oxygen difference can be calculated to examine gas exchange.

Specific Respiratory Diseases

The results of varied clinical tests can be used to delineate specific respiratory diseases/conditions, including asthma/COPD, interstitial lung disease, pulmonary vascular disease, psychogenic dyspnea, and symptom limitation.

ASTHMA OR COPD

Many patients with moderate to severe asthma or COPD exhibit al
mal cardiopulmonary exercise responses due to ventilatory limitations a
or oxygen desaturation. In patients in whom reactive airway disea:
suspected or asthma has been documented, exercise-induced bronchoc
striction frequently occurs. An exercise challenge test consisting of 6 t
minutes of strenuous running on the treadmill at a target intensity of 85
90% of the maximal heart rate is frequently used to diagnose exerci
induced bronchoconstriction. A positive test is signified by a 15% decrea:
in forced expiratory volume in 1 second ($FEV_{1.0}$) in the postexercise perio

INTERSTITIAL LUNG DISEASE

Oxygen desaturation is a common abnormality during exercise in pa
tients with interstitial lung disease. In addition, these patients usually dem
onstrate evidence of ventilatory limitation as evidenced by a low BR.

PULMONARY VASCULAR DISEASE

Patients with pulmonary vascular disease typically exhibit a low BR,
a low heart rate reserve, a high ventilatory equivalent for $\dot{V}CO_2$ ($\dot{V}_E/\dot{V}CO_2$
ratio), a low oxygen-pulse ($\dot{V}O_2/HR$), and oxygen desaturation.

PSYCHOGENIC DYSPNEA

Individuals with psychogenic dyspnea usually report breathlessness at
rest and during physical activity. The diagnosis can be made by an irregular
breathing pattern during exercise with fluctuating levels of ventilation. Psychogenic dyspnea is suspected when the patient performs a maximal effort,
the BR is normal, and there is no evidence of oxygen desaturation.

SYMPTOM LIMITATION

Patients with moderate to severe respiratory disease usually report
"severe" levels of dyspnea (e.g., 6 to 8 on the 0–10 category-ratio scale) at
peak exercise (45). These perceptual responses are similar regardless of the
specific disease. The assessment of patients should include measurement
of both ratings of dyspnea and leg discomfort during the exercise test; this
information may be useful for interpretation of the individual's primary
limitation to exercise. Some patients with respiratory disease who report
"difficulty breathing with activities" may actually report higher ratings for
leg discomfort than dyspnea at submaximal and maximal exercise intensities. Such results combined with a reduced $\dot{V}O_{2max}$ and a normal BR strongly
suggest that the individual is limited more by deconditioning and/or muscle
weakness than by respiratory disease.

References

1. Hellerstein HK, Banerja JC, Biorck G, et al. Rehabilitation of patients with cardiovascular diseases. WHO Tech Rep Series 1964:270.
2. Gibbons RA, Balady GJ, Beasely JW, et al. ACC/AHA guidelines for exercise testing. J Am Coll Cardiol 1997;30:260–315.
3. Myers J, Froelicher VF. Hemodynamic determinants of exercise capacity in chronic heart failure. Ann Intern Med 1991;115:377–386.

4. McKirnan MD, Sullivan M, Jensen D, et al. Treadmill performance and cardiac function in selected patients with coronary heart disease. J Am Coll Cardiol 1984;3:253–261.

5. Taylor HL, Buskirk ER, Henschel A. Maximal oxygen uptake as an objective measure of cardiorespiratory performance. J Appl Physiol 1955;8:73–80.

6. Londeree BR, Moeschberger ML. Influence of age and other factors on maximal heart rate. J Cardiac Rehab 1984;4:44–49.

7. Brener SJ, Pashkow FJ, Harvey SA, et al. Chronotropic response to exercise predicts angiographic severity in patients with suspected or stable coronary artery disease. Am J Cardiol 1995;76:1228–1232.

8. Ellestad MH. Chronotropic incompetence. The implications of heart rate response to exercise (compensatory parasympathetic hyperactivity?). Circulation 1996;93:1485–1487.

9. Lauer MS, Francis GS, Okin PM, et al. Impaired chronotropic response to exercise stress testing as a predictor of mortality. JAMA 1999;281:524–529.

10. Cole CR, Blackstone EH, Pashkow FJ, et al. Heart-rate recovery immediately after exercise as a predictor of mortality. N Engl J Med 1999;341:1351–1357.

11. Wolthius RA, Froelicher VF, Fischer J, et al. The response of healthy men to treadmill exercise. Circulation 1977;55:153–157.

12. Comess KA, Fenster PE. Clinical implications of the blood pressure response to exercise. Cardiology 1981;68:233–244.

13. Irving JB, Bruce RA, DeRouen TA. Variations in and significance of systolic pressure during maximal exercise (treadmill) testing: relation to severity of coronary artery disease and cardiac mortality. Am J Cardiol 1977;39:841–848.

14. Weiner DA, McCabe CH, Cutler SS, et al. Decrease in systolic blood pressure during exercise testing: reproducibility, response to coronary bypass surgery and prognostic significance. Am J Cardiol 1982;49:1627–1631.

15. Kitamura K, Jorgensen CR, Gobel FL, et al. Hemodynamic correlates of myocardial oxygen consumption during upright exercise. J Appl Physiol 1972;32:516–522.

16. Sheps DS, Ernst JC, Briese FW, et al. Exercise-induced increase in diastolic pressure: indicator of severe coronary artery disease. Am J Cardiol 1979;43:708–712.

17. Hiroyuki D, Allison TG, Squires RW, et al. Peak exercise blood pressure stratified by age and gender in apparently healthy subjects. Mayo Clin Proc 1996;71:445–452.

18. Myers J, Ahnve S, Froelicher V, et al. Spatial R wave amplitude changes during exercise: relation with left ventricular ischemia and function. J Am Coll Cardiol 1985;6:603–608.

19. Mirvis DM, Ramanathan KB, Wilson JL. Regional blood flow correlates of ST segment depression in tachycardia-induced myocardial ischemia. Circulation 1986;2:363–373.

20. Chaitman BR, Waters DD, Théroux P, et al. ST-segment elevation and coronary spasm in response to exercise. Am J Cardiol 1981;47:1350–1358.

21. Bruce RA, Fisher LD, Pettinger M, et al. ST segment elevation with exercise: a marker for poor ventricular function and poor prognosis. Circulation 1988;77:897–905.

22. Nostratian F, Froelicher VF. ST elevation during exercise testing: a review. Am J Cardiol 1989;63:986–988.

23. Lachterman B, Lehmann KG, Detrano R, et al. Comparison of ST segment: heart rate index to standard ST criteria for analysis of exercise electrocardiogram. Circulation 1990;82:44–50.

24. Lavie CJ, Oh JK, Mankin HT, et al. Significance of T-wave pseudonormalization during exercise. A radionuclide angiographic study. Chest 1988;94:512–516.

25. McHenry PL, Phillips JF, Knoebel SB. Correlation of computer-quantitated treadmill exercise electrocardiogram with arteriographic location of coronary artery disease. Am J Cardiol 1972;30:747–752.

26. Whinnery JE, Froelicher VF, Stewart AJ. The electrocardiographic response to maximal treadmill exercise in asymptomatic men with left bundle branch block. Am Heart J 1977;94:316–324.

27. Vasey CG, O'Donnell J, Morris SN, et al. Exercise-induced left bundle branch block and its relation to coronary artery disease. Am J Cardiol 1985;56:892–895.

28. Whinnery JE, Froelicher VF, Stewart AJ. The electrocardiographic response to maximal treadmill exercise in asymptomatic men with right bundle branch block. Chest 1977;71:335–340.

29. Califf RM, McKinnis RA, McNear JF, et al. Prognostic value of ventricular arrhythmias associated with treadmill exercise testing in patients studied with cardiac catheterization for suspected ischemic heart disease. J Am Coll Cardiol 1983;2:1060–1067.

30. Ellestad MH, Cooke BM, Greenberg PS. Stress testing: clinical application and predictive capacity. Prog Cardiovasc Dis 1979;21:431–460.

31. Fuller T, Movahed A. Current review of exercise testing: application and interpretation. Clin Cardiol 1987;10:189–200.

32. Busby MJ, Shefrin EA, Fleg JL. Prevalence and long-term significance of exercise-induced frequent or repetitive ventricular ectopic beats in apparently healthy volunteers. J Am Coll Cardiol 1989;14:1659–1665.

33. Yang JC, Wesley RC, Froelicher VF. Ventricular tachycardia during routine treadmill testing. Risk and prognosis. Arch Intern Med 1991;151:349–352.

34. Weiner DA. Correlations among history of angina, ST segment response and preval coronary artery disease in the Coronary Artery Surgery Study. N Engl J Med 1979;301:23

35. Cole JP, Ellestad MH. Significance of chest pain during treadmill exercise: correlation coronary events. Am J Cardiol 1978;41:227–232.

36. Barthélémy J-C, Roche F, Gaspoz J-M, et al. Maximal blood lactate level acts as a discriminant variable in exercise testing for coronary artery disease detection in men. Circ tion 1996;93:246–252.

37. Michaelides AP, Psomadaki ZD, Dilaveris PE, et al. Improved detection of coronary ar disease by exercise electrocardiography with the use of right precordial leads. N Eng Med 1999;340:340–345.

38. Chetlin MD, Alpert JS, Armstrong WF, et al. ACC/AHA guidelines for the clinical applicati of echocardiography: a report of the American College of Cardiology/American Heart Asso ation Task Force on Practice Guidelines (Committee on Clinical Application of Echocardiogr phy). J Am Coll Cardiol 1997;29:862–879.

39. Sawada SG, Ryan T, Conley MJ, et al. Prognostic value of a normal exercise echocardiograr Am Heart J 1990;120:49–55.

40. Berman DS, Kiat H, Leppo J, et al. Technetium-99m myocardial perfusion imaging agent. In: Marcus ML, Schelbert HR, Skorton DJ, et al., eds. Cardiac Imaging, A Companion t Baunwald's Heart Disease. Philadelphia: WB Saunders, 1991:1097–1109.

41. Ritchie JL, Bateman TM, Bonow RO, et al. Guidelines for clinical use of cardiac radionuclid imaging. Report of the American College of Cardiology/American Heart Association Task Force on Assessment of Diagnostic and Therapeutic Cardiovascular Procedures (Subcommit tee on Coronary Artery Bypass Graft Surgery). J Am Coll Cardiol 1991;17(3):543–589.

42. Morrow K, Morris CK, Froelicher VF, et al. Prediction of cardiovascular death in men undergo ing noninvasive evaluation for coronary artery disease. Ann Intern Med 1993;118(9):689–695.

43. Mark DB, Hlatky MA, Harrell FE, et al. Exercise treadmill score for predicting prognosis in coronary artery disease. Ann Intern Med 1987;106:793–800.

44. Wasserman K, Hansen JE, Sue DY, et al. Principles of Exercise Testing and Interpretation. 2nd ed. Malvern: Lea & Febiger, 1994:132–144.

45. Hamilton AL, Killian KJ, Summers E, et al. Symptom intensity and subjective limitation to exercise in patients with cardiorespiratory disorders. Chest 1996;110:1255–1263.

SECTION III

Exercise Prescription

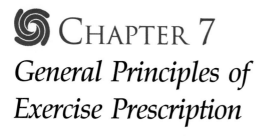

CHAPTER 7
General Principles of Exercise Prescription

Increases in physical activity (1) and cardiorespiratory fitness (2) are associated with a reduced risk of death from coronary heart disease as well as from all causes. The primary focus on achieving health-related goals has been on prescribing exercise for improvements in cardiorespiratory fitness, body composition, and most recently, strength. In 1995, the Centers for Disease Control and Prevention (CDC) and the American College of Sports Medicine (ACSM) suggested that the focus should be broadened to address the needs of all sedentary individuals, especially those who cannot or will not engage in structured exercise programs. Increasing evidence has shown that regular participation in moderate-intensity physical activity (3 to 6 metabolic equivalents [METs]) is associated with health benefits, even when aerobic fitness (e.g., maximal oxygen uptake, $\dot{V}O_{2max}$) remains unchanged. To promote this message, the CDC and ACSM recommended that "every US adult should accumulate 30 min[utes] or more of moderate-intensity physical activity on most, preferably all, days of the week" (3). The Activity Pyramid has been suggested as one way to facilitate this objective (Fig. 7-1).

Some fitness professionals viewed this recommendation as a major departure from the traditional ACSM fitness programming recommendations published in previous editions of this text and in various ACSM position stands. Others saw the new recommendation as part of a continuum of physical activity recommendations that meets the needs of almost all individuals to improve health status. For example, the upper end of the intensity range for moderate physical activity (3 to 6 METs) in the ACSM/CDC recommendation represents the lower end of the intensity scale to improve fitness for many sedentary, overweight, asymptomatic individuals. Consequently, the combined ACSM/CDC and traditional ACSM recommendations represent a true continuum for one of the primary variables in exercise prescription, that is, the intensity of exercise. Those who follow the more recent recommendation (3) will experience many of the health-related benefits of physical activity, and if they are interested in achieving higher levels of fitness, they will be ready to do so. This chapter describes how to structure exercise prescriptions to achieve and maintain fitness goals.

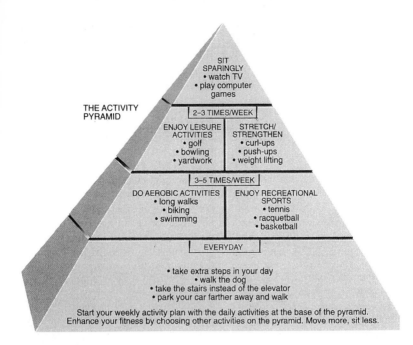

FIGURE 7-1. The Activity Pyramid, analogous to the USDA's Food Guide Pyramid, has been suggested as a model to facilitate public and patient education for the adoption of a progressively more active lifestyle. (Copyright 1997 Park Nicollet Health Source® Institute for Research and Education. Reprinted by permission.)

PRINCIPLES OF TRAINING

The fitness components identified and evaluated in Chapter 4 included body composition, cardiorespiratory fitness ($\dot{V}O_{2max}$), muscular strength and endurance, and flexibility. Improvements in the latter three components follow the two major principles of training: overload and specificity. The principle of overload states that for a tissue or organ to improve its function, it must be exposed to a load to which it is not normally accustomed. Repeated exposure is associated with an adaptation by the tissue or organ that leads to improved functional capacity. An exercise prescription specifies the intensity, duration, and frequency of training, and it is the interaction of these three variables that results in the cumulative overload to which the tissue or organ must adapt. The principle of specificity states that training effects derived from an exercise program are specific to the exercise performed and muscles involved. For example, low-resistance, high-repetition exercises cause increases in the number of mitochondria in the active muscles, leading to improvements in muscular endurance with little change in strength. In contrast, heavy resistance exercise promotes increases in strength, with little or no change in endurance. An additional example of specificity is seen in the varied cardiovascular responses to different modes of exercise even when the intensity is set at the same %$\dot{V}O_{2max}$ or rating of perceived exertion

(RPE) (4). This is due, in part, to training status of the muscles involved in each exercise. Consequently, a fitness program that involves a wide variety of exercises recruits most of the major muscle groups and increases the likelihood that the training effect may transfer to vocational and recreational activities.

OVERVIEW OF THE EXERCISE PRESCRIPTION

Exercise prescriptions are designed to enhance physical fitness, promote health by reducing risk factors for chronic disease (e.g., high blood pressure, glucose intolerance), and ensure safety during exercise participation. Based on individual interests, health needs, and clinical status, these common purposes do not carry equal or consistent weight. For the sedentary person at risk for premature chronic disease, adopting a moderately active lifestyle (i.e., the ACSM/CDC recommendation) may provide important health benefits and represent a more attainable goal than achievement of a high $\dot{V}O_{2max}$. However, enhancing physical fitness, whenever possible, is a desirable feature of exercise prescriptions. In all cases, specific outcomes identified for a particular person should be the ultimate target of the exercise prescription.

The essential components of a systematic, individualized exercise prescription include the appropriate mode(s), intensity, duration, frequency, and progression of physical activity. These five components apply when developing exercise prescriptions for persons of all ages and fitness levels, regardless of the presence or absence of risk factors and disease. The optimal exercise prescription for an individual is determined from an objective evaluation of that individual's response to exercise, including observations of heart rate (HR), blood pressure (BP), RPE, subjective response to exercise, electrocardiogram (ECG) when applicable, and $\dot{V}O_{2max}$ measured directly or estimated during a graded exercise test. As discussed in Chapter 2, an exercise test is not required for all individuals before beginning a physical conditioning program. The exercise prescription, however, should be developed with careful consideration of the individual's health status (including medications), risk factor profile, behavioral characteristics, personal goals, and exercise preferences.

THE ART OF EXERCISE PRESCRIPTION

The guidelines for exercise prescription presented in this book are based on a solid foundation of scientific information. Given the diverse nature and health needs of the population, these guidelines cannot be implemented in an overly rigid fashion by simply applying mathematical calculations to test data. The recommendations presented should be used with careful attention to the goals of the individual. Exercise prescriptions will require modification in accordance with observed individual responses and adaptations because of the following:

- Physiologic and perceptual responses to acute exercise vary among individuals and within an individual performing different types of exercise. There is a need to titrate the intensity and duration of exercise and monitor HR, BP, RPE, and, where appropriate, ECG responses to achieve a safe and effective exercise stimulus.
- Adaptations to exercise training vary in terms of magnitude and rate of development. Progress should be monitored by checking HR and RPE responses to allow fine-tuning of the exercise stimulus.
- Desired outcomes based on individual need(s) may be achieved with exercise programs that vary considerably in structure, so one should address individual interests, abilities, and limitations in the design of the program.

A fundamental objective of exercise prescription is to bring about a change in personal health behavior to include habitual physical activity. Thus, the most appropriate exercise prescription for a particular **individual** is the one that is most helpful in achieving this behavioral change. *The art of exercise prescription is the successful integration of exercise science with behavioral techniques that result in long-term program compliance and attainment of the individual's goals.* As such, knowledge of methods to change health behaviors is essential (see Chapter 12). While an abundance of literature exists on this topic, an excellent source is Section 12 of the *ACSM's Resource Manual for Guidelines for Exercise Testing and Prescription*, 3rd edition (5).

COMPONENTS OF THE TRAINING SESSION

Once the exercise prescription has been formulated, it is integrated into a comprehensive physical conditioning program, which is generally complemented by an overall health improvement plan. The exercise program consists of the following components: warm-up, endurance phase, recreational activities (optional); and a cool-down. While endurance training activities should be performed 3 to 5 d·wk^{-1}, complementary flexibility and resistance training may be undertaken at a slightly reduced frequency (2 to 3 d·wk^{-1}) (6). Flexibility training can be included as part of the warm-up or cool-down, or undertaken at a separate time. Resistance training is often performed on alternate days when endurance training is not; however, both activities can be combined into the same workout. Recently, the ACSM included flexibility and resistance training in its recommendations (position stand) for a general health and fitness program (6).

The format for the exercise session should include a warm-up period (approximately 10 minutes), a stimulus or endurance phase (20 to 60 minutes), an optional recreational game, and a cool-down period (5 to 10 minutes) (Fig. 7-2). Endurance and resistance training should be prescribed in specific terms of intensity (load), duration, frequency, and type of activities.

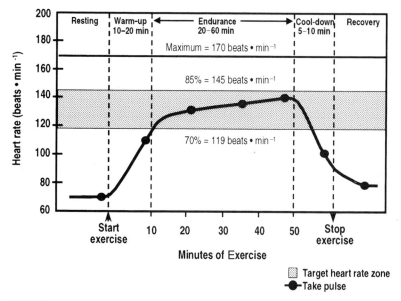

FIGURE 7-2. Format of a typical aerobic exercise session illustrating the warm-up, endurance, and cool-down phases along with a representative heart rate response. At the conclusion of warm-up, heart rate approached the lower limit of the target zone for training, corresponding to 70 to 85% of the peak heart rate achieved during maximal exercise testing.

Warm-up

Warm-up facilitates the transition from rest to exercise, stretches postural muscles, augments blood flow, and increases the metabolic rate from the resting level (1 MET) to the aerobic requirements for endurance training. A warm-up may reduce the susceptibility to musculoskeletal injury by increasing connective tissue extensibility, improving joint range of motion and function, and enhancing muscular performance (6). A preliminary warm-up may also have preventive value, decreasing the occurrence of ischemic ST-segment depression (7,8), threatening ventricular arrhythmias, and transient global left ventricular dysfunction following sudden strenuous exertion (9,10). However, studies in healthy subjects and post-myocardial infarction patients who were taking β-blockers have failed to confirm these cardiovascular abnormalities during sudden strenuous exercise (11,12).

The exercise session should begin with 5 to 10 minutes of low-intensity calisthenic-type and stretching exercises and 5 to 10 minutes of progressive aerobic activity sufficient to approach the lower limit of the prescribed heart rate for endurance training. For example, participants who use brisk walking during the endurance phase might conclude the warm-up period with slow walking. Similarly, brisk walking (e.g., 3.5 to 4.5 mi·h^{-1}) serves as an ideal warm-up for participants who jog slowly during the endurance phase. The stretching activities should exercise the major muscle groups using static, ballistic, or modified proprioceptive neuromuscular facilitation techniques or combinations thereof (6). Although it was previously recommended that stretching and flexibility exercises be performed before the endurance phase (i.e., during the warm-up), it has been suggested that the muscles, tendons, ligaments, and joints may be more responsive to these activities after the endurance phase. However, studies to confirm this hypothesis are lacking.

Endurance Phase

The stimulus or endurance phase develops cardiorespiratory fitness and includes 20 to 60 minutes of continuous or intermittent (minimum of 10-minute bouts accumulated throughout the day) aerobic activity. Duration depends on the intensity of the activity; thus, moderate-intensity activity should be conducted over a longer period of time (30 minutes or more), and, conversely, individuals training at higher levels of intensity (i.e., vigorous exercise) should train for at least 20 minutes or more (6). The most effective exercises for the endurance phase employ large muscle groups in activities that are rhythmic or dynamic in nature. Sports such as tennis, racquetball, handball, and basketball also have aerobic conditioning potential if they are pursued for a sufficient period of time. On the other hand, activities like golf and bowling are unlikely to elicit a cardiovascular training effect, but are enjoyable, have definite recreational value, and may yield health-related benefits. Duration is inversely related to the intensity of the activity (e.g., lower-intensity activity should be done for a longer period of time [30 minutes or more]). This phase of the exercise session may be complemented by recreational games, resistance training, or both.

Recreational Activities

The inclusion of enjoyable recreational activities during (or immediately after) the endurance phase often enhances adherence. However, game rules may be modified to decrease skill requirements, competition, and the energy cost and heart rate responses to play. Game modifications should maximize the experience of successful participation; winning or losing should be of lesser importance (13). Because of a potential discordance between RPE and HR during game activities, the latter should be monitored periodically to adjust the intensity of play.

The imaginative exercise leader may suggest a smaller court size, lowered net height, frequent player-position rotation, intermittent rest periods, minor rule changes, and adjusted scoring. For example, playing volleyball allowing one bounce of the ball per side facilitates longer rallies, provides additional fun, and reduces the skill required to play the game successfully. Many other team games and individual sports can be modified in a similar fashion (13).

Cool-down

The cool-down period provides a gradual recovery from the endurance/ games phase and includes exercises of diminishing intensities; for example, slower walking or jogging, calisthenics and stretching exercises, and in some cases, alternate activities (yoga, tai chi, relaxation training). The cool-down permits appropriate circulatory adjustments and return of the HR and BP to near resting values; enhances venous return, thereby reducing the potential for postexercise hypotension and dizziness; facilitates the dissipation of body heat; promotes more rapid removal of lactic acid than stationary recovery (14); and combats the potential, deleterious effects of the postexercise rise in plasma catecholamines (15). The latter, especially in patients with heart disease, may reduce the likelihood of threatening ventricular arrhythmias—potential harbingers of sudden cardiac death.

Omission of a cool-down in the immediate postexercise period has been associated with an increased incidence of cardiovascular complications. Presumably, it results in a transient decrease in venous return, possibly reducing coronary blood flow when HR and myocardial oxygen demands may still be high. Consequences may include ischemic ST-segment depression, with or without anginal symptoms, serious ventricular arrhythmias, or combinations thereof. Of 61 cardiovascular complications reported during the exercise training of cardiac patients, at least 44 (72%) occurred during either the warm-up or cool-down phases (16).

CARDIORESPIRATORY FITNESS

Improvements in the ability of the heart to deliver oxygen (O_2) to the working muscles and in the muscle's ability to generate energy with O_2 result in increased endurance performance. Improvement in cardiorespiratory fitness is measured by assessing the change in $\dot{V}O_{2max}$, which is directly related to the frequency, duration, and intensity of exercise. When exercise is performed above a minimum threshold, the volume of training (kcal) is an important determinant of the increase in $\dot{V}O_{2max}$, which generally ranges from 10 to 30%. Individuals with low initial levels of fitness, such as cardiac patients and those experiencing concomitant reductions in body weight and fat stores, generally demonstrate the greatest percent increase in $\dot{V}O_{2max}$. In contrast, more modest increases occur in healthy individuals with high initial levels of fitness and in those whose body weight remains unchanged (6).

Mode of Exercise

The greatest improvement in $\dot{V}O_{2max}$ occurs when exercise involves the use of large muscle groups over prolonged periods in activities that are rhythmic and aerobic in nature (e.g., walking, hiking, running, machine-based stair climbing, swimming, cycling, rowing, combined arm and leg ergometry, dancing, skating, cross-country skiing, rope skipping, or endurance games).

Clearly, this wide range of activities provides for individual variability relative to skill and enjoyment, factors which influence compliance to the exercise program and thus desired outcomes (see Chapter 12). Box 7-1 groups commonly prescribed activities. In the development of the exercise prescription for the novice exerciser, it may be useful to begin with group 1 activities and progress depending on the individual's interest, adaptation, and clinical status. Walking may be the activity of choice for many individuals because it is readily accessible and offers an easily tolerable exercise intensity. In contrast, other individuals might logically progress through walking and jogging programs before engaging in group 3 activities. Resistance training does little to increase the $\dot{V}O_{2max}$; however, it facilitates improvements in muscular strength and endurance, maintains or augments fat free mass, and enhances the ability to perform activities of daily living. Circuit weight training, which involves 10 to 15 repetitions with 15 to 30 seconds of rest between weight stations, results in an average improvement in $\dot{V}O_{2max}$ of about 6%. Thus, it is not generally recommended as an activity for improving cardiorespiratory endurance (6).

The risk of injury associated with high-impact activities or high-intensity weight training must also be considered when prescribing exercise modalities, especially for the overweight or novice exerciser. It may be desirable to have the individual engage in several different activities to reduce repetitive orthopedic stresses and involve a greater number of muscle groups. Because improvement in muscular endurance is largely specific to the muscles involved in exercise, it is important to consider unique vocational or recreational objectives of the exercise program when recommending activities. Finally, if possible, one should design programs to eliminate or attenuate barriers that might decrease the likelihood of compliance with, or adherence to, the exercise program (e.g., travel, schedule flexibility, childcare concerns).

BOX 7-1. Grouping of Cardiorespiratory Endurance Activities

Group 1   Activities that can be readily maintained at a constant intensity and interindividual variation in energy expenditure is relatively low. Desirable for more precise control of exercise intensity, as in the early stages of a rehabilitation program.
Examples of these activities are walking and cycling, especially treadmill and cycle ergometry.

Group 2   Activities in which the rate of energy expenditure is highly related to skill, but for a given individual can provide a constant intensity. Such activities may also be useful in early stages of conditioning, but individual skill levels must be considered.
Examples include swimming and cross-country skiing.

Group 3   Activities where both skill and intensity of exercise are highly variable. Such activities can be very useful to provide group interaction and variety in exercise, but must be cautiously employed for high-risk, low-fit, and/or symptomatic individuals. Competitive factors must also be considered and minimized. Examples of these activities are racquet sports and basketball.

Exercise Intensity

Intensity and duration of exercise determine the total caloric expenditure during a training session, and are inversely related. For example, similar improvements in cardiorespiratory endurance may be achieved by a low-intensity, longer-duration regimen as with a higher-intensity, shorter-duration program. The risk of orthopedic injury may be increased with the latter; however, programs emphasizing moderate-to-vigorous exercise with a longer training duration are recommended for most individuals (6). The ACSM recommends an intensity of exercise corresponding to between 55 and 65% (55/65%) to 90% of maximum heart rate (HR_{max}), or between 40 and 50% (40/50%) to 85% of oxygen uptake reserve ($\dot{V}O_2R$) or HR reserve (HRR) (6). The $\dot{V}O_2R$ is the difference between $\dot{V}O_{2max}$ and resting $\dot{V}O_2$. Similarly, the HRR is the difference between HR_{max} and resting HR. When exercise intensities are set according to $\dot{V}O_2R$, the percent values are approximately equal to the percent values for the HRR (6,17). Consequently, use of the $\dot{V}O_2R$ improves the accuracy of calculating a target $\dot{V}O_2$ from a HRR prescription, especially for low-fit clients, but does not alter the current methods of calculating target heart rates.

The intensity range to increase and maintain cardiorespiratory fitness is intentionally broad and reflects the fact that low-fit or deconditioned individuals may demonstrate increases in cardiorespiratory fitness with exercise intensities of only 40 to 49% HRR or 55 to 64% HR_{max}. In contrast, those who are already physically active require exercise intensities at the high end of the continuum to further augment their cardiorespiratory fitness. For most individuals, intensities within the range of 70 to 85% HR_{max} or 60 to 80% HRR are sufficient to achieve improvements in cardiorespiratory fitness, when combined with an appropriate frequency and duration of training. These ranges of exercise intensities have been used for nearly 30 years to increase $\dot{V}O_{2max}$ favorably in participants in primary and secondary prevention programs (18–20).

Factors to consider before determining the level of exercise intensity include the following:

- Individual's level of fitness: low-fit, very sedentary and clinical populations can improve fitness with lower-intensity, longer-duration exercise sessions. Higher fit individuals need to work at the higher end of the intensity continuum to improve and maintain their fitness.
- Medications (see Appendix A) that may influence HR require special attention when defining the initial target HR range and when the dose or timing is changed.
- Risk of cardiovascular and orthopedic injuries is higher and adherence is lower with higher-intensity exercise programs.
- Individual preferences for exercise must be considered to improve the likelihood that the individual will adhere to the exercise program.
- Individual program objectives (lower BP; lower body fatness; increased $\dot{V}O_{2max}$) help define the characteristics of the exercise prescription.

INTENSITY PRESCRIPTION IN METs

Traditionally, the range of exercise training intensities (in METs or $mL \cdot kg^{-1} \cdot min^{-1}$) has been based on a straight percentage of $\dot{V}O_{2max}$. For example, if an individual had a measured $\dot{V}O_{2max}$ of 10 METs, the prescribed intensity could be set at 6 to 8 METs, corresponding to 60% and 80% of $\dot{V}O_{2max}$, respectively. In the recent position stand of the ACSM, the exercise intensity has been expressed as a percentage of oxygen uptake reserve (%$\dot{V}O_2$R) (6). To calculate the target $\dot{V}O_2$ based on $\dot{V}O_2$R, the following equation is used:

$$\text{Target } \dot{V}O_2 = (\text{exercise intensity}) (\dot{V}O_{2max} - \dot{V}O_{2rest}) + \dot{V}O_{2rest}$$

This equation has the same form as the heart rate reserve (HRR) calculation of target heart rate (see below). In the target $\dot{V}O_2$ equation, $\dot{V}O_{2rest}$ is 3.5 $mL \cdot kg^{-1} \cdot min^{-1}$ (1 MET) and the exercise intensity is 50 to 85% (or as low as 40% for very deconditioned individuals). Intensity is expressed as a fraction in the equation. For example, what is the target $\dot{V}O_2$ at 40% of $\dot{V}O_2$R for a patient with a 5-MET capacity, i.e., a $\dot{V}O_{2max}$ of 17.5 $mL \cdot kg^{-1} \cdot min^{-1}$?

$$\text{Target } \dot{V}O_2 = (0.40) (17.5 - 3.5) + 3.5$$
$$\text{Target } \dot{V}O_2 = (0.40) (14.0) + 3.5$$
$$\text{Target } \dot{V}O_2 = 5.6 + 3.5$$
$$\text{Target } \dot{V}O_2 = 9.1 \ mL \cdot kg^{-1} \cdot min^{-1}$$

Once a $\dot{V}O_2$ (MET) level is identified, a corresponding work rate may be calculated through the use of metabolic equations (Appendix D) or by selecting an activity with a corresponding MET level from published tables (21). However, there are limitations to the use of $\dot{V}O_2$ in prescribing exercise:

- The caloric cost for activities in groups 2 and 3 (see Box 7-1) are quite variable and depend on the skill of the participant and/or the level of competition.
- The caloric cost of activities can provide a starting point for prescribing exercise intensity for individuals with cardiac and/or pulmonary disease, and for individuals with low functional capacities, but the load should be titrated depending on the physiologic responses, perceived exertion, and signs and symptoms.
- The caloric cost of an activity does not take into consideration the effect of environment (e.g., heat, humidity, altitude, pollution), level of hydration, and other variables that can alter the HR and RPE responses to exercise. The ability of individuals to undertake exercise successfully at a given absolute intensity is directly related to their relative effort as reflected by HR and RPE.

Consequently, the most common methods of setting the intensity of exercise to improve or maintain cardiorespiratory fitness use HR and RPE.

HEART RATE METHODS

Heart rate is used as a guide to set exercise intensity because of the relatively linear relationship between HR and $\%\dot{V}O_{2max}$. It is best to measure maximal HR (HR_{max}) during a progressive exercise test whenever possible because HR_{max} declines with age (e.g., estimated $HR_{max} = 220 - \text{age}$) and the variance for any given age is considerable (1 SD = 10–12 beats·min^{-1}). During an exercise session, the assumption is that the individual will achieve a steady-state HR response in the prescribed range; in reality (and certainly during discontinuous exercise) HR is likely to be both above and below the prescribed intensity. The goal should be to maintain an average HR close to the midpoint of the prescribed range. There are several approaches to determining a target HR range for prescriptive purposes:

- Using a plot of HR versus $\dot{V}O_2$ or exercise intensity data collected during a graded exercise test
- Using a straight percentage of HR_{max}
- Using the HR reserve (HRR) method

Direct Method   The direct method of obtaining the target HR range involves plotting measured HR against either measured $\dot{V}O_2$ (Fig. 7-3) or exercise intensity (as discussed in Chapter 4). If RPE data are available, the HR-$\dot{V}O_2$ relationship can be evaluated further in relation to the individual's RPE, which is helpful in modulating the exercise intensity. This method is appropriate for setting exercise intensity for persons with low fitness levels, those with cardiovascular and/or pulmonary disease, and those taking medications (e.g., β-blockers) that affect the HR response to exercise. The direct method allows one to prescribe an appropriate training HR range below the point of adverse signs or symptoms experienced by the individual during exercise testing.

Percent of HR_{max}   One of the oldest methods of setting the target HR range uses a straight percentage of the HR_{max}. Early researchers and clinicians used 70 to 85% of an individual's HR_{max} as the prescribed exercise intensity. This range of exercise intensities approximates 55 to 75% $\dot{V}O_{2max}$ (22) and provides the stimulus needed to improve or maintain $\dot{V}O_{2max}$ in individuals exercising in clinical and adult fitness settings (18–20). It is also simple to compute. If an individual's HR_{max} is 180 beats·min^{-1}, the target HR range is 126 to 153 beats·min^{-1}.

HR Reserve Method   The HR reserve (HRR) method is also known as the Karvonen method (23). In this method, resting heart rate (HR_{rest}) is subtracted from the maximal heart rate (HR_{max}) to obtain HRR: 180 beats·min^{-1} minus 60 beats·min^{-1} = 120 beats·min^{-1}. One then takes 60 and 80% of the HRR and adds each of these values to resting HR to obtain the target HR range:

$$\text{Target HR range} = ([HR_{max} - HR_{rest}] \times 0.60 \text{ and } 0.80) + HR_{rest}$$

The HRR method yields a target HR range of 132 to 156 beats·min^{-1} for

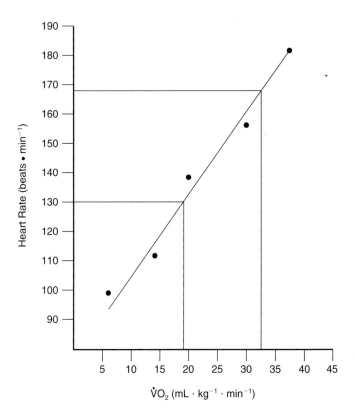

FIGURE 7-3. A line of best fit has been drawn through the data points on this plot of heart rate and oxygen consumption data observed during a hypothetical maximal exercise test in which $\dot{V}O_{2max}$ was observed to be 38 mL·kg^{-1}·min^{-1} and maximal heart rate was 184 beats·min^{-1}. A target heart rate range was determined by finding the heart rates that correspond to 50 and 85% of $\dot{V}O_{2max}$. For this individual, 50% of $\dot{V}O_{2max}$ was approximately 19 mL·kg^{-1}·min^{-1}, and 85% of $\dot{V}O_{2max}$ was approximately 32 mL·kg^{-1}·min^{-1}. The corresponding target heart rates are approximately 130 and 168 beats·min^{-1}.

this subject, similar to the target HR range calculated by the percent of maximal HR method. Sixty to 80% of the HRR is equal to about 60 to 80% of $\dot{V}O_{2max}$ for most fit individuals, but is more closely linked to the %$\dot{V}O_2R$ across the entire range of fitness levels. The latter point is most important when working with low-fit clients. Table 7-1 shows the target HR range for the %HR$_{max}$ and the HRR methods, with different resting heart rates used in the latter calculation (19). The small but systematic differences between the two HR methods are because the %HR$_{max}$ method represents about 55 to 75% $\dot{V}O_{2max}$, and the %HRR method represents about 60 to 80% $\dot{V}O_2R$. Either method can be used to approximate the range of exercise intensities known to increase or maintain $\dot{V}O_{2max}$.

As "the art of exercise prescription" suggested earlier, the target HR range is only a *guideline* used in setting the exercise intensity:

TABLE 7-1. Training Heart Rates*

HR$_{max}$ (beats·min^{-1})	HR$_{max}$ Method		Resting Heart Rate					
			60 beats·min^{-1}		70 beats·min^{-1}		80 beats·min^{-1}	
			Heart Rate Reserve Method					
	70%	85%	60%	80%	60%	80%	60%	80%
140	98	119	108	124	112	126	116	128
150	105	128	114	132	118	134	122	136
160	112	136	120	140	124	142	128	144
170	119	145	126	148	130	150	134	152
180	126	153	132	156	136	158	140	160
190	133	162	138	164	142	166	146	168
200	140	170	144	172	148	174	152	176

*Calculated for age adjusted estimates of maximal heart rates for 20 to 80 year olds (220 − age) using both the percent of maximal heart rate and the heart rate reserve methods, with 3 different resting heart rates (60, 70, 80 beats·min^{-1}) used in the latter calculation.

- Some individuals will prefer to exercise at the low end of the target HR range and focus on long duration to accomplish fitness goals. Reinforcing this option may encourage continued participation, a primary goal of a fitness program.
- Due to the specificity of training and the fact that *measured* maximal heart rate is different for different modes of exercise, an individual's perception of effort will vary among exercise modes when exercising at exactly the same HR (4).
- Conversion of a %HR$_{max}$ (or %HRR) value to a %$\dot{V}O_{2max}$ value carries with it a standard error of estimate of ±6% $\dot{V}O_{2max}$ (22).
- If an estimate of HR$_{max}$ (e.g., 220 − age) is used in the above calculations rather than measured HR, the error inherent in that estimate is carried over to the calculated target HR range. This must be considered when an individual begins an exercise program. The RPE can be helpful in adjusting the exercise intensity in such situations.

RATING OF PERCEIVED EXERTION

Commonly used RPE scales are found in Chapter 4. Use of RPE is considered an adjunct to monitoring HR because RPE determined during a graded exercise test may not consistently translate to the same intensity during an exercise session or for different modes of exercise (4). However, the RPE has proven to be a valuable aid in prescribing exercise for individuals who have difficulty with HR palpation, and in cases where the HR response to exercise may have been altered due to a change in medication. The average RPE range associated with physiologic adaptation to exercise is 12 to 16 ("somewhat hard" to "hard") on the category Borg scale (see Chapter 4). However, due to significant inter-individual variability in the psychophysiologic relationship, one should suit the RPE to the individual on a specific mode of exercise and not expect an exact matching of the RPE to a $\%HR_{max}$ or $\%HRR$ (24). Consequently, the RPE should be used as a *guideline* in setting the exercise intensity.

Table 7-2 summarizes the above information on exercise intensity (6). In the final analysis, the appropriate exercise intensity is one that is safe, is compatible with a long-term active lifestyle for that individual, and achieves the desired caloric output given the time constraints of the exercise session.

Exercise Duration

The duration of an exercise session interacts with the intensity to result in the expenditure of a sufficient number of calories to achieve heath, fitness, and weight management goals. When exercise intensity is above a minimum threshold (lower for low-fit and higher for high-fit) the total volume of exercise is important in achieving and maintaining fitness. The duration of exercise recommended by the ACSM reflects that interaction (20 to 60 minutes of continuous or intermittent [minimum of 10-minute bouts] aerobic activity accumulated throughout the day). However, the risk of both cardiovascular and orthopedic injuries increases at the higher intensities. Consequently, exercising at 70 to 85% HR_{max} or 60 to 80% HRR for 20 to 30 minutes, excluding time spent warming up and cooling down, enables most individuals to achieve health, fitness, and weight management goals (6). Consistent with the manner in which the intensity of a session is gradually increased over weeks of training, the duration (e.g., 30 minutes) can begin with as little as 4 to 6, 5-minute bouts with rest periods between bouts for those with low levels of cardiorespiratory fitness. The duration of the exercise bout can be increased progressively over time until the goal is achieved.

 TABLE 7-2. Classification of Physical Activity Intensity Based on Physical Activity Lasting up to 60 Minutes*

		Relative Intensity	
Intensity	%HRR or %VO$_2$R	%HR$_{max}$	RPE†
Very light	<20	<35	<10
Light	20–39	35–54	10–11
Moderate	40–59	55–69	12–13
Hard	60–84	70–89	14–16
Very hard	≥85	≥90	17–19
Maximal	100	100	20

*Adapted from Pollock ML, Gaesser GA, Butcher JD, et al. The recommended quantity and quality of exercise for developing and maintaining cardiorespiratory and muscular fitness, and flexibility in healthy adults. Med Sci Sports Exerc 1998;30(6):975–991.

†Borg rating of perceived exertion, 6–20 scale.

Increases in exercise duration should be made as the individual adapts to training without evidence of undue fatigue or injury. The rate of progression of exercise is discussed later in the chapter.

Exercise Frequency

Although deconditioned persons may improve cardiorespiratory fitness with only twice-weekly exercise, optimal training frequency appears to be achieved with 3 to 5 workouts per week. The additional benefits of more frequent training appear to be minimal, whereas the incidence of lower extremity injuries increases abruptly. Consequently, the ACSM recommends an exercise frequency of 3 to 5 $d \cdot wk^{-1}$. For those exercising at 60 to 80% HRR or 70 to 85% HR_{max}, an exercise frequency of 3 $d \cdot wk^{-1}$ is sufficient to improve or maintain $\dot{V}O_{2max}$. For those exercising at the lower end of the intensity continuum, exercising more than 3 $d \cdot wk^{-1}$ may be needed to achieve the caloric expenditure associated with weight loss and fitness goals. Patients with functional capacities of less than 3 METs may benefit from multiple brief daily exercise sessions; 1 to 2 short sessions per day are most appropriate for those with 3 to 5 MET capacities; and 3 to 5 sessions per week are recommended for individuals with functional capacities of more than 5 METs. Clearly, the number of exercise sessions per week varies depending on the caloric goals, participant preferences, and limitations imposed by the participant's lifestyle.

ENERGY EXPENDITURE GOALS

The interaction of physical activity intensity, duration, and frequency determines net caloric expenditure from the activity. It is generally accepted that many of the health benefits and training adaptations associated with increased physical activity are related to the total amount of work accomplished during training (3,25,26). However, the caloric thresholds necessary to elicit significant improvements in $\dot{V}O_{2max}$, weight loss, or a reduced risk of premature chronic disease may be different. Therefore, individualized exercise prescriptions should be designed with energy expenditure goals in mind. The ACSM recommends a target range of 150 to 400 kcal of energy expenditure per day in physical activity and/or exercise (25,26). The lower end of this range represents a minimal caloric threshold of approximately 1000 kcal per week from physical activity and should be the initial goal for previously sedentary individuals. Based on the dose-response relationships between physical activity and health and fitness, individuals should be encouraged to move toward attainment of the upper end of the recommended range (e.g., 300 to 400 kcal per day from activity) as their fitness levels improve during the training program.

Estimating caloric expenditure during exercise has been problematic for exercise professionals, and developing an exercise plan based on caloric thresholds should not be viewed as an exact science. Interindividual differences in skill, coordination, and exercise economy (the $\dot{V}O_2$ at a given submaximal work rate) and the variable intensities within each available

TABLE 7-3. Leisure Activities in METs: Sports, Exercise Classes, Games, Dancing

	Mean	Range
Archery	3.9	3–4
Backpacking	—	5–11
Badminton	5.8	4–9+
Basketball		
Game play	8.3	7–12+
Nongame play	—	3–9
Billiards	2.5	—
Bowling	—	2–4
Boxing		
In-ring	13.3	—
Sparring	8.3	—
Canoeing, rowing, and kayaking	—	3–8
Conditioning exercise	—	3–8+
Climbing hills	7.2	5–10+
Cricket	5.2	4–8
Croquet	3.5	—
Cycling		
Pleasure or to work	—	3–8+
10 mph	7.0	—
Dancing (social, square, tap)	—	3–8
Dancing (aerobic)	—	6–9
Fencing	—	6–10+
Field hockey	8.0	—
Fishing		
From bank	3.7	2–4
Wading in stream	—	5–6
Football (touch)	7.9	6–10
Golf		
Power cart	—	2–3
Walking (carrying bag or pulling cart)	5.1	4–7
Handball	—	8–12+
Hiking (cross-country)	—	3–7
Horseback riding		
Galloping	8.2	—
Trotting	6.6	—
Walking	2.4	—
Horseshoe pitching	—	2–3
Hunting (bow or gun)		
Small game (walking, carrying light load)	—	3–7
Big game (dragging carcass, walking)	—	3–14
Judo	13.5	—
Mountain climbing	—	5–10+
Music playing	—	2–3
Paddleball, racquetball	9	8–12
Rope jumping	11	—
60–80 skips/min	9	—
120–140 skips/min	—	11–12

	Mean	Range
TABLE 7-3. (*continued*)		
Running		
12 min per mile	8.7	—
11 min per mile	9.4	—
10 min per mile	10.2	—
9 min per mile	11.2	—
8 min per mile	12.5	—
7 min per mile	14.1	—
6 min per mile	16.3	—
Sailing	—	2–5
Scuba diving	—	5–10
Shuffleboard	—	2–3
Skating, ice and roller	—	5–8
Skiing, snow		
Downhill	—	5–8
Cross-country	—	6–12+
Skiing, water	—	5–7
Sledding, tobogganing	—	4–8
Snowshoeing	9.9	7–14
Squash	—	8–12+
Soccer	—	5–12+
Stair climbing	—	4–8
Swimming	—	4–8+
Table tennis	4.1	3–5
Tennis	6.5	4–9+
Volleyball	—	3–6

activity strongly influence estimation of caloric expenditure during exercise. One useful method to approximate the caloric cost of exercise is by using the following equation based on the MET level of the activity:

$$(\text{METs} \times 3.5 \times \text{body weight in kg})/200 = \text{kcal/min}$$

This formula helps an individual understand the components of the exercise prescription and the volume of exercise necessary to achieve the caloric goals of the program. Consider the following example. The weekly goal of the exercise program has been set at 1000 kilocalories for an individual who weighs 70 kg, and the MET level of the prescribed activity is 6 METs. In this example, the *net* caloric expenditure from the exercise would be 5 METs because 1 MET of the activity represents resting metabolic rate. Therefore, the *net* caloric expenditure from the exercise is 6 kcal/min, requiring 167 minutes per week to attain the 1000 kilocalorie threshold. Given a 4 d·wk^{-1} program, the individual would require approximately 42 minutes per day to achieve the 1000 kcal goal (or 33 minutes per day, 5 d·wk^{-1}). Working backward from the caloric goal to determine the volume of exercise needed to reach the goal is useful in determining the appropriate exercise prescription components. Table 7-3 lists the aerobic requirements, expressed as

METs, for selected vocational and recreational activities. For information on MET values for over 500 physical activities, see Ainsworth et al. (21).

RATE OF PROGRESSION

The recommended rate of progression in an exercise conditioning program depends on functional capacity, medical and health status, age, individual activity preferences and goals, and an individual's tolerance to the current level of training. For apparently healthy adults, the endurance aspect of the exercise prescription has three stages of progression: initial, improvement, and maintenance (Table 7-4). Exercise professionals should recognize that recent physical activity recommendations from the ACSM/CDC (3) and the Surgeon General (26) include 30 minutes of *moderate* physical activity on most, if not all, days of the week. While some apparently healthy but sedentary individuals may not be able to attain this initial level of activity, they should be encouraged to progress to this goal during the first few weeks of the training program.

Initial Conditioning Stage

The initial stage should include light muscular endurance exercises and moderate level aerobic activities (40 to 60% of HR reserve), exercises that are compatible with minimal muscle soreness, discomfort, and injury. Exercise

TABLE 7-4. Example: Training Progression for the Apparently Healthy Participant

Program Stage	Week	Exercise Frequency (Sessions/wk)	Exercise Intensity (%HRR)	Exercise Duration (min)
Initial stage	1	3	40–50	15–20
	2	3–4	40–50	20–25
	3	3–4	50–60	20–25
	4	3–4	50–60	25–30
Improvement stage	5–7	3–4	60–70	25–30
	8–10	3–4	60–70	30–35
	11–13	3–4	65–75	30–35
	14–16	3–5	65–75	30–35
	17–20	3–5	70–85	35–40
	21–24	3–5	70–85	35–40
Maintenance stage	24+	3–5	70–85	30–45

adherence may decrease if the program is initiated too aggressively. This stage may last up to 4 weeks, but the length depends on the adaptation of the individual to the exercise program. The duration of the exercise session during the initial stage may begin with approximately 15 to 20 minutes and progress to 30 minutes. It is recommended that individuals who are starting a moderate-intensity conditioning program should exercise 3 to 4 times per week.

Individual goals should be established early in the exercise program. They should be developed by the participant with the guidance of an exercise professional. The goals must be realistic, and a system of rewards—intrinsic or extrinsic—should be established at that time.

Improvement Stage

The goal of this stage of training is to provide a gradual increase in the overall exercise stimulus to allow for significant improvements in cardiorespiratory fitness. The improvement stage of the exercise conditioning program differs from the initial stage in that the participant is progressed at a more rapid rate. This stage typically lasts 4 to 5 months, during which intensity is progressively increased within the upper half of the target range of 50 to 85% of HR reserve. Duration is increased consistently every 2 to 3 weeks until participants are able to exercise at a moderate-to-vigorous intensity for 20 to 30 minutes continuously. The frequency and magnitude of the increments are dictated by the rate at which the participant adapts to the conditioning program. Deconditioned individuals should be permitted more time for adaptation at each stage of conditioning. Age also should be taken into consideration when progressions are recommended; experience suggests that adaptation to conditioning may take longer in older individuals (6).

Maintenance Stage

The goal of this stage of training is the long-term maintenance of cardiorespiratory fitness developed during the improvement stage. This stage of the exercise program usually begins after the first 5 or 6 months of training, but may begin at any time the participant has reached preestablished fitness goals. During this stage, the participant may no longer be interested in further increasing the conditioning stimulus. Further improvement may be minimal, but continuing the same workout routine enables individuals to maintain their fitness levels.

At this point, the goals of the program should be reviewed and new goals set. To maintain cardiorespiratory fitness, an exercise prescription should incorporate an intensity, frequency, and duration consistent with the participant's long-term goals, and should also meet, and preferably exceed, the minimal caloric thresholds identified earlier in the chapter. If there is the need for further weight loss during this phase of the program, a moderate intensity is recommended. Such programs, however, are usually associated with an increased exercise duration, frequency, or both. It is important to include exercises and recreational activities (Box 7-1, Group 3 activities) that the individual finds enjoyable.

Training Specificity

Numerous studies have investigated the cardiorespiratory and metabolic responses of trained versus untrained muscles to chronic aerobic conditioning. For example, arm or leg training resulted in only minor improvements in submaximal and maximal leg or arm exercise responses, respectively. Thus, subjects trained by leg exercise failed to demonstrate a conditioning bradycardia during arm work, and vice versa (Fig. 7-4) (27). Similar muscle-specific adaptations have been shown for blood lactate (28) and pulmonary ventilation (29). These findings suggest that a substantial portion of the training effect derives from peripheral rather than central changes, including cellular and enzymatic adaptations that increase the oxidative capacity of chronically exercised skeletal muscle (30).

Some *transfer-of-training effects* have been reported, however, including increased $\dot{V}O_{2max}$ or reduced submaximal heart rate with untrained limbs, providing evidence for central circulatory adaptations to chronic endurance exercise (31,32). It has been suggested that approximately half of the increase in trained limb performance is due to a centralized training effect and that half is due to peripheral adaptations, specifically alterations in trained skeletal muscle (33). However, the latter may predominate in some patient subsets, for example, cardiac patients with left ventricular dysfunction (34). Although the conditions under which the interchangeability of arm and leg training effects may vary, there is evidence to suggest that the initial fitness of the subjects as well as the intensity, frequency, and duration of training may be important variables in determining the extent of cross-training benefits (35).

The limited degree of cardiovascular and metabolic crossover benefits of training from one set of limbs to another appears to discredit the general practice of limiting exercise training to the legs alone. Many recreational and occupational activities require sustained arm work to a greater extent than leg work. Consequently, individuals who rely on their upper extremities should be advised to train the arms as well as the legs, with the expectation of improved cardiorespiratory, hemodynamic, and perceived exertion responses to both forms of effort. Such programs should serve to maximize the conditioning response through increased crossover of training benefits to real life situations.

Musculoskeletal Flexibility

Optimal musculoskeletal function requires that an adequate range of motion be maintained in all joints. Of particular importance is maintenance of

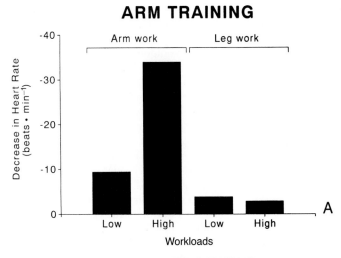

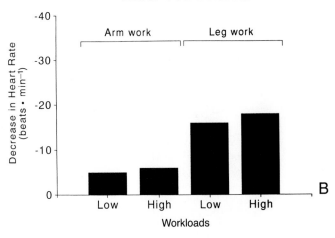

FIGURE 7-4. Importance of peripheral adaptation to training of the arms **(A)** and legs **(B)**. Arm training on the cycle ergometer reduced the heart rate during arm work but not during leg work. Similarly, leg training was associated with a lower heart rate response during leg exercise but not during arm exercise. (Adapted from Clausen JP, Trap-Jensen J, Lassen NA. The effects of training on the heart rate during arm and leg exercise. Scand J Clin Lab Invest 1970;26:295–301.)

flexibility in the lower back and posterior thigh regions. Lack of flexibility in this area may be associated with an increased risk for the development of chronic lower back pain. Therefore, preventive and rehabilitative exercise programs should include activities that promote the maintenance of flexibility. Lack of flexibility is prevalent in the elderly, among whom this condition often contributes to a reduced ability to perform activities of daily living.

Accordingly, exercise programs for the elderly should emphasize proper stretching, especially for the arm and shoulder, upper and lower trunk, neck, and hip regions.

Different types of stretching techniques (e.g., static, ballistic, and proprioceptive neuromuscular facilitation [PNF]) can be performed. Static stretching involves slowly stretching a muscle to the point of mild discomfort and then holding that position for an extended period of time (usually 10 to 30 seconds). The risk of injury is low, it requires little time and assistance, and it is quite effective. For these reasons, static stretching is the most commonly recommended method. Ballistic stretching uses the momentum created by repetitive bouncing movements to produce muscle stretch. This type of stretch can result in muscle soreness or injury if the forces generated by the ballistic movements are too great. PNF stretching involves a combination of alternating contraction and relaxation of both agonist and antagonist muscles through a designated series of motions. While research has suggested that PNF stretching produces the largest improvements in flexibility, this technique typically causes some degree of muscle soreness. Moreover, it typically requires a partner trained in the technique and is more time-consuming than alternative methods.

Properly performed stretching exercises can aid in improving and maintaining range of motion in a joint or series of joints. Flexibility exercises should be performed in a slow, controlled manner with a gradual progression to greater ranges of motion. A general exercise prescription for achieving and maintaining flexibility should adhere to the following guidelines (6):

Type:	A general stretching routine that exercises the major muscle and/or tendon groups using static or PNF techniques
Frequency:	A minimum of 2 to 3 d·wk^{-1}
Intensity:	To a position of mild discomfort
Duration:	10 to 30 seconds for static; 6-second contraction followed by 10 to 30 seconds assisted stretch for PNF
Repetitions:	3 to 4 for each stretch

A series of easy-to-understand stretches are published in the *ACSM Fitness Book.* Yoga and tai chi movements may also be used to improve flexibility, balance, and agility, when appropriate. Stretching exercises can be effectively included in the warm-up and/or cool-down periods that precede and follow the aerobic conditioning phase of an exercise session. It is recommended that an active warm-up precede vigorous stretching exercises. Some commonly employed stretching exercises may not be appropriate for some participants who may—through prior injury, joint insufficiency, or other conditions—be at greater risk for musculoskeletal injuries. Although research evidence concerning the risks of specific exercises is lacking, those activities that require substantial flexibility and/or skill are not recommended for older, less flexible, and less experienced participants.

For additional information on the topic, refer to the *ACSM's Resource Manual for Guidelines for Exercise Testing and Prescription* (36–38).

MUSCULAR FITNESS

Although aerobic activities have been shown to be effective for developing cardiorespiratory fitness, most have little influence on muscular strength or muscular endurance, especially of the upper body. Every activity—including activities of daily living—requires a certain percentage of an individual's maximal strength and endurance. The maintenance or enhancement of muscular strength and muscular endurance enables any individual to perform such tasks with less physiologic stress and will aid in maintaining functional independence throughout the life span. The cardiovascular stress of lifting or holding a given weight is proportional to the percentage of maximal strength involved.

Resistance training of moderate intensity (i.e., sufficient to develop and maintain muscular fitness and fat-free mass) should be an integral part of adult fitness and rehabilitative exercise programs. In addition to the development and maintenance of muscular strength and muscle mass, the physiologic benefits of resistance training include increases in bone mass and in the strength of connective tissue. These adaptations are beneficial for middle-aged and older adults, and, in particular, postmenopausal women who may experience a more rapid loss of bone mineral density.

Muscular strength and endurance are developed by the overload principle—by increasing the resistance to movement or the frequency or duration of activity to levels above those normally experienced. Muscular strength is best developed by using weights that evoke maximal or nearly maximal muscle tension with relatively few repetitions. Muscular endurance is best developed by using lighter weights with a greater number of repetitions. To elicit improvement in both muscular strength and endurance, most experts recommend 8 to 12 repetitions for healthy participants under 50 to 60 years of age and 10 to 15 repetitions for individuals older than 50 to 60 years of age.

Any overload will result in strength development, but higher-intensity effort at or near maximal effort will produce a significantly greater effect. The intensity of resistance training can be manipulated by varying the weight, the number of repetitions, the length of the rest interval between exercises, or the number of sets of exercises completed. Caution is advised for training that emphasizes lengthening (eccentric) contractions, compared to shortening (concentric) or isometric contractions, because the potential for skeletal muscle soreness is accentuated.

Muscular strength and endurance can be developed by means of static or dynamic exercises. Although each type of training has advantages and limitations, dynamic resistance exercises are recommended for most adults. Resistance training for the average participant should be rhythmic, performed at a moderate-to-slow speed, involve a full range of motion, and not interfere with normal breathing. Heavy resistance exercise combined with breath-holding (Valsalva maneuver) can cause a dramatic, acute increase in both systolic and diastolic blood pressure.

The following resistance training guidelines are recommended for the apparently healthy adult (6):

- Perform a minimum of 8 to 10 separate exercises that train the major muscle groups (arms, shoulders, chest, abdomen, back, hips, and legs).
  —A primary goal of the program should be to develop total body strength and endurance in a relatively time-efficient manner. Programs lasting longer than 1 hour per session are associated with higher dropout rates.
- Perform a minimum of 1 set of 8 to 12 repetitions of each of these exercises to the point of volitional fatigue. For individuals primarily interested in developing muscular endurance as well as older (approximately 50 to 60 years of age) or more frail persons, 10 to 15 repetitions may be more appropriate.
- Perform these exercises 2 to 3 $d\cdot wk^{-1}$.
  —Although more frequent training and additional sets or combinations of sets and repetitions may elicit larger strength gains, the additional improvement is relatively small for previously sedentary individuals training in the typical fitness setting.
- Adhere as closely as possible to the specific techniques for performing a given exercise.
- Perform every exercise through a full range of motion.
- Perform both the lifting (concentric phase) and lowering (eccentric phase) portion of the resistance exercises in a controlled manner.
- Maintain a normal breathing pattern: breath-holding can induce excessive increases in blood pressure.
- If possible, exercise with a training partner who can provide feedback, assistance, and motivation.

For additional information on the topic, see the *ACSM's Resource Manual for Guidelines for Exercise Testing and Prescription* (39).

MAINTENANCE OF THE TRAINING EFFECT

Numerous studies have investigated the physiologic consequences of a reduced exercise dosage or complete cessation of training in physically conditioned persons. A significant reduction in cardiorespiratory fitness occurs within 2 weeks of stopping intense endurance training (40), with participants returning to pretraining levels of aerobic fitness after 10 weeks (41) to 8 months of detraining (42). During periods of inactivity, initial improvements in $\dot{V}O_{2max}$ will decrease over time, with half of the gains lost after only 4 to 12 weeks of detraining (41,43). Maintenance of the training effect generally shows a direct relationship to the length of time in training

(40) but may be modulated by the level of fitness, age, intervening illness or injury, and specific conditioning practices.

A related series of studies examined the relative effects of decreased exercise frequency (44), duration (45), or intensity (46) on the maintenance of $\dot{V}O_{2max}$ during a period of reduced training. All three studies trained young men and women for 40 minutes, 6 d·wk^{-1} for 10 weeks at a moderate-to-high exercise intensity, followed by 15 weeks of reduced training at one-third and two-third reductions in the frequency, duration, or intensity of training. Only when the intensity of training was reduced was there a significant decrease in $\dot{V}O_{2max}$; moreover, most of the reduction occurred within the first 5 weeks of reduced training (46). In contrast, decreasing the frequency or duration of training had little influence on the postconditioning $\dot{V}O_{2max}$, provided that the intensity was maintained. Similarly, restricted walk training resulted in rapid deconditioning in cardiac patients who had been jogging, despite an unchanged exercise frequency and duration (47). Collectively, these findings suggest that exercise intensity is especially important in maintaining a cardiovascular training response.

The preservation of resistance training effects has also been examined relative to a reduced exercise frequency. In these studies, strength gains were maintained for 12 weeks with 1 training session per week (48) and only 1 training session every 2 to 4 weeks (49), provided that the weight training loads remained constant. Thus, it appears that a reduced training frequency or duration will not adversely affect $\dot{V}O_{2max}$ or muscular strength if the training intensity is maintained.

Additional evidence, relevant to the maintenance of training effects, suggests that arm training per se has little influence on the retention of leg training effects (50), further reinforcing the principle of training specificity. However, an alternate training modality augments energy expenditure and serves to maintain health benefits.

PROGRAM SUPERVISION

Information from health screening, medical evaluation, and exercise testing allow the exercise professional to determine those individuals for whom supervised exercise programs are suggested. Exercise professionals should recognize that most individuals can exercise safely at a moderate intensity without supervision. However, for those who wish to increase their fitness levels by following the exercise prescription guidelines within this chapter, Table 7-5 provides general criteria for participation in unsupervised versus supervised programs.

Supervised exercise programs are recommended for symptomatic and cardiorespiratory disease patients who are considered by their physicians to be clinically stable and who have been medically cleared for participation in such programs. It is recommended that supervised exercise programs for such individuals be under the combined overall guidance of a physician, appropriate nursing staff, and an ACSM-certified Program Director$_{SM}$ or Exercise Specialist$_{SM}$. Direct supervision of each session by a physician, however, is not necessarily required to ensure safety (51). These programs

TABLE 7-5. General Guidelines for Participation in Unsupervised and Supervised Exercise Programs

	Program	
	Unsupervised	**Supervised**
Health status	Apparently healthy (low risk)	≥2 major CAD risk factors (Table 2-1) Major signs/symptoms (Box 2-1) Known cardiopulmonary or metabolic disease
Functional capacity	≥8 METs	<8 METs*

CAD, coronary artery disease.

*For functional capacity of less than 5 METs, a small staff-to-patient ratio (i.e., 1 professional staff member for every 5 to 8 patients) is also recommended.

can be useful for those who need instruction in proper exercise techniques. For some participants, direct supervision may enhance compliance with an exercise program.

References

1. Paffenbarger RS, Hyde RT, Wing AL, et al. The association of changes in physical-activity level and other lifestyle characteristics with mortality among men. N Engl J Med 1993;328:538–545.
2. Blair SN, Kohl HW, Barlow CE, et al. Changes in physical fitness and all-cause mortality: a prospective study of healthy and unhealthy men. JAMA 1995;273:1093–1098.
3. Pate RR, Pratt M, Blair SN, et al. Physical activity and public health: a recommendation from the Centers for Disease Control and Prevention and the American College of Sports Medicine. JAMA 1995;273:402–407.
4. Thomas TR, Ziogas G, Smith T, et al. Physiological and perceived exertion responses to six modes of submaximal exercise. Res Q Exerc Sport 1995;66:239–246.
5. Southard DR. Modifications of health behavior. In: Roitman JL, ed. ACSM's Resource Manual for Guidelines for Exercise Testing and Prescription. 3rd ed. Baltimore: Williams & Wilkins, 1998:523–584.
6. Pollock ML, Gaesser GA, Butcher JD, et al. The recommended quantity and quality of exercise for developing and maintaining cardiorespiratory and muscular fitness, and flexibility in healthy adults. Med Sci Sports Exerc 1998;30(6):975–991.
7. Barnard RJ, Gardner GW, Diaco NV, et al. Cardiovascular responses to sudden strenuous exercise: heart rate, blood pressure, and ECG. J Appl Physiol 1973;34:833–837.
8. Barnard RJ, MacAlpin R, Kattus AA, et al. Ischemic response to sudden strenuous exercise in healthy men. Circulation 1973;48:936–942.
9. Foster C, Anholm JD, Hellman CK, et al. Left ventricular function during sudden strenuous exercise. Circulation 1981;63:592–596.
10. Foster C, Dymond DS, Carpenter J, et al. Effect of warm-up on left ventricular response to sudden strenuous exercise. J Appl Physiol 1982;53:380–383.
11. Chesler RM, Michielli DW, Aron M, et al. Cardiovascular response to sudden strenuous exercise: an exercise echocardiographic study. Med Sci Sports Exerc 1997;29(10):1299–1303.
12. Stein RA, Berger HJ, Zaret BL. The cardiac response to sudden strenuous exercise in the post-myocardial infarction patient receiving beta blockers. J Cardiopulm Rehabil 1986;6:336–342.
13. Franklin BA, Stoedefalke KG. Games-as-aerobics: activities for adult fitness and cardiac reha-

bilitation programs. In: Fardy PS, ed. Current Issues in Cardiac Rehabilitation: Training Techniques. Champaign, IL: Human Kinetics, 1998:106–136.

14. Belcastro AN, Bonen A. Lactic acid removal rates during controlled and uncontrolled recovery exercise. J Appl Physiol 1975;39:932–936.

15. Dimsdale JE, Hartley H, Guiney T, et al. Postexercise peril: plasma catecholamines and exercise. JAMA 1984;251:630–632.

16. Haskell WL. Cardiovascular complications during exercise training of cardiac patients. Circulation 1978;57:920–924.

17. Swain DP, Leutholtz BC. Heart rate reserve is equivalent to $\dot{V}O_2$ reserve, not to %$\dot{V}O_{2max}$. Med Sci Sports Exerc 1997;29:410–414.

18. Fox SM, Naughton JP, Gorman PA. Physical activity and cardiovascular health. III. The exercise prescription: frequency and type of activity. Mod Concepts Cardiovasc Dis 1972; 41(6):25–30.

19. Haskell WL. Design and implementation of cardiac conditioning programs. In: Wenger NK, Hellerstein HK, eds. Rehabilitation of the Coronary Patient. New York: John Wiley & Sons, 1978:203–241.

20. Hellerstein HK, Franklin BA. Exercise testing and prescription. In: Wenger NK, Hellerstein HK, eds. Rehabilitation of the Coronary Patient. New York: John Wiley & Sons, 1978:149–202.

21. Ainsworth BE, Haskell WL, Leon AS, et al. Compendium of physical activities: classification of energy costs of human physical activities. Med Sci Sports Exerc 1993;25:71–80.

22. Londeree BR, Ames SA. Trend analysis of the %$\dot{V}O_{2max}$-HR regression. Med Sci Sports Exerc 1976;8:122–125.

23. Karvonen M, Kentala K, Mustala O. The effects of training on heart rate: a longitudinal study. Annales Medicinae Experimentalis et Biologial Fennial 1957;35:307–315.

24. Whaley MH, Brubaker PH, Kaminsky LA, et al. Validity of rating of perceived exertion during graded exercise testing in apparently healthy adults and cardiac patients. J Cardiopulm Rehabil 1997;17:261–267.

25. Haskell WL. Health consequences of physical activity: understanding and challenges regarding dose-response. Med Sci Sports Exerc 1994;26:649–660.

26. US Department of Health and Human Services. Physical activity and health: a report of the Surgeon General. Atlanta, GA: US Department of Health and Human Services, Centers for Disease Control and Prevention, National Center for Chronic Disease Prevention and Health Promotion; 1996.

27. Clausen JP, Trap-Jensen J, Lassen NA. The effects of training on the heart rate during arm and leg exercise. Scand J Clin Lab Invest 1970;26:295–301.

28. Klausen K, Rasmussen B, Clausen JP, et al. Blood lactate from exercising extremities before and after arm or leg training. Am J Physiol 1974;227:67–72.

29. Rasmussen B, Klausen K, Clausen JP, et al. Pulmonary ventilation, blood gases and blood pH after training of the arms or the legs. J Appl Physiol 1975;38:250–256.

30. Henriksson J, Reitman JS. Time course of changes in human skeletal muscle succinate dehydrogenase and cytochrome oxidase activities and maximal oxygen uptake with physical activity and inactivity. Acta Physiol Scand 1977;99:91–97.

31. Clausen JP, Klausen K, Rasmussen B, et al. Central and peripheral circulatory changes after training of the arms or legs. Am J Physiol 1973;225:675–682.

32. McKenzie DC, Fox EL, Cohen K. Specificity of metabolic and circulatory responses to arm or leg interval training. Eur J Appl Physiol 1978;39:241–248.

33. Thompson PD, Cullinane E, Lazarus B, et al. Effect of exercise training on the untrained limb exercise performance of men with angina pectoris. Am J Cardiol 1981;48:844–850.

34. Detry JM, Rousseau M, Vandenbroucke G, et al. Increased arteriovenous oxygen difference after physical training in coronary heart disease. Circulation 1971;44:109–118.

35. Lewis S, Thompson P, Areskog NH, et al. Transfer effects of endurance training to exercise with untrained limbs. Eur J Appl Physiol 1980;44:25–34.

36. Fredette DM. Exercise recommendations for flexibility and range of motion. In: Roitman JL, ed. ACSM's Resource Manual for Guidelines for Exercise Testing and Prescription. 3rd ed. Baltimore: Williams & Wilkins, 1998:456–465.

37. McGill SM. Low back exercises: prescription for the healthy back and when recovering from injury. In: Roitman JL, ed. ACSM's Resource Manual for Guidelines for Exercise Testing and Prescription. 3rd ed. Baltimore: Williams & Wilkins, 1998:116–126.

38. Protas EJ. Flexibility and range of motion. In: Roitman JL, ed. ACSM's Resource Manual for Guidelines for Exercise Testing and Prescription. 3rd ed. Baltimore: Williams & Wilkins, 1998:368–377.

39. Bryant CX, Peterson JA, Graves JE. Muscular strength and endurance. In: Roitman JL, ed. ACSM's Resource Manual for Guidelines for Exercise Testing and Prescription. 3rd ed. Baltimore: Williams & Wilkins, 1998:448–455.

40. Coyle EF, Martin WH, Sinacore DR, et al. Time course of loss of adaptation after stopping prolonged intense endurance training. J Appl Physiol 1984;57:1857–1864.

41. Fringer MN, Stull AG. Changes in cardiorespiratory parameters during periods of training and detraining in young female adults. Med Sci Sports 1974;6:20–25.
42. Knuttgen HG, Nordesjö LO, Ollander B, et al. Physical conditioning through interval training with young male adults. Med Sci Sports 1973;5:220–226.
43. Kendrick ZB, Pollock ML, Hickman TN, et al. Effects of training and detraining on cardiovascular efficiency. Am Correct Ther J 1971;25:79–83.
44. Hickson RC, Rosenkoetter MA. Reduced training frequencies and maintenance of increased aerobic power. Med Sci Sports Exerc 1981;13:13–16.
45. Hickson RC, Kanakis C, Davis JR, et al. Reduced training duration effects on aerobic power, endurance, and cardiac growth. J Appl Physiol 1982;53:225–229.
46. Hickson RC, Foster C, Pollock ML, et al. Reduced training intensities and loss of aerobic power, endurance, and cardiac growth. J Appl Physiol 1985;58:492–499.
47. Dressendorfer RH, Franklin BA, Smith JL, et al. Rapid cardiac deconditioning in joggers restricted to walking: training heart rate and ischemic threshold. Chest 1997;112:1107–1111.
48. Graves JE, Pollock ML, Leggett SH, et al. Effect of reduced training frequency on muscular strength. Int J Sports Med 1988;9:316–319.
49. Tucci JT, Carpenter DM, Pollock ML, et al. Effect of reduced frequency of training and detraining on lumbar extension strength. Spine 1993;17:1497–1501.
50. Pate RR, Hughes RD, Chandler JV, et al. Effects of arm training on retention of training effects derived from leg training. Med Sci Sports Exerc 1978;10:71–74.
51. Franklin BA, Bonzheim K, Gordon S, et al. Safety of medically supervised outpatient cardiac rehabilitation exercise: a 16-year follow-up. Chest 1998;114:902–906.

⑤ CHAPTER 8
Exercise Prescription for Cardiac Patients

Properly prescribed exercise during hospitalization and following discharge affords numerous benefits for appropriately selected cardiac patients, in addition to those mentioned in Chapter 1. These exercises:

- Offset the deleterious psychologic and physiologic effects of bed rest during hospitalization.
- Provide additional medical surveillance of patients.
- Identify patients with significant cardiovascular, physical, or cognitive impairments that may influence prognosis.
- Enable patients to return to activities of daily living within the limits imposed by their disease.
- Prepare the patient and the support system at home to optimize recovery following hospital discharge.

Cardiac rehabilitation programs have traditionally been categorized as Phase I (inpatient), Phase II (up to 12 weeks of supervised exercise and/or education following hospital discharge), Phase III (variable length program of intermittent or no electrocardiographic [ECG] monitoring under supervision), and Phase IV (no ECG monitoring, limited supervision). New theories of risk stratification, recent data on the safety of exercise, and pressures in the era of managed, capitated health care have contributed to a change in traditional cardiac rehabilitation services. There is now movement toward a structure wherein patients follow a regimen of exercise specific to their vocational and recreational needs, with more individualization of the length of program, degree of ECG monitoring, and level of clinical supervision. Such recommendations have been published in the literature (1,2) and form the basis for the risk stratification models presented in Chapter 2. Outcome analysis is an important part of this evolution and includes not only clinical parameters and quality of life, but also recurrent cardiac events as well as physiologic, functional, and health outcomes (3).

INPATIENT PROGRAMS

Clinical indications for cardiac rehabilitation are listed in Box 8-1. Although not all patients in these categories may be suitable candidates for inpatient exercise, virtually all will benefit from some level of inpatient intervention, including risk factor assessment, activity counseling, and patient and family education. Because of the decreased length of hospital stay for most cardiac patients, traditional programs with multiple steps for increasing activity are no longer feasible. In many instances, patients are now seen for only 3 to 5 days following referral to an inpatient cardiac rehabilitation program. Assessment of tolerance to the anticipated aerobic requirements of daily living (e.g., monitoring signs and symptoms during inpatient activity programs) and emphasis on patient activity counseling and education have become major components of inpatient cardiac rehabilitation.

Inpatients should be risk-stratified as early as possible following their acute cardiac event. The AACVPR or ACP risk stratification models (1,4) (Chapter 2) are useful for inpatients because they include clinical criteria not included in other risk stratification models. Contraindications to entry into inpatient programs are included in Box 8-1, although exceptions should be considered based on sound clinical judgment. In addition to these contraindications, certain clinical characteristics appear to increase the risk of

---

BOX 8-1. Clinical Indications and Contraindications for Inpatient and Outpatient Cardiac Rehabilitation

Indications
- Medically stable post-myocardial infarction
- Stable angina
- Coronary artery bypass graft surgery
- Percutaneous transluminal coronary angioplasty
- Compensated congestive heart failure
- Cardiomyopathy
- Heart or other organ transplantation
- Other cardiac surgery including valvular and pacemaker insertion (including implantable cardioverter defibrillator)
- Peripheral vascular disease
- High-risk cardiovascular disease ineligible for surgical intervention
- Sudden cardiac death syndrome
- End-stage renal disease
- At risk for coronary artery disease, with diagnoses of diabetes mellitus, hyperlipidemia, hypertension, etc.
- Other patients who may benefit from structured exercise and/or patient education (based on physician referral and consensus of the rehabilitation team)

Contraindications
- Unstable angina
- Resting systolic blood pressure of >200 mm Hg or resting diastolic blood pressure of >110 mm Hg should be evaluated on a case-by-case basis
- Orthostatic blood pressure drop of >20 mm Hg with symptoms
- Critical aortic stenosis (peak systolic pressure gradient of >50 mm Hg with an aortic valve orifice area of <0.75 cm^2 in an average size adult)
- Acute systemic illness or fever
- Uncontrolled atrial or ventricular arrhythmias
- Uncontrolled sinus tachycardia (>120 beats·min^{-1})
- Uncompensated congestive heart failure
- 3° AV block (without pacemaker)
- Active pericarditis or myocarditis
- Recent embolism
- Thrombophlebitis
- Resting ST segment displacement (>2 mm)
- Uncontrolled diabetes (resting blood glucose of >400 mg/dL)
- Severe orthopedic conditions that would prohibit exercise
- Other metabolic conditions, such as acute thyroiditis, hypokalemia or hyperkalemia, hypovolemia, etc.

exercise-related complications (see Chapter 1). Box 8-2 details complicating factors following acute myocardial infarction (MI) to assist the clinician in identifying inpatients at increased risk (5). Premorbid status and course of hospitalization influence the patient's functional status, perhaps on a daily basis.

Activities during the first 48 hours following MI and/or cardiac surgery should logically be restricted to self-care activities, arm and leg range of

BOX 8-2. Complicating Factors After Myocardial Infarction

Low-risk patients
- No complicating factors by day 4

Moderate-risk patients
- Poor ventricular function (EF of <30%), or
- Significant myocardial ischemia with low-level activity (2–3 METs) beyond day 4

High-risk patients
- Continued myocardial ischemia
- Left ventricular failure
- Episode of shock
- Serious arrhythmias

motion, and postural change. Simple exposure to orthostatic or gravitational stress, such as intermittent sitting or standing during hospital convalescence, may prevent much of the deterioration in exercise performance that follows an acute cardiac event (6). Structured, formalized, in-hospital exercise programs after acute MI appear to offer little additional physiologic or behavioral (self-efficacy) benefits over routine medical care (7,8). Nevertheless, use of treadmills and cycle ergometers for uncomplicated patients, usually 3 to 5 days after the event, provides more precise quantification of their exercise tolerance. To assist the clinician further, Box 8-3 suggests an activity classification guide. In general, the criteria for terminating an inpatient exercise session are similar to or slightly more conservative than those for terminating a low-level exercise test.

BOX 8-3. Activity Classification Guide for Inpatient Activities

Activity Class I
- Sits up in bed with assistance
- Does own self-care activities—seated, or may need assistance
- Stands at bedside with assistance
- Sits up in chair 15 to 30 minutes, 2 to 3 times per day

Activity Class II
- Sits up in bed independently
- Stands independently
- Does self-care activities in bathroom—seated
- Walks in room and to bathroom (may need assistance)

Activity Class III
- Sits and stands independently
- Does own self-care activities in bathroom, seated or standing
- Walks in halls with assistance short distances (50 to 100 ft) as tolerated, up to 3 times per day

Activity Class IV
- Does own self-care and bathes
- Walks in halls short distances (150 to 200 ft) with minimal assistance, 3 to 4 times per day

Activity Class V
- Walks in halls independently, moderate distances (250 to 500 ft), 3 to 4 times per day

Activity Class VI
- Independent ambulation on unit, 3 to 6 times per day

The optimal dosage of exercise for inpatients depends in part on medical history, clinical status, and symptoms. Upper limits to exercise should be physician-directed. The rating of perceived exertion (RPE) provides a useful and complementary guide to heart rate (HR) to gauge exercise intensity. Recommendations for inpatient exercise programming include the following:

Intensity
- RPE less than 13 (6–20 scale)
- Post-MI: HR less than 120 beats·min^{-1} or HR$_{rest}$ + 20 beats·min^{-1} (arbitrary upper limit)
- Postsurgery: HR$_{rest}$ + 30 beats·min^{-1} (arbitrary upper limit)
- To tolerance if asymptomatic

Duration
- Intermittent bouts lasting 3 to 5 minutes
- Rest periods
  —at patient's discretion
  —lasting 1 to 2 minutes
  —shorter than exercise bout duration
- Total duration of up to 20 minutes

Frequency
- Early mobilization: 3 to 4 times per day (days 1 to 3)
- Later mobilization: 2 times per day (beginning on day 4)

Progression
- Initially increase duration to 10 to 15 minutes of exercise, then increase intensity

By hospital discharge, the patient should demonstrate a knowledge of activities that may be inappropriate or excessive. Moreover, a safe, progressive plan of exercise and optimal risk reduction should be formulated for them to take home. The patient should also be apprised of outpatient exercise program options and provided with information regarding the use of home exercise equipment. Selected moderate- to high-risk patients should be strongly encouraged to participate in outpatient rehabilitation programs and, at a minimum, to be able to manage their discharge rehabilitation plan and report cardiovascular symptoms promptly, should they occur.

OUTPATIENT PROGRAMS

Presuming that the goals for inpatient cardiac rehabilitation are met, the goals for outpatient programs are as follows:

- Provide appropriate patient monitoring and supervision to detect a deterioration in clinical status and provide timely feedback to the referring physician to enhance effective medical management.
- Contingent on patient clinical status, return the patient to premorbid vocational and/or recreational activities, modify these activities as necessary, or find alternate activities.

- Develop and help the patient implement a safe and effective home exercise program and recreational lifestyle.
- Provide patient and family education and therapies to maximize secondary prevention.

Use of a risk stratification model permits classification of patients according to their subsequent risk of cardiovascular events. Risk stratification, however, should be only one factor to consider when making recommendations for outpatient medical supervision and the extent of ECG telemetry monitoring during exercise.

Whenever possible, patients should be encouraged to engage in multiple activities to promote total physical conditioning, including range-of-motion exercise and resistance training. Where possible, use of a variety of equipment (treadmills, cycle and arm ergometers, stair-climbers, and rowing machines) is encouraged to maximize the carry-over of training benefits to real-life activities. Prescriptive techniques for determining the amount of exercise, that is, frequency, intensity, and duration, are detailed in Chapter 7 and summarized later in this chapter, with specific reference to cardiac patients.

Intensity

The prescribed exercise intensity should be above a minimal level required to induce a "training effect," yet below the metabolic load that evokes abnormal clinical signs or symptoms (9–14). For most deconditioned cardiac patients, the threshold intensity for exercise training probably lies between 40 and 50% (40/50%) of the maximum oxygen uptake reserve ($\dot{V}O_2R$) (15). Improvement in $\dot{V}O_{2max}$ with low-to-moderate training intensities suggests that a decrease in the intensity may be partially or totally compensated for by increases in the exercise duration or frequency, or both.

Because heart rate and oxygen consumption are linearly related during dynamic exercise involving large muscle groups, a predetermined training or target heart rate (THR) has become widely used as an index of exercise intensity (10). Prescribed heart rates for aerobic conditioning are generally determined by one of two methods from data obtained during peak or symptom-limited exercise testing: 1) the maximal heart rate reserve method of Karvonen (11), in which THR = (maximal heart rate − resting heart rate) × 40–85% + resting heart rate (15), or 2) the percentage of maximal heart rate method (12). The former more closely approximates the same percentage of the oxygen uptake "reserve" (%$\dot{V}O_2R$) (13), rather than the %$\dot{V}O_{2max}$ (14). For example, a patient with a functional capacity of 10 METs would have a 9 MET "reserve," considering resting metabolism as 1 MET. If the prescribed training intensity was at 60% of his heart rate reserve, he would be working at 6.4 METs (9 METs × 60% = 5.4 METs + 1 MET), rather than 6 METs. This terminology relates heart rate reserve to a level of metabolism that starts at a resting level (i.e., 1 MET) rather than from zero (15). Additional advantages include increased accuracy in the calculation of net caloric expenditure (13). However, computing the THR as a fixed percentage of the measured peak heart rate (e.g., 55 to 90% HR_{max}) underestimates the %$\dot{V}O_2R$ by 10 to 15%, especially during light to moderate exercise intensities (15). Nevertheless, this latter approach has been in common use for decades because of the close relationship between %$\dot{V}O_{2max}$ and %HR_{max}. Moreover, one cannot simply rely on these formulas when prescribing exercise for clinical populations because other variables (e.g., ischemic ST-segment depression, anginal symptoms, arrhythmias, perceived exertion) should also be considered when establishing the exercise intensity.

The RPE also provides a useful and important adjunct to heart rate as an intensity guide for exercise training (16). It is particularly valuable when patients enter an exercise-based rehabilitation program without a preliminary exercise test, or when clinical status or medical therapy changes. Exercise rated as 11 to 13 (6–20 scale), between "fairly light" and "somewhat hard," generally corresponds to the upper limit of prescribed training heart rates during the early stages of outpatient cardiac rehabilitation (e.g., Phase II). For higher levels of training (Phases III or IV), ratings of 12 to 15 may be appropriate, which approximates 60 to 80% $\dot{V}O_2R$. However, there is considerable interindividual variation among patients in this regard (17). Although perceived exertion correlates well with exercise intensity, even in patients taking β-blockers (18), ischemic ST-segment depression and serious ventricular arrhythmias can occur at low heart rates and/or ratings of perceived effort.

For some cardiac patients, it is important to know when myocardial ischemia occurs during exercise, so that the patient can exercise below the anginal or ischemic threshold. Such patients may wish to consider using a heart rate monitor that is highly accurate and offers the advantage of alarms for the upper and lower limits of training, thereby potentially increasing the safety and effectiveness of exercise. A peak exercise heart rate 10 beats· min^{-1} or more below the threshold has been suggested, as silent myocardial ischemia has been identified as a link between lack of premonitoring symptoms and increased risk of cardiac arrest during physical stress (19). Box 8-4 outlines criteria for setting a safe upper limit for exercise intensity in cardiac patients. It is also important to consider medication effects (see Appendix A) and those clinical characteristics that place the patient at increased risk for exercise-related cardiovascular events.

Frequency

Improvement in cardiorespiratory fitness increases as a function of the frequency of training. Increases in $\dot{V}O_{2max}$, however, tend to plateau when the frequency of training exceeds 3 to 5 d·wk^{-1} (20), and the incidence of injury increases disproportionately (21). In the early weeks of Phase II cardiac rehabilitation, two exercise sessions may be as effective as three per week for cardiorespiratory conditioning, eliciting similar increases in $\dot{V}O_{2max}$ and decreases in submaximal heart rate (22). However, more frequent training may elicit greater health benefits.

> **BOX 8-4. Signs and Symptoms Below Which an Upper Limit for Exercise Intensity Should be Set***
>
> - Onset of angina or other symptoms of cardiovascular insufficiency
> - Plateau or decrease in systolic blood pressure, systolic blood pressure of >240 mm Hg, or diastolic blood pressure of >110 mm Hg
> - ≥1 mm ST-segment depression, horizontal or downsloping
> - Radionuclide evidence of left ventricular dysfunction or onset of moderate-to-severe wall motion abnormalities during exertion
> - Increased frequency of ventricular arrhythmias
> - Other significant ECG disturbances (e.g., 2° or 3° AV block, atrial fibrillation, supraventricular tachycardia, complex ventricular ectopy, etc.)
> - Other signs/symptoms of intolerance to exercise

*The peak exercise heart rate should generally be at least 10 beats·min^{-1} below the heart rate associated with any of the above-referenced criteria. Other variables (e.g., the corresponding systolic blood pressure response and perceived exertion), however, should also be considered when establishing the exercise intensity.

Duration

The duration of exercise (20 to 60 minutes of continuous or intermittent activity) required to elicit a significant training effect varies inversely with the intensity; the greater the intensity, the shorter the duration of exercise necessary to achieve favorable adaptation and improvement in cardiorespiratory fitness (15). Conversely, low-intensity exercise may be compensated by a longer exercise duration. Moreover, recent studies suggest that longer exercise sessions can be *accumulated* in shorter periods of activity (e.g., 10- to 15-minute exercise bouts), yielding similar physiologic improvements provided that the total volume of training (kcal expenditure) is comparable (23). For some patients, this exercise regimen may fit better into a busy schedule than a single long bout.

Outpatient Rate of Progression

It is important to individualize exercise progression because patients participating in outpatient cardiac rehabilitation programs have a wide range of functional capacities. It is generally prudent to progress patients over a 3- to 6-month period to a level of moderate-to-vigorous exercise that will elicit a minimal caloric output of approximately 1000 kcal/week. Progression has been traditionally divided into an initial conditioning phase, followed by improvement and maintenance stages. General principles for progressing the patient include an increase in exercise (as tolerated by the patient) every 1 to 3 weeks, with a goal of achieving 20 to 30 minutes of continuous exercise before prescribing additional increases in intensity. Patients requiring an intermittent format, such as those with peripheral vascular disease, should be progressed according to symptoms and clinical status. Intensity should be kept low until a continuous duration of 10 to 15 minutes is achieved. An example of exercise progression using an intermittent format is presented in Table 8-1. The progression should be guided by goals associated with the vocational and recreational needs within the limits imposed by disease.

A goal at the time of hospital discharge for most patients is an exercise tolerance that permits safe participation in common activities of daily living. Patients with lower functional capacities have a poorer prognosis and require a more conservative approach to exercise therapy, and thus progress more slowly. Conversely, patients with higher functional capacities respond well to more rapid progression. Fortunately, patients with low functional capacities respond favorably to lower-intensity activity emphasizing frequent short bouts of exercise with intermittent rest periods. Because these patients often have impaired cardiac function, the emphasis for adaptation shifts to peripheral mechanisms. An example of a progression from intermittent to continuous exercise is found in Table 8-1. It is important to individualize the exercise prescription based on clinical status and symptoms. Consideration should also be given to other factors that could hinder long-term adherence, compliance, and exercise progression, such as concomitant orthopedic problems.

TABLE 8-1. Example of Exercise Progression Using Intermittent Exercise

Functional Capacity (FC) > 4 METs

Wk	%FC	Total Min at %FC	Min Exercise	Min Rest	Reps
1	50–60	15–20	3–5	3–5	3–4
2	50–60	15–20	7–10	2–3	3
3	60–70	20–30	10–15	Optional	2
4	60–70	30–40	15–20	Optional	2

Functional Capacity (FC) ≤ 4 METs

Wk	%FC	Total Min at %FC	Min Exercise	Min Rest	Reps
1	40–50	10–15	3–5	3–5	3–4
2	40–50	12–20	5–7	3–5	3
3	50–60	15–25	7–10	3–5	3
4	50–60	20–30	10–15	2–3	2
5	60–70	25–40	12–20	2	2
6	Continue with 2 reps of continuous exercise, with one rest period or progress to a single continuous bout				

Types of Outpatient Programs

For most patients, progression toward an independent self-managed program is desirable, but some patients may need to remain in a clinically supervised program. These include patients at high risk for cardiovascular complications, those unable to self-monitor, or those whose adherence depends heavily on group support. As a general rule, most patients should participate in a clinically supervised rehabilitation program for at least 3 months to facilitate both exercise and lifestyle management changes. Clinically supervised programs have traditionally been divided into Phase II and Phase III, both of which are supervised by a clinically trained staff. Given the shifting parameters for classifying cardiac patients and prescribing exercise monitoring and supervision, the progression of patients from Phase II to Phase III should be based on a variety of objectives and outcomes. The shift from continuous ECG monitoring to intermittent monitoring or self-monitoring should take place on an individual basis. No specific guidelines are provided regarding the duration of continuous ECG monitoring; however, the degree of ECG surveillance should be linked inversely with the cardiac stability of the patient. The progression to independent exercise with minimal or no supervision is a decision best reached by the physician with input from the rehabilitation team. General criteria for such decisions are presented in Box 8-5.

Not all patients will be able to, or wish to, participate in a supervised program. Many choose to exercise at home, based on expense, schedule flexibility, and other factors. Advantages to exercising under supervision include group support, professional feedback and monitoring, increased access to varied training modalities, and the availability of emergency support.

BOX 8-5. Guidelines for Progression to Independent Exercise With Minimal or No Supervision

- Functional capacity of ≥8 METs or twice the level of occupational demand
- Appropriate hemodynamic response to exercise (increase in systolic blood pressure with increasing work load) and recovery
- Appropriate ECG response at peak exercise with normal or unchanged conduction, stable or benign arrhythmias, and nondiagnostic ischemic response (i.e., <1 mm ST-segment depression)
- Cardiac symptoms stable or absent
- Stable and/or controlled baseline heart rate and blood pressure
- Adequate management of risk factor intervention strategy and safe exercise participation such that the patient demonstrates independent and effective management of risk factors with favorable changes in those risk factors
- Demonstrated knowledge of the disease process, abnormal signs and symptoms, medication use, and side effects

EXERCISE PRESCRIPTION WITHOUT A PRELIMINARY EXERCISE TEST

It may not always be feasible to conduct a peak or symptom-limited exercise test before starting a cardiac rehabilitation program. In some instances, a pharmacologic stress test (e.g., dipyridamole or adenosine studies with concomitant myocardial perfusion imaging or dobutamine echocardiography) may have been recently performed. Unfortunately, the data obtained from these tests may be insufficient in formulating an exercise prescription because these evaluations do not provide an assessment of functional capacity, hemodynamic responses and/or symptoms associated with progressive physical exertion, or an ischemic ECG threshold. Furthermore, maximal exercise testing may be inappropriate for some patients at or soon after hospital discharge. Economic issues and the significance of these results are additional reasons why these evaluations may be delayed. However, the referring physician may request an accelerated, low-level exercise rehabilitation program for some patients. Such patients may include those with extreme deconditioning, orthopedic limitations, or those with left ventricular dysfunction who are limited by shortness of breath (24). In these patient subsets, the use of submaximal exercise tolerance testing (i.e., to a perceived exertion of "somewhat hard" to "hard") is being increasingly employed to assess function and prescribe exercise. Exercise programs for patients without preliminary exercise testing should be implemented conservatively with close medical surveillance; moreover, a period of continuous ECG-telemetry monitoring is highly recommended. The patient should be observed closely for signs and symptoms of exercise intolerance, and blood pressure measurements should be obtained regularly.

Dobutamine testing may, in some instances, evoke a considerable rise in heart rate. If the echocardiogram or myocardial perfusion imaging results are negative for ischemia, the highest heart rate obtained may be used as a guide to determine the prescribed THR. An abnormal test, however, may signify the need for coronary revascularization, more aggressive medical management (e.g., drug therapy), or both, before initiating a cardiac exercise training program. Because these test results may not necessarily define the ischemic ECG threshold, other complementary methods (e.g., symptoms, Holter monitoring, ECG-telemetry, heart rate monitor [watches]) should be used in conjunction with conservative heart rate guidelines to determine the exercise intensity.

Initial exercise intensities can be determined according to the length of time from the acute cardiac event and associated complications, duration since hospital discharge, and from the information obtained during the patient's preliminary outpatient assessment (e.g., activities of daily living, current home walking program, associated signs and symptoms). Patient questionnaires, such as the Duke Activity Status Index (Fig. 8-1) (25) and the Veterans Specific Activity Questionnaire (26), can be used to estimate an individual's activity status and functional capacity in the absence of a preliminary exercise stress test. Nevertheless, initial exercise intensities usually range from 2 to 3 METs, corresponding to 1 to 3 mph, 0% grade

Can you:	Weight
1) Take care of yourself, that is, eat, dress, bathe or use the toilet?	2.75
2) Walk indoors, such as around your house?	1.75
3) Walk a block or two on level ground?	2.75
4) Climb a flight of stairs or walk up a hill?	5.50
5) Run a short distance?	8.00
6) Do light work around the house like dusting or washing dishes?	2.70
7) Do moderate work around the house like vacuuming, sweeping floors or carrying groceries?	3.50
8) Do heavy work around the house like scrubbing floors or lifting or moving heavy furniture?	8.00
9) Do yard work like raking leaves, weeding or pushing a power mower?	4.50
10) Have sexual relations?	5.25
11) Participate in moderate recreational activities like golf, bowling, dancing, doubles tennis or throwing a baseball or football?	6.00
12) Participate in strenuous sports like swimming, singles tennis, football, basketball or skiing?	7.50

FIGURE 8-1. Duke Activity Status Index (DASI) = the sum of weights for "yes" replies. $\dot{V}O_{2peak}$ (mL·kg^{-1}·min^{-1}) = 0.43 × DASI + 9.6.

on the treadmill, or 100 to 300 kg·m·min^{-1} on the cycle ergometer, depending on body weight, with gradual increments of 0.5 to 1.0 METs as tolerated (1). The THR can be set at approximately 20 beats·min^{-1} above standing rest, and gradually increased using perceived exertion in the absence of symptoms, abnormal hemodynamics, threatening ventricular arrhythmias, or ECG changes signifying myocardial ischemia. If ECG-telemetry monitoring suggests new-onset ST-segment depression, this should be confirmed with 12-lead electrocardiography during a simulated exercise session.

One study compared the rehabilitation outcomes in 229 post-MI and coronary artery bypass patients who had undergone preliminary symptom-limited exercise testing with 271 matched patients who did not (27). All subjects underwent a 12-week, exercise-based cardiac rehabilitation program, including ECG-telemetry monitoring for the first 3 to 6 weeks. The group with no preliminary exercise test started at a training intensity of 2 to 3 METs and progressed using heart rate and perceived exertion. Both groups showed similar physiologic improvements, and there were no cardiovascular events in either group.

RESISTANCE TRAINING

Traditionally, cardiac rehabilitation programs have emphasized dynamic aerobic exercise to physically condition individuals with cardiovascular disease. However, many patients lack the physical strength and/or self-confidence to perform common activities of daily living. Resistance training provides an effective method for improving muscular strength and endurance, preventing and managing a variety of chronic medical conditions, modifying coronary risk factors, and enhancing independence in elderly patients (28). Because increased muscle mass correlates with an increased basal metabolic rate, a major component of daily energy expenditure, it complements aerobic exercise for weight control. Strength training has also been shown to attenuate the rate-pressure product when lifting any given load (29). Thus, resistance training appears to decrease cardiac demands during daily activities like carrying groceries or lifting moderate-to-heavy objects, while simultaneously increasing the endurance capacity to sustain these submaximal endeavors (30).

Eligibility and Exclusion Criteria

Many low-to-moderate risk patients should be encouraged to incorporate resistance training into their physical conditioning program, especially those who rely on their upper extremities for work or recreational pursuits. However, the safety and effectiveness of resistance training in other populations of coronary patients (e.g., women, older patients with low aerobic fitness, patients with severe left ventricular dysfunction) have not been well studied (31). Accordingly, these patient subsets may require more careful evaluation, initial monitoring, and progression.

Contraindications to resistance training are similar to those used for the aerobic component of cardiac exercise programs. Patients are generally excluded from participation for any of the following conditions (28): unstable angina, uncontrolled arrhythmias, left ventricular outflow obstruction (e.g., hypertrophic cardiomyopathy with obstruction), a recent history of congestive heart failure that has not been evaluated and effectively treated, severe valvular disease, and uncontrolled hypertension (systolic blood pressure ≥ 160 mm Hg and/or diastolic blood pressure ≥ 105 mm Hg). Because patients with myocardial ischemia and poor left ventricular function may develop wall motion abnormalities or threatening ventricular arrhythmias during resistance training, moderate-to-good left ventricular function and an exercise capacity of greater than 5 METs without anginal symptoms or ischemic ST-segment depression have been suggested as additional prerequisites for participation in traditional resistance training programs (32). Nevertheless, these include both absolute and relative contraindications, and a patient's participation in resistance training should be contingent on approval of the medical director and/or his or her personal physician. Many deconditioned patients at low risk may safely participate in resistance training if modest weight loads are employed.

Certain patient subsets may derive added benefits from resistance training. Older patients often demonstrate dramatic improvements in muscular strength and endurance, gait speed, and bone mineral density, thus reducing the potential for debilitating osteoporosis and falls (33,34). Similarly, cardiac transplant recipients who participate in low- to moderate-intensity resistance training may offset the deleterious effects of prednisone therapy on muscle mass and bone density (35). Women may also experience remarkable improvements in physical function following a resistance training program.

Time Course to Resistance Training

Although previous participation guidelines suggested that cardiac patients should avoid moderate-to-heavy resistance training for several months (36), many patients can safely perform static-dynamic activity equivalent to carrying up to 30 pounds by 3 weeks after acute MI (37). Thus, it is possible that resistance exercise could be initiated sooner if a continuum of modalities are employed. A traditional resistance training program has been defined as one in which patients lift weights corresponding to 50% or more of the maximum weight that could be used to complete one repetition (i.e., 1-repetition maximum, 1 RM) (1). However, the use of elastic bands, light (1- to 5-pound) cuff and hand weights, light free weights, and wall pulleys may be initiated in a progressive fashion at immediate outpatient program entry (i.e., Phase II) in the absence of contraindications.

Low-level resistance training (e.g., use of elastic bands, very light hand weights) should not begin until 2 to 3 weeks post-MI. Once the patient completes the convalescence stage of recovery, usually 4 to 6 weeks after the event, regular barbells and/or weight machines may be initiated. Surgical patients are encouraged to use range-of-motion activities and very light (i.e., 1- to 3-pound) hand weights during convalescence and recovery. However, these patients should probably avoid traditional resistance training exercises (with moderate-to-heavy weights), which may cause pulling on the sternum within 3 months of coronary artery bypass surgery and sternotomy (28). Moreover, the sternum should be checked for stability by an experienced health care professional before a traditional resistance training regimen is initiated.

Appropriately selected cardiac patients who wish to initiate a traditional resistance training program may benefit by first participating in an aerobic exercise regimen for 2 weeks or more (1). These patients include those who have undergone percutaneous transluminal coronary angioplasty. Although scientific data to support this recommendation are lacking, this time period permits sufficient observation of the patient in a supervised setting and allows the cardiorespiratory and musculoskeletal adaptations needed to progress to more intense exercise.

Prescriptive Guidelines

Range-of-motion exercises of the upper and lower extremities are recommended for most cardiac inpatients. Bypass surgery patients who experience sternal movement or have surgical sternal wound complications would perform lower extremity exercises only. Nevertheless, significant soft tissue and bone damage of the chest wall can occur during surgery. If this area does not receive range-of-motion exercise, adhesions may develop and the musculature can become weaker and foreshorten, accentuating postural problems and hindering strength gains. Stretching or flexibility activities can begin as early as 24 and 48 hours after bypass surgery or uncomplicated MI, respectively. Patients may be seen once daily and perform 10 to 15 repetitions of each exercise.

Although a traditional resistance training prescription involves performing each exercise 3 times (e.g., 3 sets of 8 to 15 repetitions per set), a single set of 8 to 10 different exercises (e.g., chest press, shoulder press, triceps extension, biceps curl, pull-down [upper back], lower back extension, abdominal crunch/curl-up, quadriceps extension or leg press, leg curls [hamstrings], calf raise) that train the major muscle groups, performed 2 to 3 d· wk^{-1}, will elicit favorable adaptations and improvements (38). Greater frequencies of training and more sets may be used, but the additional gains are usually small. To achieve a balanced increase in both muscular strength and endurance a repetition range of 8 to 12 is recommended for healthy participants under 50 to 60 years of age, and 10 to 15 repetitions at a lower relative resistance for cardiac patients and healthy participants older than 50 to 60 years of age (Table 8-2; Fig. 8-2) (1,2,15,23,39–41). The reason for the increased repetition range at a lower relative effort for the older, more frail patient is injury prevention.

The cardiac patient should start at a low weight and perform 1 set of 10 to 15 repetitions to moderate fatigue using 8 to 10 different exercises. Weight is increased slowly as the patient adapts to the program (approximately 2 to 5 pounds per week for arms and 5 to 10 pounds per week for legs). The rate-pressure product should not exceed that during prescribed endurance exercise, and perceived exertion should range from 11 to 14 ("fairly light" to "somewhat hard") on the Borg category scale (16). Additionally, patients should be counseled to raise weights with slow, controlled movements to full extension, exhale during the exertion phase of the lift, avoid straining and the Valsalva maneuver, minimize rest periods between

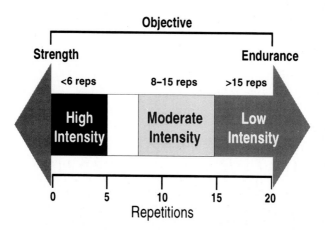

FIGURE 8-2. Classification of weight training intensity (resistance). Using weight loads that permit 8 to 15 repetitions (reps) will generally facilitate improvements in muscular strength and endurance, considering age and health status.

TABLE 8-2. Standards, Guidelines, and Position Statements Regarding Resistance Training

Population (Reference)	Sets; Reps	Stations/Devices	Frequency
Healthy/Sedentary Adults			
1995 ACSM Guidelines (39)	1 set; 8–12 reps	8–10 exercises*	2 d·wk^{-1}, min^{+}
1998 ACSM Position Stand (15)	1 set; 8–12 reps (persons under 50–60 yrs) 10–15 reps (persons 50–60 yrs and older)	8–10 exercises	2–3 d·wk^{-1}
1995 CDC/ACSM Public Health Statement (23)	addressed, not specified		
1996 Surgeon General's Report (40)	1–2 sets; 8–12 reps	8–10 exercises	2 d·wk^{-1}, min^{+}
Elderly Persons			
Pollock et al. (41)	1 set; 10–15 reps	8–10 exercises	2 d·wk^{-1}, min^{+}
Cardiac Patients			
1995 AHA Exercise Standards (2)	1 set; 10–15 reps	8–10 exercises	2–3 d·wk^{-1}
1999 AACVPR Guidelines (1)	1 set; 12–15 reps	8–10 exercises	2–3 d·wk^{-1}
2000 AHA Advisory (28)	1 set; 10–15 reps	8–10 exercises	2–3 d·wk^{-1}

ACSM, American College of Sports Medicine; AHA, American Heart Association; CDC, Centers for Disease Control and Prevention; AACVPR, American Association of Cardiovascular and Pulmonary Rehabilitation; reps, repetitions.

*Minimum one exercise per major muscle group: e.g., chest press, shoulder press, triceps extension, biceps curl, pull-down (upper back), lower back extension, abdominal crunch/curl-up, quadriceps extension or leg press, leg curls (hamstrings), calf raise.

$^{+}$min = minimum.

exercises to maximize muscular endurance, and stop exercise in the event of warning signs and symptoms (1). Tight gripping of the weight handles or bar should be avoided to prevent an excessive blood pressure response to lifting.

Arm Exercise Prescription

Guidelines for arm exercise prescription should include recommendations regarding three variables: 1) the prescribed heart rate for training; 2) the power output (kg·m·min^{-1} or Watts) that will elicit the required metabolic load for training; and 3) the appropriate training equipment or modalities.

Arm Exercise Training Heart Rate

Although the prescribed heart rate for arm training should ideally be based on the maximal heart rate (HR$_{max}$) obtained during a progressive multistage arm ergometer test, this is rarely practical. Research indicates that a slightly lower HR$_{max}$ is generally obtained during arm than during leg exercise testing, except among persons with severe arteriosclerosis of the lower extremities (42). A review comparing the HR$_{max}$ during arm and leg ergometry in men and women with and without heart disease revealed consistently lower heart rates during arm ergometry (3 to 23 beats·min^{-1}, $\bar{x}$ = 11 beats·min^{-1}), equivalent to 88 to 98% of the HR$_{max}$ during leg ergometry, with a mean value of 94% (43). Consequently, an arm exercise prescription based on a maximal heart rate obtained during leg ergometry may result in an overestimation of the training heart rate.

Exercise training at approximately 60 to 80% of $\dot{V}O_{2max}$, equivalent to approximately 70 to 85% HR$_{max}$, has been shown to elicit favorable adaptations and improvements in the oxidative capacity of skeletal muscle (44). Because the relationships between relative oxygen uptake (%$\dot{V}O_{2max}$) and relative heart rate (%HR$_{max}$) are nearly identical for arm and leg exercise, it appears that a given percentage of the HR$_{max}$ during arm exercise results in a percentage of arm aerobic capacity comparable to that of leg exercise (42). Moreover, the heart rate–oxygen uptake relation that is determined during a graded treadmill test can be generalized to *combined* arm and leg exercise (45).

Work Rates for Arm Training

When estimating the work rate or power output that is appropriate for arm training, it is important to emphasize that although maximal physiologic responses are generally greater during leg exercise than arm exercise, the oxygen uptake, minute ventilation, heart rate, systolic blood pressure, and perceived exertion during arm work are greater for a given external work rate. Consequently, a power output considered appropriate for leg training will generally be too high for arm training. A work rate approximating 50 to 66% of that used for leg training has been suggested for arm training (43,46). In other words, a patient using 300 kg·m·min^{-1} for leg training would use 150 to 200 kg·m·min^{-1} for arm training, demonstrating similar heart rates and perceived exertion ratings at these work rates. These findings suggest that arm training work rates can be estimated from those used during leg training, even in the absence of a preliminary arm ergometer evaluation.

Arm Exercise Equipment and Training Modalities

Equipment suitable for upper extremity training includes arm ergometers, resistance training apparatus, rowing machines, light dumbbells, vertical climbing devices, cross-country skiing simulators, pulleys, and arm-leg ergometers for arm exercise alone, using only the arm levers, or combined arm and leg exercise, using the levers and pedals simultaneously. Walking or jogging while pumping hand-held weights can also be used to facilitate training of the upper extremities, eliciting significantly greater increases in heart rate, oxygen consumption, and caloric expenditure over conventional walking or jogging at comparable speeds (47).

Various calisthenics and recreational activities can also be used to condition the upper extremities. The latter include volleyball, racquetball, tennis, basketball, canoeing, cross-country skiing, kayaking, and swimming. However, several of these may be difficult to prescribe, particularly for unfit subjects or cardiac patients, because the associated energy expenditure is highly dependent on competition, skill, and efficiency.

Exercise Training for Return to Work

Failure to return to work after a cardiac event can stem from a variety of factors, including low work capacity, poor prognosis, low self-efficacy, or inappropriate perceptions of actual job demands (48). Exercise training may enhance the return to work decision and long-term employment by helping selected patients to improve their work capacity and self-efficacy for physical work. Nevertheless, it appears that exercise-based cardiac rehabilitation exerts less of an influence on the rates of return to work than many nonexercise variables, including employer attitudes, prior employment status, and economic incentives (31).

A progressive dynamic exercise program during early convalescence serves an important role in the return to work process as it helps patients to retain or improve tolerance for physical work. Long-term participation in an aerobic exercise training program further promotes a higher work capacity and lower rate-pressure product at an absolute level of submaximal physical work. These adaptations may be especially beneficial for patients with low to marginal work capacity or with exercise-induced myocardial ischemia because it may allow them to resume their jobs within a reasonable level of myocardial demand.

A substantial portion of the improvement in work tolerance with exercise training results from peripheral adaptations within the trained muscles. Because many job tasks require a component of static and/or arm muscular work, inclusion of progressive resistance exercise and/or arm dynamic exercise within a training program may enhance occupational work potential. In designing a program to promote peripheral adaptations for work resumption, the program should be individualized according to job demands because peripheral adaptations often are specific to the muscle and muscle action taken during training (43).

In addition to enhancing work capacity, exercise training may help patients gain a better appreciation of their ability to perform physical work within reasonable levels of safety. Monitoring the physiologic responses to a simulated work environment may also be helpful in this regard. Enhanced self-efficacy, in turn, may lead to a greater willingness on the part of patients to resume work and/or more willingness to remain employed long-term following a cardiac event.

Patients who plan to resume work combined with environmental heat stress should consider a gradual exposure to an outdoor exercise program during convalescence rather than restricting all exercise to an air-conditioned environment (48). A few days of relatively short periods of mild-to-moderate exercise in a warm environment can enhance thermoregulation which, in turn, can lower the cardiovascular demand of work combined with heat stress (49). Importantly, work combined with heat/humidity stress can increase cardiovascular strain as reflected by a disproportionate increase in heart rate. Thus, the absolute exercise level (e.g., walking speed) often needs to be lower than in a thermoneutral environment when exercising within the prescribed THR, especially if the individual is not heat acclimated. Fluid intake should always be encouraged during work in a hot environment.

Optimal Exercise Dosage? Pathophysiologic Considerations

Exercise training as a sole intervention does not necessarily halt the progression of coronary artery disease (CAD) or, for that matter, prevent restenosis or reinfarction. Conventional exercise training does little to improve left ventricular ejection fraction, regional wall motion abnormalities, and cardiac hemodynamic measurements at cardiac catheterization (31). However, in patients with heart failure and left ventricular dysfunction, exercise training may result in improved hemodynamics secondary to an enhanced oxidative capacity of skeletal muscle functioning. Studies describing changes in ventricular arrhythmias following exercise rehabilitation have also produced inconsistent results (31). Some investigators have used thallium exercise testing and multiple-gated image acquisition scans on subjects before and after exercise training to assess changes in cardiac function. Although the findings have been generally unimpressive, modest improvements have been reported with and without vigorous exercise training regimens (50).

Nevertheless, angiographic studies in group trials have, without exception, failed to confirm the appearance of new coronary collateral vessels following conventional exercise training programs (51).

Intensive multifactorial intervention (including exercise) can result in regression or limitation of progression of angiographically documented coronary atherosclerosis (52,53). One study (54), which included a low-fat, low-cholesterol diet (fat less than 20% of energy; cholesterol less than 200 mg/day) showed that a minimum of 1533 kcal/week of physical activity may halt the progression of CAD, whereas regression may be achieved with an energy expenditure of 2204 kcal/week (Fig. 8-3). For many patients, these goals would require walking 24 and 32 km (15 and 20 miles) per week, respectively.

A consensus statement on preventing heart attack and death in patients with coronary disease extolled the importance of a minimum of 30 to 60 minutes of moderate-intensity activity 3 or 4 times weekly supplemented by an increase in daily lifestyle activities (e.g., walking breaks at work, using stairs, gardening, household chores); 5 to 6 hours a week was suggested for maximum cardioprotective benefits (55). Increasing physical activity in daily living can be helpful in this regard (see Fig. 7-1).

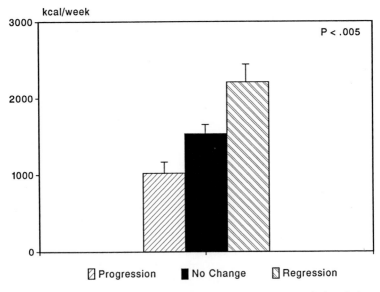

FIGURE 8-3. Effects of leisure-time physical activity on coronary morphology in intervention and control groups combined. The lowest activity level was noted in patients with progression of coronary artery disease (1022 ± 142 kcal/week) compared with patients with no change (1533 ± 122 kcal/week) or regression (2204 ± 237 kcal/week). (Adapted from Hambrecht R, Niebauer J, Marburger C, et al. Various intensities of leisure time physical activity in patients with coronary artery disease: effects on cardiorespiratory fitness and progression of coronary atherosclerotic lesions. J Am Coll Cardiol 1993;22:468–477.)

SPECIAL PATIENT POPULATIONS

The exercise prescription uses objective information obtained from a recent exercise stress test such as heart rate, blood pressure, perceived exertion, symptoms, ECG changes, and functional capacity. This approach is adequate for most cardiac patients; however, patients who have specific needs to consider when formulating the exercise prescription include those with angina or silent ischemia, congestive heart failure, pacemakers, implantable cardioverter defibrillators (ICDs), and transplant recipients. A more comprehensive description of exercise testing and training protocols for these patient subsets is available elsewhere (56).

Angina or Silent Ischemia

Coronary atherosclerosis involves a localized accumulation of fibrous tissue and, to a lesser extent, lipid within the coronary artery, progressively narrowing the lumen of the vessel. Ischemia occurs when clinically significant lesions (i.e., 70% or more of the vessel's cross-sectional area) result in blood flow inadequate to meet myocardial oxygen demands, causing significant ST-segment depression, angina pectoris, or both. When the former occurs in the absence of symptoms it is referred to as silent ischemia. For a given patient, stable angina predictably occurs with progressive exercise at approximately the same rate-pressure product. In contrast, unstable angina may be characterized by an abrupt increase in the frequency of angina, angina at rest, or both. This acceleration of symptoms may herald an impending cardiovascular event and serves as a contraindication to exercise. Accordingly, such patients generally require immediate medical attention.

Patients with stable angina pectoris for whom revascularization is not appropriate and/or those with an anginal threshold of 4 METs or more are candidates for exercise programs. However, exercise may be inappropriate for those who experience exertional angina at aerobic requirements of less than 3 METs. The primary goal for persons with angina is to increase the anginal and ischemic ECG threshold by decreasing the rate-pressure product at any given level of submaximal exertion. The patient should be evaluated for evidence of myocardial ischemia before (i.e., during the history), during, and after the exercise test. Especially important are symptoms that may represent classic angina pectoris, such as substernal pressure radiating across the chest and/or down the left arm, back, jaw, or stomach, or lower neck pain or discomfort. Such symptoms can be subjectively rated by the patient on a scale of 1 to 4: 1 = perceptible but mild; 2 = moderate; 3 = moderately severe; and 4 = severe. Teaching the patient to grade anginal symptoms during the exercise test may help determine the intensity of chest discomfort ($\geq +2$) at which the exercise session should be discontinued or at least decreased in intensity until resolved. Patients with stable angina should be counseled regarding the potential exacerbation of symptoms while exercising in the cold.

The exercise session should include a prolonged warm-up and cool down ($\geq$10 minutes), both of which may have an antianginal effect, and consist of range of motion, stretching, and low-level aerobic activities (57). The goal is to gradually raise the heart rate response within 10 to 20 beats·min^{-1} of the lower limit prescribed for endurance training. Because symptomatic or silent ischemia may be arrhythmogenic (19), the THR for endurance exercise should be set safely below ($\geq$10 beats·min^{-1}) the ischemic ECG or anginal threshold. A heart rate monitor may be helpful in this regard. Patients with stable angina may, in selected cases, also benefit from prophylactic (preexercise) nitroglycerin and/or intermittent, shorter duration-type exercise on a more frequent basis (e.g., 4 to 6 d·wk^{-1} with 5 to 10 minutes per session and 2 or 3 sessions per day) (57). Any increase in anginal symptoms should be recorded and receive immediate medical attention. Blood pressure should be checked routinely before and after the administration of nitroglycerin to assess for hypotensive sequelae. In the event that anginal symptoms are not relieved by termination of exercise or by the use of three sublingual nitroglycerin tablets (one taken every 5 minutes), the patient should be transported to the nearest hospital emergency center.

Congestive Heart Failure

Congestive heart failure (CHF) is characterized by the inability of the heart to adequately deliver oxygenated blood to metabolizing tissues, secondary to impairment in cardiac output, depressed left ventricular systolic function, diastolic dysfunction, abnormalities in skeletal muscle metabolism or pulmonary function, or combinations thereof. Associated central hemodynamic responses include a decreased cardiac output at rest and/or during exercise, elevated left ventricular filling pressures, compensatory ventricular volume overload, and increased pulmonary and central venous pressures. This scenario often leads to a hyperventilatory response to exercise, lactate accumulation in the blood at low work rates, and early fatigue. Catecholamine levels are usually elevated in this patient subset, and abnormalities in β-receptor density probably contribute to reduced myocardial contractility. In addition, concomitant skeletal muscle abnormalities often result in greater glycolysis, reduced oxidative phosphorylation, and increased metabolic acidosis (58).

Traditionally, heart failure was treated with bed rest and restricted physical activity. Although this treatment is still appropriate for acute or unstable conditions, exercise can be safe and beneficial for those with chronic heart failure. Physical conditioning in patients with heart failure and moderate-to-severe left ventricular dysfunction results in improved functional capacity and quality of life, and reduced symptoms, mortality, and hospital readmission rates for heart failure (31,59). Peripheral (skeletal muscle) adaptations are largely responsible for the increase in exercise tolerance (50).

Concerns have been raised regarding the potential deleterious effects of early exercise training for patients recovering from large anterior wall MI, causing abnormal ventricular remodeling and infarct expansion. One nonrandomized controlled study of patients with anterior MI and diminished ejection fraction showed a significantly greater deterioration in global and regional left ventricular function in exercising patients compared with nonexercising patients (60). However, two randomized controlled trials in patients with anterior Q-wave MI and decreased ejection fraction showed no significant difference in left ventricular dysfunction between exercise and control patients (61,62).

CHF patients who are selected for exercise training should be stable on medical therapy without absolute contraindications (particularly obstruction to left ventricular outflow, decompensated CHF, or threatening arrhythmias) and have an exercise capacity of more than 3 METs. If possible, oxygen consumption should be determined by direct gas exchange measurements because aerobic capacity may be markedly overestimated from treadmill exercise time in CHF patients (58). Many of these patients may also be taking multiple medications, including digoxin, diuretics, vasodilators, ACE inhibitors, and antiarrhythmics which have the potential to augment ST-segment changes, lower blood pressure, increase heart rate, and improve performance. Moreover, hypokalemia commonly results from chronic diuretic therapy. The combination of digoxin and altered electrolytes may precipitate malignant ventricular dysrhythmias, which are the most common cause of sudden cardiac death in CHF patients. Thus, supervisory staff should be especially vigilant of signs and/or symptoms that suggest a deterioration in clinical status: increasing fatigue, worse-than-usual dyspnea or shortness of breath or angina on exertion, edema, sudden weight gain, or increases in dysrhythmias. Serial ECG and blood pressure monitoring may be helpful in this regard.

The exercise intensity should be based on a symptom-limited treadmill or cycle ergometer evaluation, using a THR range corresponding to approximately 40 to 75% $\dot{V}O_{2max}$, 3 to 7 $d \cdot wk^{-1}$, 20 to 40 min/session (58). If possible, ancillary study data (exercise echocardiogram, radionuclide studies, gas analysis) may be helpful when formulating the exercise intensity to avoid work rates that produce ischemic wall motion abnormalities (19), a drop in ejection fraction, a pulmonary wedge pressure greater than 20 mm Hg, or exceed the ventilatory threshold (58). Warm-up and cool-down periods should be lengthened to a minimum of 10 to 15 minutes each, and patients should be advised to avoid isometric exertion. Training sessions should initially be brief (e.g., 10 to 20 minutes), including exercise for intervals of 2 to 6 minutes separated by 1 to 2 minutes of rest, and progressively lengthened as the patient's tolerance improves. Recently, interval exercise training has been used in patients with chronic CHF, applying short bouts of intense muscular loading, with good clinical results and accelerated rehabilitation outcomes (63). Walking, stationary cycling, and other aerobic activities, including arm exercise training, are recommended. These activities may be complemented by resistance training (high repetitions, low resistance) and range-of-motion exercises 2 to 3 $d \cdot wk^{-1}$. Because the chronotropic response may be impaired, perceived exertion and dyspnea may be used preferentially over heart rate or workload targets. Perceived exertion ratings of 11 to 14 (on the 6–20 scale) are useful guides.

Position	I	II	III	IV	V
Category	Chamber(s) Paced	Chambers Sensed	Response to Sensing	Programmability/ Modulation	Antitachyarrhythmia Functioning
	0 = None	0 = None	0 = None	0 = None	0 = None
	A = Atrium	A = Atrium	T = Triggered	P = Simple programmable	P = Pacing (antitachyarrhythmia)
	V = Ventricle	V = Ventricle	I = Inhibited	M = Multiprogram	S = Shock
	D = Dual (A&V)	D = Dual (A&V)	D = Dual (T&I)	C = Communicating	D = Dual (P&S)
				R = Rate modulation	

TABLE 8-3. NASPE/BPEG Generic Pacemaker Code

Pacemaker and Implantable Cardioverter Defibrillators

Patients with a history of resuscitated sudden cardiac death, threatening ventricular dysrhythmias, or disease of the sinus node or conduction system with permanent pacemakers or an implantable cardioverter defibrillator (ICD), are being increasingly referred to exercise-based cardiac rehabilitation programs (64). Although these patients were traditionally cautioned to avoid vigorous physical activity because of the pacemaker's fixed rate, advances in technology now enable dual chamber pacing with atrioventricular (AV) synchrony as well as dynamic adjustment of the heart rate to match increasing levels of metabolic demand (65). Contemporary pacemakers use sensors that respond to physiologic, mechanical, or electrical signals to facilitate pacing in a more "physiologic" manner.

Most pacemakers are employed to manage bradydysrhythmias that may be secondary to acquired AV block, persistent advanced AV block after MI, or sick sinus syndrome with symptomatic bradycardia. Other less common indications are in individuals with hypertrophic cardiomyopathy, those with dilated cardiomyopathy and symptoms of low cardiac output, and those with ablative mediated AV block (64). ICDs, however, are designed to electrically terminate ventricular tachydysrhythmias that are potentially life-threatening.

A pacing system includes a pulse generator that consists of a battery, electronic circuitry, and one or more leads. In 1987, the North American Society of Pacing and Electrophysiology (NASPE)/British Pacing and Electrophysiology Group (BPEG) proposed a standard international five-letter code to provide a universal description of pacemaker characteristics (Table 8-3). Pacemakers are categorized by these codes (e.g., AAI, VVI, DDD, VVIR, and AATOP). The first letter position represents the chamber(s) paced, the second letter position describes the chamber(s) sensed, and the third letter position signifies the response of the pacemaker to a sensed event. The fourth letter represents rate-responsive properties, and the fifth position denotes any antitachyarrhythmia function of the pacemaker.

For many patients, the pacemaker is programmed in VVI to manage ventricular bradycardias effectively (66). However, limitations of VVI pacing include the lack of AV synchronization, absence of an atrial contribution to end-diastolic volume, and intermittent valvular regurgitation. Consequently, the patient demonstrates an attenuated rise in cardiac output during physical activity, and functional capacity may be severely compromised. Other individuals with VVI pacemakers may have little or no chronotropic reserve. Although it was previously believed that exercise training programs would be ineffective for patients with a fixed heart rate response, it appears that these patients adapt to physical conditioning in a manner similar to patients with CAD who are heart rate-responsive (67). In this patient subset, the exercise intensity can be determined by modifying the Karvonen (11) equation from heart rate (HR) to systolic blood pressure (SBP), as follows:

Standard Karvonen Formula

$$THR = (HR_{max} - HR_{rest}) \, (50\text{--}80\%) + HR_{rest}$$

Modified Karvonen Formula

$$TSBP = (SBP_{max} - SBP_{rest})(50-80\%) + SBP_{rest}$$

where THR equals training heart rate and TSBP equals training systolic blood pressure. However, extended warm-up and cool-down periods are recommended, and systolic blood pressure should be monitored throughout exercise to ensure a safe and effective exercise intensity. Such patients should also work at a markedly reduced intensity for the first few minutes of exercise to avoid dyspnea or premature fatigue (66). Finally, it should be emphasized that without rate adaptive pacing, the functional capacity of VVI-paced patients may be greatly reduced when compared to those with rate modulation and AV synchrony.

Rate responsiveness to exercise can be achieved in patients with chronotropic incompetence with VVIR or DDD pacing. For these pacing modalities, the pacing rate is determined by physiologic variables or atrial tracking. For patients with adequate sinus node function but high-grade AV block, the DDD pacemaker offers the advantage of AV synchrony as well as rate responsiveness during activity via atrial tracking. Pacing in the VVIR mode provides rate responsiveness to activity, but without AV synchrony. Nevertheless, it should augment cardiac output during activity in appropriately selected patients. Finally, the DDDR pacemaker most closely resembles the normal heart's conduction system because it provides AV synchrony and uses sinus rhythm for the sensor-driven heart rate.

The R in the pacemaker coding system indicates that physiologic or nonphysiologic sensors are used for rate modulation. Exercise intensity for patients with rate-modulating pacemakers can be prescribed using several methods, alone, or in combination (66): the maximal heart rate reserve method of Karvonen (11); a fixed percentage of the maximal heart rate (12); rating of perceived exertion (16); and by METs. If either of the heart rate methods are used, consideration should be given to the upper- and lower-rate limits of the pacemaker device. If signs or symptoms of myocardial ischemia occur during exercise, the upper limit for prescribed heart rate in DDD and VVIR pacemakers should be set at 10 beats·min^{-1} or more below the person's ischemic threshold. Reprogramming of maximum heart rate below the ischemic threshold should also be considered.

Various rate-responsive sensors have relative advantages and disadvantages. Exercise recommendations for patients with nonphysiologic sensors, such as a motion sensitive piezoelectric crystal device or accelerometer, should be carefully designed with respect to the type and intensity of activity. For example, treadmill exercise should use speed increments more than gradient changes because these units may respond at an inappropriately slower rate during uphill walking, despite comparable aerobic requirements. Similarly, stationary cycle ergometry may not produce sufficient motion of the thorax to yield an adequate rise in heart rate. A combined arm-leg ergometer that uses the levers and pedals simultaneously may elicit a more appropriate chronotropic response (66).

Antitachycardia pacemakers and ICDs are commonly used to manage tachyarrhythmias (usually with burst pacing or shock). An ICD consists of a cardioverter device and a lead system. The unit is designed to recognize rapid rhythms and respond in a tiered fashion. Because the device is programmed to detect arrhythmias using heart rate and intervals as the main criteria, it is critical to know the cutoff rate. Persons with ICDs are at risk of receiving inappropriate shocks during exercise if the sinus heart rate exceeds the programmed threshold or the patient develops an exercise-induced supraventricular tachycardia (64). For this reason, patients with ICDs should be closely monitored using continuous or instantaneous ECG telemetry monitoring, pulse palpation, or both, to titrate a safe and effective exercise dose. A magnet should be readily available to override or inactivate the device should it malfunction.

Exercise prescription for pacemaker patients should be based on a recent exercise test, with specific reference to the workload achieved, ECG response, hemodynamics, perceived exertion, and symptoms. The exercise intensity should approximate 50 to 85% of HR reserve, 4 to 7 d·wk^{-1}, 20 to 60 min/session (64). Because of the nonlinear relationship between oxygen consumption and heart rate, especially in patients without rate-adaptive pacemakers, adjunctive target MET levels and perceived exertion limits should be provided. Endurance exercise should be complemented with low- to moderate-intensity resistance training and range-of-motion activities 2 to 3 d·wk^{-1}. For the pacemaker-dependent patient, ST-segment changes that develop during exercise may be uninterpretable with respect to myocardial ischemia. Alternative diagnostic tests that use myocardial perfusion imaging, such as thallous (thallium) chloride-201 or technetium-Tc99m sestamibi (Cardiolite, Dupont Medical, North Billerica, MA), or exercise echocardiography, may be helpful in this regard.

Because some upper body movements may dislodge implanted leads, there is a brief period (approximately 2 to 3 weeks) following pacemaker implantation during which the patient should avoid raising the arm on the affected side above the shoulder. Thereafter, patients may participate in physical activities that are compatible with their functional capacity. Although vigorous upper body activities and contact sports are not advised for patients with pacemakers, most physicians permit routine activities involving the upper extremities. Initial ECG telemetry monitoring may be useful to ensure proper functioning of the pacemaker during progressive physical activity. Particularly important is maintenance of the proper emergency and resuscitation equipment, including a cardioverter/defibrillator with R-wave synchronizing capability (65).

Cardiac Transplant

Cardiac transplantation represents a therapeutic alternative for nearly 3000 patients each year with end-stage heart failure. Moreover, 1- and 3-year survival rates for transplant recipients now approximate 83 and 77%, respectively (68). Despite surgery, cardiac transplant patients continue to experience exercise intolerance due to extended inactivity and convalescence, associated skeletal muscle derangements, loss of muscle mass and strength, and the absence of autonomic cardiac innervation. Because of the adverse side effects of immunosuppressive drug therapy (cyclosporine and prednisone), such as hyperlipidemia, hypertension, obesity, and diabetes, these individuals are at increased risk of developing coronary atherosclerosis of the donor heart. As a result, increasing numbers of patients are being referred to exercise rehabilitation early after cardiac transplantation to improve functional capacity, coronary risk factors, and quality of life (69).

Due to the orthoptic procedure, the ventricle is no longer innervated by the autonomic system. In other words, except for parasympathetic, postganglionic nerve fibers that are left intact, there is a loss of autonomic modulation (e.g., the heart is decentralized). Consequently, there are numerous differences in the cardiorespiratory, ECG (e.g., two separate P waves may be apparent), hemodynamic, and neuroendocrine responses at rest and during exercise when comparing transplant recipients with age and gender matched healthy individuals. Resting sinus tachycardia (90 to 110 beats·min^{-1}) is common, and systolic and diastolic hypertension may be due to elevated catecholamine levels, the effects of immunosuppressive medications, altered baroreceptor sensitivity, or combinations thereof. The cardiovascular response of the denervated heart to exercise is also different.

In the normally innervated heart, the increase in cardiac output during exercise is elicited by a significant increase in heart rate, and, to a lesser extent, in stroke volume. In the denervated heart, the cardioacceleratory response to exercise is delayed, yet cardiac output increases to support the metabolic demand. Studies in cardiac transplant recipients have shown that the initial increase in cardiac output with submaximal exercise is achieved by an increase in stroke volume via the Frank-Starling mechanism because immediate cardioacceleratory stimulation is lacking. At higher work rates, however, the myocardium responds with tachycardia to humoral adrenergic stimulation, specifically to rising plasma norepinephrine levels (70).

The response of cardiac transplant recipients to symptom-limited treadmill or cycle ergometer testing, compared with that of age-matched controls, is characterized by an increase in the respiratory exchange ratio, minute ventilation, and plasma norepinephrine levels at submaximal exercise, increased peak values for ventilatory equivalent and blood lactate, and decreased peak values for heart rate, blood pressure, oxygen uptake, ventilatory threshold, stroke volume, cardiac output, and exercise time (70). Peak oxygen consumption in untrained cardiac transplant recipients generally approximates 17 ± 5 mL·kg^{-1}·min^{-1} (68). In the early postexercise recovery period, elevated catecholamine levels exert a positive chronotropic effect. As a result, heart rate declines slowly. Collectively, these data indicate an earlier onset of anaerobiosis among transplant recipients than in healthy individuals.

Cardiac transplant patients respond to isometric exercise with a normal increase in systolic and diastolic blood pressure and an unchanged heart rate (71), in contrast to the increased heart rate response reported in normal individuals. The mechanism for the isometric-induced blood pressure increase among transplant recipients appears primarily due to increased peripheral vascular resistance, as opposed to enhanced myocardial contractility or an elevated cardiac output.

The exercise prescription for the cardiac transplant recipient should be based on data derived from exercise testing to volitional fatigue, using ramping or steady-state protocols with 1 to 2 MET increments per 3-minute stage (68). Although isolated cases of chest pain have been reported in cardiac transplant recipients, there is generally an absence of anginal symptoms due to denervation. The sensitivity of the exercise ECG in this patient subset is extremely low relative to the detection of myocardial ischemia. Consequently, radionuclide testing or exercise echocardiography may be more appropriate in assessing atherosclerotic heart disease.

Current recommendations to guide exercise intensity in cardiac transplant recipients include: 50 to 75% $\dot{V}O_2$ peak; rating of perceived exertion (11 to 15 on the 6 to 20 scale); METs; ventilatory threshold (when available); and use of the dyspnea scale. Because the initial heart rate response is attenuated and may not correspond with exercise intensity, predetermined work rates or MET loads may be preferred, using perceived exertion and dyspnea ratings as adjunctive guides for training. However, large interindividual variations in RPE at a given oxygen uptake have been reported in this patient population (72). With continued exercise it is not uncommon for cardiac transplant patients to approach or exceed the maximal heart rate achieved on a previous exercise test (68). Longer periods of warm-up and cool-down are indicated because the physiologic responses to exercise and recovery take longer. Cardiac transplant recipients should perform aerobic exercises 4 to 6 d·wk^{-1} while progressively increasing the duration of training from 15 to 60 min/session (68). Low- to moderate-intensity resistance training and range-of-motion activities performed 2 to 3 d·wk^{-1} may be used to complement this regimen. Moreover, 6 months of resistance training prevents glucocorticoid-induced myopathy in heart transplant recipients and restores fat-free mass to levels greater than before transplantation surgery (73).

Surveillance of the transplant patient should focus on resting and exercise blood pressures, possible adverse effects of immunosuppressive drug therapy, and evidence of rejection. Blood pressure should be monitored carefully because hypertension is a common side effect of cyclosporin. Moreover, prednisone therapy may result in numerous side effects, including sodium and fluid retention; loss of muscle mass; glucose intolerance and/or diabetes mellitus; osteoporosis; fat redistribution from the extremities to the torso; gastric irritation; increased appetite; increased susceptibility to infection; predisposition to peptic ulcers; and increased potassium excretion. Finally, knowledge of the most recent cardiac biopsy score is important because rejection exacerbates exercise intolerance. If evidence of rejection is present, the prescribed exercise regimen should be discontinued until this is reversed.

Exercise: An Integral Component of a Comprehensive Treatment Approach

Until the late 1960s, secondary prevention of coronary atherosclerosis focused primarily on early ambulation and exercise training. These regimens generally resulted in improved functional capacity, reduced myocardial demands at submaximal work rates, and modest decreases in cardiovascular mortality. However, reinfarction rates and the course of atherosclerotic heart disease remained largely unchanged. Since then, the treatment of CAD has evolved to an array of costly medical and surgical interventions (Fig. 8-4) that too often fail to address the underlying causes—high-fat and high-cholesterol diets, cigarette smoking, hypertension, obesity, and physical inactivity.

Contemporary studies now suggest that aggressive coronary risk factor modification, and especially more intensive measures to control hyperlipidemia with diet, drugs, and exercise, especially in combination, may slow, halt, and even reverse the otherwise inexorable progression of atherosclerotic CAD (74). Added benefits include a reduction in anginal symptoms, decreases in exercise-induced myocardial ischemia, fewer recurrent cardiac events, and a diminished need for coronary revascularization. Several mechanisms may contribute to these improved clinical outcomes, including partial (albeit small) anatomic regression of coronary artery stenoses, a reduced incidence of plaque rupture, and improved coronary artery vasomotor function. These findings suggest a new paradigm in the treatment of patients with CAD.

An American Heart Association expert panel published a set of comprehensive risk-reduction strategies designed to extend overall survival, improve quality of life, decrease the need for revascularization, and reduce subsequent cardiovascular events in patients with coronary heart and vascular disease (55). These consensus strategies were endorsed by the American College of Cardiology and, when amplified to include homocysteine interventions (B vitamins) and psychosocial counseling, can be summarized as the "ABCDE'Ss" of secondary prevention (Box 8-6). Each letter represents one or more specific interventions. Today, exercise remains an integral component of a comprehensive approach to treating heart disease (Fig. 8-5)—an approach that also includes psychosocial and/or vocational coun-

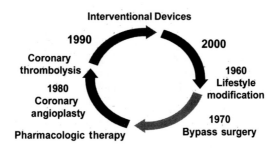

FIGURE 8-4. In the 1960s, treatment of heart disease largely involved early ambulation and exercise training. Since then, bypass surgery, intensive pharmacotherapy, angioplasty, thrombolytics, and interventional devices (e.g., coronary stents) have emerged. However, recent studies have shown that aggressive risk factor reduction, including exercise training, can stabilize and even reverse the atherosclerotic process.

BOX 8-6. ABCDE's of Secondary Prevention: Comprehensive Risk Reduction Strategies for Patients With Coronary and Other Vascular Disease*

Risk Intervention   **Recommendations**

Antiplatelet agents/anticoagulants—Start aspirin 80 to 325 mg/d if not contraindicated. Consider warfarin to international normalized ratio = 2 to 3.5 for post-MI patients not able to take aspirin.

ACE inhibitors post-MI—Start early post-MI in stable high-risk patients (e.g., anterior MI). Continue indefinitely for all patients with left ventricular dysfunction (ejection fraction ≤ 40%) or symptoms of failure.

β-Blockers—Start in high-risk post-MI patients at 5 to 28 days for ≥6 months. Observe usual contraindications.

B vitamins—Ensure adequate intake of folate (≥0.4 mg/day), vitamin B_6 (≥2 mg/day for men and 1.6 mg/day for women) and vitamin B_{12} (≥0.002 mg/day for men and women) to reduce elevated homocysteine levels.

Blood pressure control—Initiate lifestyle modification in all patients with BP >140 mm Hg systolic or 90 mm Hg diastolic. Add BP medications if these goals are not achieved in 3 months or if initial BP is >160 mm Hg systolic or 100 mm Hg diastolic.

Cholesterol management—Primary goal, LDL < 100 mg/dL; Secondary goals, HDL > 35 mg/dL; TG < 200 mg/dL. Initiate lifestyle modifications (e.g., low-fat, low-cholesterol diet, exercise, smoking cessation) and, if needed to achieve LDL goals, consider niacin, statin, fibrate.

Diet—At a minimum, start AHA Step II Diet in all patients: ≤30% fat, <7% saturated fat, <200 mg/d cholesterol. Modify as necessary.

Exercise—Encourage minimum of 30 to 60 min of moderate-intensity activity 3 or 4 times weekly supplemented by an increase in daily lifestyle activities. Maximum benefit 5 to 6 hours a week.

Estrogen therapy—Consider estrogen replacement in all post-menopausal women. Individualize recommendation consistent with other health risks.

Social support—Numerous studies now suggest that social support (via the spouse, family, friends, and health care professionals) is helpful in combating the deleterious effects of heart disease.

Stop smoking—Strongly encourage patient and family to stop smoking. Provide counseling, nicotine replacement and formal smoking cessation programs as appropriate. Such programs are generally effective in ~20 ± 5% of all patients.

Stress series—Patients should be encouraged to participate in a well-structured stress reduction series involving education, counseling, and psychosocial interventions, as these have been shown to be effective in lowering levels of self-reported emotional stress, depression, hypochondriasis, and social isolation and in favorably modifying Type-A behavior.

*Adapted from Smith SC, Blair SN, Criqui MH, et al. Preventing heart attack and death in patients with coronary disease. Circulation 1995;92:2–4.

MI, myocardial infarction; BP, blood pressure; LDL, low-density lipoprotein cholesterol; HDL, high-density lipoprotein cholesterol; TG, triglycerides; AHA, American Heart Association.

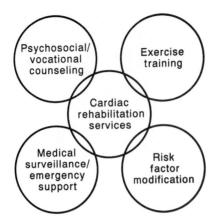

FIGURE 8-5. Core components of a contemporary cardiac rehabilitation program.

seling, medical surveillance and/or emergency support, and aggressive coronary risk factor modification.

References

1. American Association of Cardiovascular and Pulmonary Rehabilitation. Guidelines for Cardiac Rehabilitation and Secondary Prevention Programs. 3rd ed. Champaign, IL: Human Kinetics, 1999.
2. Fletcher GA, Balady G, Froelicher VF, et al. Exercise standards: a statement for healthcare professionals from the American Heart Association. Circulation 1995;91:580–615.
3. Franklin BA, Hall L, Timmis GC. Contemporary cardiac rehabilitation services. Am J Cardiol 1997;79:1075–1077.
4. Health and Public Policy Committee, American College of Physicians. Cardiac rehabilitation services. Ann Intern Med 1988;15:671–673.
5. Hillegass EA, Sadowsky HS, eds. Essentials of Cardiopulmonary Physical Therapy. Philadelphia: WB Saunders, 1994.
6. Convertino VA. Effect of orthostatic stress on exercise performance after bed rest: relation to in-hospital rehabilitation. J Cardiac Rehabil 1983;3:660–663.
7. Sivarajan ES, Bruce RA, Almes MJ, et al. In-hospital exercise after myocardial infarction does not improve treadmill performance. N Engl J Med 1981;305:357–362.
8. Oldridge NB, Rogowski BL. Self-efficacy and in-patient cardiac rehabilitation. Am J Cardiol 1990;66:362–365.
9. Franklin BA, Gordon S, Timmis GC. Amount of exercise necessary for the patient with coronary artery disease. Am J Cardiol 1992;69:1426–1432.
10. Wilmore JH. Exercise prescription: role of the physiatrist and allied health professional. Arch Phys Med Rehabil 1976;57:315–319.
11. Karvonen M, Kentala K, Mustala O. The effects of training on heart rate: a longitudinal study. Annales Medicinae Experimentalis et Biologiae Fenniae 1957;35:307–315.
12. American Heart Association. Exercise testing and training of individuals with heart disease or at high risk for its development: a handbook for physicians. Dallas: American Heart Association, 1975.
13. Swain DP, Leutholtz BC. Heart rate reserve is equivalent to $\dot{V}O_2$ reserve, not to $\dot{V}O_{2max}$. Med Sci Sports Exerc 1997;29:837–843.
14. Davis JA, Convertino VA. A comparison of heart rate methods for predicting endurance training intensity. Med Sci Sports 1975;7:295–298.
15. Pollock ML, Gaesser GA, Butcher JD, et al. The recommended quantity and quality of exercise for developing and maintaining cardiorespiratory and muscular fitness, and flexibility in healthy adults. Med Sci Sports Exerc 1998;30:975–991.
16. Borg G. Borg's Perceived Exertion and Pain Scales. Champaign, IL: Human Kinetics, 1998.
17. Whaley MH, Brubaker PH, Kaminsky LA, et al. Validity of rating of perceived exertion during

graded exercise testing in apparently healthy adults and cardiac patients. J Cardiopulm Rehabil 1997;17:261–267.

18. Pollock ML, Lowenthal DT, Foster C, et al. Acute and chronic responses to exercise in patients treated with beta-blockers. J Cardiopulm Rehabil 1991;11:132–144.

19. Hoberg E, Schuler G, Kunze B, et al. Silent myocardial ischemia as a potential link between lack of premonitoring symptoms and increased risk of cardiac arrest during physical stress. Am J Cardiol 1990;65:583–589.

20. American College of Sports Medicine Position Stand. Exercise for patients with coronary artery disease. Med Sci Sports Exerc 1994;26(3):i–v.

21. Pollock ML, Gettman LR, Milesis CA, et al. Effects of frequency and duration of training on attrition and incidence of injury. Med Sci Sports 1977;9:31–36.

22. Dressendorfer RH, Franklin BA, Cameron JL, et al. Exercise training frequency in early post infarction cardiac rehabilitation: influence on aerobic conditioning. J Cardiopulm Rehabil 1995;15:269–276.

23. Pate RR, Pratt M, Blair SN, et al. Physical activity and public health: a recommendation from the Centers for Disease Control and Prevention and the American College of Sports Medicine. JAMA 1995;273:402–407.

24. McConnell TR. Exercise prescription: when the guidelines do not work. J Cardiopulm Rehabil 1996;16:34–37.

25. Hlatky MA, Boineau RE, Higginbotham MB, et al. A brief self-administered questionnaire to determine functional capacity (the Duke Activity Status Index). Am J Cardiol 1989;64:651–654.

26. Myers JN, Do D, Herbert W, et al. A nomogram to predict exercise capacity from a specific activity questionnaire and clinical data. Am J Cardiol 1994;73:591–596.

27. McConnell TR, Klinger TA, Gardner JK, et al. Cardiac rehabilitation without exercise tests for post-myocardial infarction and post-bypass surgery patients. J Cardiopulm Rehabil 1998;18:458–463.

28. Pollock ML, Franklin BA, Balady GJ, et al. Resistance exercise in individuals with and without cardiovascular disease: benefits, rationale, safety, and prescription. Circulation (in press).

29. McCartney N, McKelvie RS, Martin J, et al. Weight-training-induced attenuation of the circulatory response of older males to weight lifting. J Appl Physiol 1993;74:1056–1060.

30. Hickson RC, Rosenkoetter MA, Brown MM. Strength training effects on aerobic power and short-term endurance. Med Sci Sports Exerc 1980;12:336–339.

31. Wenger NK, Froelicher ES, Smith LK, et al. Cardiac rehabilitation as secondary prevention. Clinical practice guideline No. 17. Rockville, MD: US Department of Health and Human Services, Public Health Service, Agency for Health Care Policy and Research and the National Heart, Lung, and Blood Institute; October 1995. AHCPR Publication No. 96-0672.

32. Franklin BA, Bonzheim K, Gordon S, et al. Resistance training in cardiac rehabilitation. J Cardiopulm Rehabil 1991;11:99–107.

33. Fiatarone MA, Marks EC, Ryan ND, et al. High-intensity strength training in nonagenarians. JAMA 1990;263:3029–3034.

34. Fragnoli-Munn K, Savage PD, Ades PA. Combined resistive-aerobic training in older patients with coronary artery disease early after myocardial infarction. J Cardiopulm Rehabil 1998;18:416–420.

35. Verrill DE, Ribisl PM. Resistive exercise training in cardiac rehabilitation: an update. Sports Med 1996;21:347–383.

36. Kelemen MH. Resistive training safety and assessment guidelines for cardiac and coronary prone patients. Med Sci Sports Exerc 1989;21:675–677.

37. Wilke NA, Sheldahl LM, Tristani FE, et al. The safety of static-dynamic effort soon after myocardial infarction. Am Heart J 1985;110:542–545.

38. Feigenbaum MS, Pollock ML. Strength training: rationale for current guidelines for adult fitness programs. Physician Sportsmed 1997;24:44–64.

39. American College of Sports Medicine. Guidelines for Exercise Testing and Prescription. 5th ed. Baltimore: Williams & Wilkins, 1995.

40. US Department of Health and Human Services. Physical activity and health: a report of the Surgeon General. Atlanta: US Deptartment of Health and Human Services, Centers for Disease Control and Prevention, National Center for Chronic Disease Prevention and Health Promotion; 1996.

41. Pollock ML, Graves JE, Swart DL, et al. Exercise training and prescription for the elderly. South Med J 1994;87:S88–S95.

42. Fardy PS, Webb D, Hellerstein HK. Benefits of arm exercise in cardiac rehabilitation. Physician Sportsmed 1977;5:30–41.

43. Franklin BA. Exercise testing, training and arm ergometry. Sports Med 1985;2:100–119.

44. Hellerstein HK, Hirsch EZ, Ader R, et al. Principles of exercise prescription for normals and cardiac subjects. In: Naughton JP, Hellerstein HK, eds. Exercise Testing and Exercise Training in Coronary Heart Disease. New York: Academic Press, 1973:129–167.

45. Goss FL, Robertson RJ, Auble TE, et al. Are treadmill-based exercise prescriptions generalizable to combined arm and leg exercise? J Cardiopulm Rehabil 1987;7:551–555.

46. Wetherbee S, Franklin BA, Hollingsworth V, et al. Relationship between arm and leg training work loads in men with heart disease: implications for exercise prescription. Chest 1991;99:1271–1273.

47. Makalous SL, Araujo J, Thomas TR. Energy expenditure during walking with hand weights. Physician Sportsmed 1988;16:139–148.

48. Sheldahl LM, Wilke NA, Tristani FE. Evaluation and training for resumption of occupational and leisure-time physical activities in patients after a major cardiac event. Med Exerc Nutr Health 1995;4:273–289.

49. Folinsbee LJ. Heat and air pollution: In: Pollock ML, Schmidt DH, eds. Heart Disease and Rehabilitation. 3rd ed. Champaign, IL: Human Kinetics, 1995;327–342.

50. Balady GJ, Fletcher BJ, Froelicher ES, et al. Cardiac rehabilitation programs. A statement for healthcare professionals from the American Heart Association. Circulation 1994;90:1602–1610.

51. Franklin BA. Exercise training and coronary collateral circulation. Med Sci Sports Exerc 1991;23:648–653.

52. Ornish D, Brown SE, Scherwitz LW, et al. Can lifestyle changes reverse coronary heart disease? Lancet 1990;336:129–133.

53. Haskell WL, Alderman EL, Fair JM, et al. Effects of intensive multiple risk factor reduction on coronary atherosclerosis and clinical cardiac events in men and women with coronary artery disease: the Stanford Coronary Risk Intervention Project (SCRIP). Circulation 1994; 89:975–990.

54. Hambrecht R, Niebauer J, Marburger C, et al. Various intensities of leisure time physical activity in patients with coronary artery disease: effects on cardiorespiratory fitness and progression of coronary atherosclerotic lesions. J Am Coll Cardiol 1993;22:468–477.

55. Smith SC, Blair SN, Criqui MH, et al. Preventing heart attack and death in patients with coronary disease. Circulation 1995;92:2–4.

56. American College of Sports Medicine. In: Durstine JL, ed. ACSM's Exercise Management for Persons With Chronic Diseases and Disabilities. Champaign, IL: Human Kinetics, 1997.

57. Friedman D. Angina and silent ischemia. In: Durstine JL, ed. ACSM's Exercise Management for Persons With Chronic Diseases and Disabilities. Champaign, IL: Human Kinetics, 1997: 32–36.

58. Myers JN. Congestive heart failure. In: Durstine JL, ed. ACSM's Exercise Management for Persons With Chronic Diseases and Disabilities. Champaign, IL: Human Kinetics, 1997: 48–53.

59. Belardinelli R, Georgiou D, Cianci G, et al. Randomized, controlled trial of long-term moderate exercise training in chronic heart failure. Circulation 1999;99:1173–1182.

60. Jugdutt BI, Michorowski BL, Kappagoda CT. Exercise training after anterior Q wave myocardial infarction: importance of regional left ventricular function and topography. J Am Coll Cardiol 1988;12:362–372.

61. Giannuzzi P, Temporelli PL, Tavazzi L, et al. EAMI-exercise training in anterior myocardial infarction: an ongoing multicenter randomized study: preliminary results on left ventricular function and remodeling. Chest 1992;101(suppl 5):315S–321S.

62. Giannuzzi P, Tavazzi L, Temporelli PL, et al. Long-term physical training and left ventricular remodeling after anterior myocardial infarction: results of the Exercise in Anterior Myocardial Infarction (EAMI) trial. J Am Coll Cardiol 1993;22:1821–1829.

63. Meyer K, Samek L, Schwaibold M, et al. Interval training in patients with severe chronic heart failure: analysis and recommendation procedures. Med Sci Sports Exerc 1997;29:306–312.

64. West M, Johnson T, Roberts SO. Pacemakers and implantable cardioverter defibrillators. In: Durstine JL, ed. ACSM's Exercise Management for Persons With Chronic Diseases and Disabilities. Champaign, IL: Human Kinetics, 1997:37–41.

65. Schweikert RA, Pashkow FJ, Wilkoff BL. Rehabilitation of patients with arrhythmias, pacemakers, and defibrillators. In: Pashkow FJ, Dafoe WA, eds. Clinical Cardiac Rehabilitation: A Cardiologist's Guide. 2nd ed. Baltimore: Williams & Wilkins, 1999:192–203.

66. Sharp CT, Busse EF, Burgess JJ, et al. Exercise prescription for patients with pacemakers. J Cardiopulm Rehabil 1998;18:421–431.

67. Superko HR. Effects of cardiac rehabilitation in permanently paced patients with third-degree heart block. J Cardiac Rehabil 1983;3:561–568.

68. Keteyian SJ, Brawner C. Cardiac transplant. In: Durstine JL, ed. ACSM's Exercise Management for Persons With Chronic Diseases and Disabilities. Champaign, IL: Human Kinetics, 1997:54–58.

69. Kobashigawa JA, Leaf DA, Lee N, et al. A controlled trial of exercise rehabilitation after heart transplantation. N Engl J Med 1999;340:272–277.

70. Shepard RJ. Responses of the cardiac transplant patient to exercise and training. Exerc Sport Sci Rev 1992;7:297–320.

71. Savin WM, Alderman EL, Haskell WL, et al. Left ventricular response to isometric exercise in patients with denervated and innervated hearts. Circulation 1980;61:897–901.

72. Shephard RJ, Kavanagh T, Mertens DJ, et al. The place of perceived exertion ratings in exercise prescription for cardiac transplant patients before and after training. Br J Sports Med 1996;30:116–121.
73. Braith RW, Welsch MA, Mills RM, et al. Resistance exercise prevents glucocorticoid-induced myopathy in heart transplant recipients. Med Sci Sports Exerc 1998;30:483–489.
74. Franklin BA, Kahn JK. Delayed progression or regression of coronary atherosclerosis with intensive risk factor modification: effects of diet, drugs, and exercise. Sports Med 1996; 22:306–320.

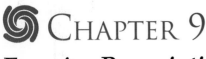 CHAPTER 9

Exercise Prescription for Pulmonary Patients

Exercise training is a key component of pulmonary rehabilitation programs. Documented benefits of exercise training in patients with respiratory disease include increased exercise capacity (endurance), increased functional status, decreased severity of dyspnea, and improved quality of life (1,2). These improvements can be expected from patients regardless of the severity of preexisting lung dysfunction. Although exercise prescription should be individualized for healthy subjects and for patients with coronary artery disease, this concept is even more important for patients with pulmonary disease.

EXERCISE PRESCRIPTION

Current evidence suggests that the standard principles of exercise prescription (mode, frequency, intensity, and duration) can be applied to patients with respiratory diseases, including asthma, chronic obstructive pulmonary disease (COPD), and interstitial lung disease. However, the majority of published data has been obtained from those with COPD.

Mode of Exercise

Any mode of aerobic exercise training involving large muscle groups is appropriate for pulmonary patients. Walking is strongly recommended because it is involved in most activities of daily living. Alternative modes of exercise include cycle ergometry and rowing. It is important that patients have activities—either primary or alternative activities—that can be performed indoors in case of inclement weather.

Frequency

The recommended minimal goal for exercise frequency is 3 to 5 $d \cdot wk^{-1}$. For some individuals, an every other day exercise schedule provides flexibility and time for recovery. Individuals with a reduced functional capacity may require more frequent (i.e., daily) exercise training for optimal improvement.

Intensity

Intensity and duration of exercise training are closely interrelated. At present there is no consensus as to the "optimal" intensity of exercise training for pulmonary patients. The two major approaches are described in Box 9-1 (3,4). Either of these strategies may be used for an individual patient. The exercise professional should closely monitor initial exercise sessions and be ready to adjust intensity and/or duration according to patient responses.

In general, most, if not all, patients with chronic respiratory disease are deconditioned. There is evidence of muscular dysfunction in the lower extremities in patients with COPD (5). Therefore, any training program should improve exercise capacity and reduce dyspnea. Although a higher intensity should lead to greater improvements (e.g., "more is better") (6), this approach should be supervised and may adversely affect patient motivation and compliance. The prescribed intensity for a patient with lung disease should be based on clinical and graded exercise test (GXT) data as well as the patient's specific goals. Early sessions should be supervised so that appropriate adjustments can be made to the exercise intensity, duration, or frequency.

Duration

It is probably unrealistic for most patients with chronic respiratory disease to perform 20 to 30 minutes of continuous exercise at the start of a physical

---

BOX 9-1. Strategies for Selecting Exercise Intensity for Pulmonary Patients

1. **Exercise at 50% of peak oxygen uptake**
   This intensity is consistent with the minimal intensity recommended for healthy adults. Because most patients with moderate-to-severe lung disease are deconditioned, training at this intensity should improve exercise performance and reduce dyspnea. Adherence may be enhanced and the risk of injury reduced at this moderate exercise intensity.

2. **Maximal limits as tolerated by symptoms**
   The principle of high-intensity exercise training is based on the observation that patients with moderate-to-severe COPD can sustain ventilation at a high percentage of their maximal minute ventilatory volume (3). Although most individuals can sustain this intensity for only a few minutes, patients can eventually increase their exercise endurance over time (4).

training program. Therefore, some patients may be able to exercise only at a specified intensity for a few minutes because of dyspnea, leg discomfort, or other symptoms. Intermittent exercise, that is, repetitive exercise-rest periods, may be necessary for the initial training sessions until the patient can achieve sustained physical exertion.

SPECIAL CONSIDERATIONS

Patients with obstructive airway disease (in particular, asthma, COPD, and cystic fibrosis) should be instructed in pursed-lips breathing during exercise, as well as the use of supplemental oxygen.

Pursed-Lips Breathing

Simple patient instructions for pursed-lips breathing are to breathe in through your nose, keep your lips firmly together except at the very center, breathe out twice as long as you breathe in, and when exhaling, "blow the air" out with a firm steady effort. The benefits of pursed-lips breathing are decreased frequency of respiration, increased tidal volume, improved sense of control for oxygenation, and a sense of control for the patient over breathing distress.

Supplemental Oxygen

Some measure of the blood oxygenation, that is, partial pressure of arterial oxygen (P_aO_2) or percent saturation of arterial oxygen (S_aO_2), should be made during the initial GXT. In addition, oximetry is recommended for the initial exercise training sessions to evaluate possible exercise-induced O_2 desaturation. Based on the recommendations of the Nocturnal Oxygen Therapy Trial (7), supplemental O_2 is indicated for patients with a P_aO_2 of 55 mm Hg or less, or an S_aO_2 of 88% or less while breathing room air.

Those same guidelines apply when considering supplemental oxygen during exercise training. The flow rate for O_2 should be titrated to maintain S_aO_2 at 90% or more throughout the exercise period. A trial of oxygen therapy may help evaluate the benefits of oxygen in patients who are extremely breathless during activities despite adequate blood oxygenation. It is unclear whether the addition of supplemental O_2 alters the magnitude of the training effect.

ALTERNATIVE MODES OF EXERCISE TRAINING

Traditional aerobic exercise training may be complemented and enhanced by other therapeutic interventions, including continuous positive airway pressure (CPAP), upper body resistance training, and ventilatory muscle training (VMT).

Continuous Positive Airway Pressure

Dynamic hyperinflation is a physiologic consequence of physical exertion in many patients with obstructive airway disease. Dynamic hyperinflation increases the elastic recoil of the lung parenchyma; the added elastic load must be overcome by the work of the respiratory muscles to begin inspiration. CPAP has been shown to counterbalance the added elastic recoil and thereby "unload" the respiratory muscles and reduce the sense of dyspnea.

The use of CPAP (usually at a pressure of 5 to 10 cm H_2O) can increase exercise duration and/or decrease breathlessness in patients with COPD and those with cystic fibrosis (8,9). Therefore, a trial of CPAP may be considered in individual patients during exercise training because it may allow patients to exercise longer with less dyspnea. CPAP can be delivered to the patient via face mask or mouthpiece and can be titrated upward from an initial level of 2 to 3 cm H_2O, increasing by 2 to 3 cm H_2O based on the patient's subjective ratings of dyspnea or breathing discomfort. Additional studies are required before CPAP can be routinely applied for exercise training purposes.

Upper Body Resistance Training

Resistance training of the upper extremities is an integral part of many pulmonary rehabilitation programs (1,10). Typical exercises include high repetition, low intensity efforts of the arm and shoulder muscles (10,11). These exercises can be done using manual resistance or light weights (1 to 2 kg). Patients should be encouraged to coordinate breathing with upper extremity movement; usually expiration is linked with the motion of the arms requiring the greatest effort.

Ventilatory Muscle Training

Respiratory muscle strength and/or endurance can be specifically increased with ventilatory muscle training. For strength training, high inspiratory resistances with few repetitions are used (e.g., near maximal or maximal inspiratory effort against an occluded airway). For endurance training, low-to-moderate inspiratory resistances are used for 15 to 30 minutes. Resistive inspiratory muscle training may be considered in conjunction with or following an exercise training program. The major indications for VMT are as follows:

- Patients who remain symptomatic and functionally limited despite otherwise optimal therapy
- Patients with decreased respiratory muscle strength (decreased values for inspiratory [PI_{max}] and expiratory [PE_{max}] mouth pressures)
- Absence of severe hyperinflation on chest radiograph

Various studies have demonstrated that respiratory muscle strength and endurance can be increased with VMT. However, it is unclear whether these physiologic changes contribute to consistent improvements in clinical outcomes. In a small number of controlled studies, dyspnea has been shown to be reduced with VMT in patients with COPD (12,13). VMT may be considered in an individual patient using guidelines outlined in Box 9-2. Appropriate clinical measures such as dyspnea ratings, PI_{max} and PE_{max}, and exercise performance should be measured before and after a trial of VMT.

PROGRAM DESIGN AND SUPERVISION

The design and supervision of an exercise training program for patients with respiratory disease depends on multiple factors, including staff availability, facilities for testing and training, and number of patients. Inpatient exercise-based rehabilitation programs should be considered for patients who have a very limited functional status and for those with unstable disease. Inpatient exercise sessions also provide an excellent setting for instruction of both the patient and family members.

There is tremendous variability in current outpatient programs. These vary from patients participating in supervised exercise sessions 5 d·wk^{-1} at a clinic, hospital, or community-based rehabilitation setting, to one supervised session per week with additional unsupervised training in the patient's home, a public facility, or a fitness center. It is essential that program design and supervision be flexible and adapted to local conditions, opportunities, and constraints.

Most formal exercise training programs for pulmonary patients last 6 to 8 weeks, with physiologic, psychologic, and/or clinical benefits noticeable by the end of the program. Exercise prescription, especially intensity, can be modified at any time during the 6- to 8-week period. Upon completion of the program, each patient should be given a written exercise prescription with clear and concise instructions to maintain their improved status. Longer-term community-based programs are beneficial in this population in encouraging continued participation. Ideally, periodic clinical follow-up with repeat testing should be scheduled to enhance the patient's compliance with his or her exercise training. However, geographic and financial considerations may limit this possibility.

Monitoring Exercise Training Intensity

The traditional method for monitoring the training intensity has been heart rate. A pulse oximeter or electrocardiographic telemetry surveillance can

---

BOX 9-2. Guidelines for Ventilatory Muscle Training

1. Frequency—Minimum of 4 to 5 d·wk^{-1}
2. Intensity—30% of PI_{max} measured at functional residual capacity
3. Duration—Two 15-minute sessions or one 30-minute session per day. If this cannot be achieved, the intensity should be reduced.

be readily used during supervised training sessions to verify that the patient's effort matches the desired S_aO_2/heart rate response. However, patients need some guideline for monitoring their training intensity when exercise is unsupervised. Self-palpation of the radial or carotid pulse has been the traditional method for monitoring the appropriate intensity. However, patients usually need to stop exercise to palpate their pulse, and there are inherent inaccuracies with this method, even in healthy adults. An alternative approach is to use a dyspnea rating obtained from a GXT as a "target" for exercise training. Most patients with COPD can accurately and reliably produce a desired exercise intensity using a dyspnea target of approximately 5 ("severe") on the 0–10 category-ratio scale during submaximal exercise of 10 minutes (14). Additional information on exercise in chronic lung disease can be found in *ACSM's Resource Manual for Guidelines for Exercise Testing and Prescription* (15).

References

1. ACCP/AACVPR Pulmonary Rehabilitation Guidelines Panel. Pulmonary rehabilitation: Joint ACCP/AACVPR evidence-based guidelines. Chest 1997;112:1363–1396.
2. Report of the European Respiratory Society Rehabilitation and Chronic Care Scientific Group. Pulmonary rehabilitation in chronic obstructive pulmonary disease (COPD) with recommendations for its use, prepared by C Donner and P Howard. Eur Respir J 1992;5:266–275.
3. Punzal PA, Ries AL, Kaplan RM, et al. Maximum intensity exercise training in patients with chronic obstructive pulmonary disease. Chest 1991;100:618–623.
4. Ries AL, Kaplan RM, Limberg TM, et al. Effects of pulmonary rehabilitation on physiologic and psychosocial outcomes in patients with chronic obstructive pulmonary disease. Ann Intern Med 1995;122:823–832.
5. Maltais F, Simard AA, Simard C, et al. Oxidative capacity of the skeletal muscle and lactic acid kinetics during exercise in normal subjects and in patients with COPD. Am J Respir Crit Care Med 1996;153:288–293.
6. Casaburi R, Patessio A, Ioli F, et al. Reductions in exercise lactic acidosis and ventilation as a result of exercise training in patients with obstructive lung disease. Am Rev Respir Dis 1991;143:9–18.
7. Nocturnal Oxygen Therapy Trial Group. Continuous or nocturnal oxygen therapy in hypoxemic chronic obstructive lung disease: a clinical trial. Ann Intern Med 1980;93:391–398.
8. Henke KG, Regnis JA, Bye PTP. Benefits of continuous positive airway pressure during exercise in cystic fibrosis and relationship to disease severity. Am Rev Respir Dis 1993; 148:1272–1276.
9. O'Donnell DE, Sanii R, Younes M. Improvement in exercise endurance in patients with chronic airflow limitation using continuous positive airway pressure. Am Rev Respir Dis 1988;133:1510–1514.
10. Lake FR, Henderson K, Briffa T, et al. Upper-limb and lower-limb exercise training in patients with chronic airflow obstruction. Chest 1990;97:1077–1082.
11. Simpson K, Killian K, McCartney N, et al. Randomized controlled trial of weightlifting exercise in patients with chronic airflow limitation. Thorax 1992;47:70–75.
12. Harver A, Mahler DA, Daubenspeck JA. Targeted inspiratory muscle training improves respiratory muscle function and reduces dyspnea in patients with chronic obstructive pulmonary disease. Ann Intern Med 1989;111:117–124.
13. Lisboa C, Munoz V, Beroiza T, et al. Inspiratory muscle training in chronic airflow limitation: comparison of two different training loads with a threshold device. Eur Respir J 1994;7:1266–1274.
14. Horowitz MB, Lettenberg B, Mahler DA. Dyspnea ratings for prescribing exercise intensity in patients with COPD. Chest 1996;109:1169–1175.
15. Casaburi R. Special considerations for exercise training in chronic lung disease. In: Roitman J, Kelsey M, eds. ACSM's Resource Manual for Guidelines for Exercise Testing and Prescription. 3rd ed. Baltimore: Williams & Wilkins, 1998:334–338.

⑥ CHAPTER 10
Other Clinical Conditions Influencing Exercise Prescription

Although the general principles of exercise prescription apply to persons with and without chronic disease, certain clinical conditions may require differences in programming to maximize effectiveness and avoid complications. These include persons with hypertension, lower-extremity peripheral vascular disease, diabetes mellitus, and obesity, or those with multiple comorbid conditions.

HYPERTENSION

More than 50 million Americans are hypertensive, as defined by either a resting blood pressure (BP) of 140/90 mm Hg or higher and/or current use of antihypertensive medication (1). The prevalence of hypertension rises sharply with age and is higher in men than in women and in blacks compared with whites. It may be categorized as primary (cause unknown) or secondary (caused by identifiable endocrine or structural disorders). The 1997 classification system recommended by the Joint National Committee on Prevention, Detection, Evaluation, and Treatment of Hypertension (JNC VI) presented in Table 3-1 describes the stages of hypertension. Although stage 1 hypertension is the most common form of high BP in the adult population, all stages are associated with increased risk of nonfatal cardiovascular events and renal disease. Moreover, high-normal BP (i.e., systolic BP of 130 to 139 mm Hg and/or diastolic BP of 85 to 89 mm Hg) is now known to be associated with an accentuated risk for the development of hypertension and target organ damage (1).

Blood pressure is determined by cardiac output and total peripheral resistance. Consequently, it can be augmented by elevations in either, or both, of these variables. The goal of prevention and management of hypertension is to reduce morbidity and mortality by the least intrusive means possible. This may be accomplished by achieving and maintaining a systolic BP below 140 mm Hg and diastolic BP below 90 mm Hg and lower if tolerated, while controlling other cardiovascular disease risk factors (1). To accomplish this, the following lifestyle modifications are recommended, alone or with pharmacologic treatment, by JNC VI:

- Lose weight if overweight.
- Limit alcohol intake to no more than 1 oz (30 mL) of ethanol (e.g., 24 oz [720 mL] of beer, 10 oz [300 mL] of wine, or 2 oz [60 mL] of 100-proof whiskey) per day or 0.5 oz (15 mL) of ethanol per day for women and lighter-weight people.
- Increase aerobic physical activity (accumulate 30 to 45 minutes most days of the week).
- Reduce sodium intake to no more than 100 mmol/d (<2.4 g of sodium or <6 g of sodium chloride).
- Maintain adequate intake of dietary potassium (approximately 90 mmol/d or 3.5 g/d).
- Maintain adequate intake of dietary calcium and magnesium for general health.
- Stop smoking.
- Reduce intake of dietary saturated fat and cholesterol for overall cardiovascular health.

Recently, the effectiveness of dietary intervention in the management of borderline ("high normal") and mild ("stage I") hypertension has been demonstrated (2). The decision to initiate pharmacologic therapy requires consideration of several variables, in particular, the degree of BP elevation, the presence of target organ damage, and the presence of clinical cardiovascular disease or other risk factors (Table 3-2). Specific antihypertensive medications and their effects on the exercise response are outlined in Appendix A.

ACSM makes the following recommendations regarding exercise testing and training of persons with hypertension (3,4):

- Mass exercise testing is not advocated to determine those individuals at high risk for developing hypertension in the future as a result of an exaggerated exercise BP response. However, if exercise test results are available and an individual has a hypertensive response to exercise, this information does provide some indication of risk stratification for that patient and the necessity for appropriate lifestyle counseling to ameliorate this increase. In certain instances, medication changes may be appropriate.
- Endurance exercise training by individuals who are at high risk for developing hypertension will reduce the rise in BP that occurs with age, thus justifying its use as a nonpharmacologic strategy to reduce the incidence of hypertension in susceptible individuals.

- Endurance exercise training will elicit an average reduction of 10 mm Hg for both systolic and diastolic BP in individuals with stage 1 or stage 2 essential hypertension (BP in the range of 140 to 179/90 to 109 mm Hg) and even greater reductions in BP in patients with secondary hypertension due to renal dysfunction.
- The recommended mode, frequency, duration, and intensity of exercise are generally the same as those for low risk individuals. Exercise training at somewhat lower intensities (e.g., 40 to 70% $\dot{V}O_{2max}$) appears to lower BP as much as, if not more than, exercise at higher intensities, which may be especially important in specific hypertensive populations, such as the elderly.
- Based on the high number of exercise-related health benefits and low risk for morbidity and/or mortality, it seems reasonable to recommend exercise as part of the initial treatment strategy for individuals with stage 1 or stage 2 essential hypertension.
- Individuals with more marked elevations in BP should add endurance exercise training to their treatment regimen only after initiating pharmacologic therapy; exercise may reduce their BP further, allow them to decrease their antihypertensive medications, and attenuate their risk for premature mortality.
- Resistance training is not recommended as the primary form of exercise training for hypertensive individuals. With the exception of circuit weight training, resistance training has not consistently been shown to lower BP. Thus, resistance training is recommended as a component of a well-rounded fitness program, but not when done independently.

See Table 10-1 for additional exercise testing and prescription guidelines.

LOWER-EXTREMITY PERIPHERAL VASCULAR DISEASE

Peripheral vascular disease (PVD) is a generic term that encompasses vascular insufficiencies such as arteriosclerosis, arterial stenosis, Raynaud's phenomenon (an abnormal vasomotor tone exacerbated by cold exposure), and Buerger disease (an inflammation of the sheath encapsulating the neurovascular bundle in the extremities). Peripheral arteriosclerosis is common in the elderly and is often associated with hypertension and hyperlipidemia. Peripheral vascular disease is frequently observed in patients with coronary artery disease, diabetes mellitus, and a long-term history of cigarette smoking.

Patients with PVD may have clinical manifestations related to arterial circulatory involvement of the lower extremities or of the brain. Patients with lower-extremity PVD may experience ischemic pain (claudication) during physical activity as a result of a mismatch between active muscle oxygen supply and demand. The various manifestations of the symptoms may be described as burning, searing, aching, tightness, or cramping. The pain is most often experienced in the calf of the leg but can begin in the buttock region and radiate down the leg. The symptoms typically disappear on cessation of exercise.

Assessment of the extent of disease is possible through many procedures, including physical examination, Doppler studies, ankle-to-arm pressure indices, nuclear medicine flow studies, and arteriography. To determine the ankle/brachial systolic pressure index (ABI), ankle systolic BP is measured and expressed relative to the brachial systolic BP. Ankle systolic BP and ABI are obtained during supine rest and following exercise. Based on the literature, an abnormal ABI has ranged from 0.80 to 0.97, with a value of 0.90 or less generally considered to be the reference criterion. The normal range of ABI is widely accepted as a value of 1.00 or higher, with values between 0.91 and 1.00 considered to represent borderline peripheral arterial occlusive disease (5). Ankle systolic BP and ABI are reduced after exercise because blood flow is shunted into the proximal leg musculature at the expense of the periphery and distal areas of the leg. Severe lower-extremity PVD is treated initially with cardiovascular disease risk factor modification, exercise training, and medications that decrease blood viscosity (such as pentoxifylline or Trental, dipyridamole or Persantine [Boehringer Ingelheim, Inc., Ridgefield, CT], warfarin or Coumadin [Dupont, Wilmington, DE], and aspirin) (6). Treatment with angioplasty (with or without stenting) or bypass grafting may also be indicated. Weight-bearing exercise (i.e., walking) is preferred to facilitate greater functional changes (7) but may not be well-tolerated initially. As such, prescription of non–weight-bearing exercise (which may permit a greater intensity or longer duration) is a suitable alternative. See Table 10-1 for exercise testing and prescription guidelines. A subjective grading scale for PVD pain is as follows:

- Grade 1   Definite discomfort or pain, but only of initial or modest levels (established, but minimal)
- Grade 2   Moderate discomfort or pain from which the patient's attention can be diverted, for example by conversation
- Grade 3   Intense pain (short of grade 4) from which the patient's attention cannot be diverted
- Grade 4   Excruciating and unbearable pain

If treadmill testing in patients with PVD is prematurely stopped due to ischemic leg pain, an arm ergometer evaluation should be considered to establish the prescribed heart rate for arm exercise training (e.g., arm ergometry, rowing) because a higher peak heart rate may be achieved (8). As functional capacity improves with less peripheral limitations, central cardiac responses may assume greater importance, and angina may be revealed. This may require further modification of the program in terms of supervision, intensity, and duration.

TABLE 10-1. Recommendations for Special Populations

Condition	Exercise Test Methods	Exercise Prescription	Exercise Precautions
Hypertension	Standard methods and protocols Medications should be taken at usual time relative to the exercise bout Observe for exaggerated pressor response (systolic BP >260 mm Hg or diastolic BP >115 mm Hg are indications for test termination)	Frequency: 3–7 d·wk^{-1} Duration: 30–60 min Intensity: 40–70% $\dot{V}O_{2max}$ Aim for 700–2000 kcal/week Resistance training should involve lower resistance with higher repetitions	Do not exercise if resting systolic BP > 200 mm Hg or diastolic BP > 115 mm Hg β-Blockers attenuate heart rate α_1-Blockers, α_2-blockers, calcium channel blockers, and vasodilators may cause postexertion hypotension: emphasize adequate cool-down Diuretics may cause a decrease in K$^+$, leading to arrhythmias Avoid Valsalva maneuvers during resistance training
Peripheral vascular disease	Multi-stage discontinuous protocol may be necessary to achieve peak O$_2$ consumption Use scale for subjective ratings of pain Record time of pain onset and maximal pain If symptom limited at low work rates, consider arm ergometer	Frequency: 3–7 d·wk^{-1} Duration: 20–40 min/session Intensity: 40–70% of $\dot{V}O_{2max}$. May require intermittent exercise to 3 out of 4 on claudication scale Weight bearing activities are preferred, but non–weight-bearing activities may allow longer duration and higher-intensity exercise	High-risk for coronary artery disease β-Blockers may decrease time to claudication Pentoxifylline, dipyridamole, aspirin, and warfarin may improve time to claudication Improvement in exercise tolerance may unmask myocardial ischemia

Diabetes	May require modification of standard protocols or arm ergometry. Autonomic neuropathy may be associated with silent ischemia, postural hypotension, and/or blunted heart rate response	Frequency: 4–6 d·wk^{-1}, or daily at low to moderate intensity. Duration: 20–60 min/session. Intensity: 50–85% $\dot{V}O_{2max}$. Type 2: maximize caloric expenditure if obese. May need to use perceived exertion as an adjunct to heart rate for monitoring exercise intensity	Postpone exercise if blood glucose > 300 mg/dL or > 240 mg/dL with urinary ketone bodies. Especially when beginning a program, monitor blood glucose before, during, and after exercise if taking insulin or oral agents. Adjustments in carbohydrate intake and/or insulin may be needed before testing and training; ingest carbohydrate if blood glucose is <80–100 mg/dL. Exercising late in the evening increases risk of nocturnal hypoglycemia. Exercise caution when exercising in hot weather
Obesity	Standard methods and protocols. Use of cycle or arm ergometry may enhance testing capability	Frequency: 5 d·wk^{-1} or daily. Duration: 40–60 min/session (or 2 sessions/day of 20–30 min). Intensity: 40/50–70% $\dot{V}O_{2max}$. Initially emphasize increasing duration rather than intensity with goal of optimizing caloric expenditure. Use of low-impact modes of activity. Strength training may serve as a valuable adjunct to aerobic training	Increased risk of orthopedic injury, cardiovascular disease, and hyperthermia: take appropriate precautions. Equipment modification may be necessary, e.g., wide seats on cycle ergometers and rowers

DIABETES MELLITUS

Diabetes mellitus is a group of metabolic diseases characterized by hyperglycemia resulting from defects in insulin secretion, insulin action, or both. The chronic hyperglycemia of diabetes is associated with long-term damage, dysfunction, and failure of various organs, especially the eyes, kidneys, nerves, heart, and blood vessels (9). Most cases of diabetes fall into two broad etiopathogenetic categories. In one category (type 1 diabetes), the cause is an absolute deficiency of insulin secretion. In the other, much more prevalent category (type 2 diabetes), the cause is a combination of resistance to insulin action and an inadequate compensatory insulin secretory response. Recently revised diagnostic criteria for diabetes are as follows (9):

1. Symptoms of diabetes plus casual plasma glucose concentration of >200 mg/dL (11.1 mmol/L) (*casual* is defined as any time of day without regard to time since the last meal); the classic symptoms of diabetes include polyuria, polydipsia, and unexplained weight loss; or
2. Fasting plasma glucose of >126 mg/dL (7.0 mmol/L) (*fasting* is defined as no caloric intake for at least 8 hours); or
3. Two-hour plasma glucose of >200 mg/dL during an oral glucose tolerance test; the test should be performed as described by World Health Organization, using a glucose load containing the equivalent of 75 g anhydrous glucose dissolved in water.

In the absence of unequivocal hyperglycemia with acute metabolic decompensation, the aforementioned criteria should be confirmed by repeat testing on a different day. The third measure, oral glucose tolerance testing, is not recommended for routine clinical use.

In some individuals with type 2 diabetes, adequate glycemic control can be achieved with exercise training and weight reduction. Oral hypoglycemic agents are needed to achieve adequate glycemic control in other individuals with type 2 diabetes who do not require insulin. However, there are other individuals with type 2 diabetes who have some residual insulin secretion but still require exogenous insulin for adequate glycemic control. Although these individuals can survive without exogenous insulin, individuals with type 1 diabetes have extensive β-cell destruction and require exogenous insulin for survival (9).

The response to exercise in the diabetic taking insulin depends on a variety of factors, including the adequacy of control by exogenous insulin. If the diabetic is under appropriate control or is only slightly hyperglycemic without ketosis, exercise decreases blood glucose concentration, and a lower insulin dosage may be required. However, problems can arise during exercise if the diabetic is not under adequate control. A lack of sufficient insulin before exercise may impair glucose transport into the muscles, limiting the availability of glucose as an energy substrate. To compensate, use of free fatty acids increases and ketone bodies are produced, possibly leading to the development of ketosis. In addition, the resulting greater glucose production further exacerbates the hyperglycemic state. For these reasons, diabetics must be under adequate control before beginning an exercise program. A blood glucose concentration greater than 300 mg/dL or greater than 240 mg/dL with urinary ketone bodies is considered a relative contraindication to exercise participation (10).

Because exercise has an insulin-like effect, however, exercise-induced hypoglycemia is the most common problem experienced by exercising diabetics who take exogenous insulin (or, to a lesser degree, oral hypoglycemic agents). Hypoglycemia may result when too much insulin is present, or if there is accelerated absorption of insulin from the injection site, both of which may occur with exercise. Hypoglycemia occurs not only during exercise, but may occur up to 4 to 6 hours after an exercise bout. To counteract this response, the diabetic may need to reduce his or her insulin dosage or increase carbohydrate intake before or after exercise. In persons taking insulin, consideration should be given to the ingestion of 20 to 30 grams of additional carbohydrate before exercise when the preexercise blood glucose is below 100 mg/dL.

The risk of hypoglycemic events may be minimized by taking the following precautions (11):

- Measure blood glucose before, during, and after exercise.
- Avoid exercise during periods of peak insulin activity.
- Unplanned exercise should be preceded by extra carbohydrates, e.g., 20 to 30 g/30 min of exercise; insulin may have to be decreased after exercise.
- If exercise is planned, insulin dosages must be decreased before and after exercise, according to the exercise intensity and duration as well as the personal experience of the patient; insulin dosage reductions may amount to 50 to 90% of daily insulin requirements.
- During exercise, easily absorbable carbohydrates may have to be consumed.
- After exercise, an extra carbohydrate-rich snack may be necessary.
- Be knowledgeable of the signs and symptoms of hypoglycemia.
- Exercise with a partner.

Other precautions that should be taken include 1) wearing proper footwear and practicing good foot hygiene, 2) realizing that β-blockers may attenuate cardiac demands and prevent angina and that other medications may interfere with the ability to discern hypoglycemic symptoms, and 3) recognizing that exercise in excessive heat may exacerbate the risk of heat injury in diabetics with autonomic neuropathy. Patients with advanced retinopathy should not perform activities that cause excessive jarring or marked increases in blood pressure. Patients should have physician approval to resume exercise training following laser treatment. See Table 10-1 for exercise testing and prescription guidelines (12).

OBESITY

Obesity is a serious and common public health problem. The most recent National Health and Nutrition Examination Survey (NHANES III) reported that 33.4% of Americans are overweight (13), representing an increase from the 25% prevalence found in the earlier (1976–1980) survey. Obesity may be classified as a body mass index of 30.0 kg/m² or more, and it is functionally defined as the percent body fat at which disease risk increases. Body fat is reduced when a chronic negative caloric balance exists. It is recommended that both an increase in caloric expenditure through exercise and a decrease in caloric intake be used to accomplish this goal. Exercise increases energy expenditure and slows the rate of fat-free tissue loss that occurs when a person loses weight by severe caloric restriction. Exercise also helps maintain the resting metabolic rate, which contributes significantly to the daily caloric expenditure.

Obese individuals are almost invariably sedentary and many have had poor experiences with exercise. The exercise professional should interview the obese participant to determine past exercise history, potential scheduling difficulties, and the locations where exercise might be performed (e.g., sports club, home, street, school gym, or track). This may increase adherence to an agreed upon exercise program.

The initial exercise prescription should be based on low intensity and progressively longer durations of activity. Based on each person's response to the initial exercise program, the exercise professional should eventually work toward increasing the intensity to bring the person into a target heart rate range suitable for cardiorespiratory conditioning. The higher intensity will allow for a shorter duration per session, or fewer sessions per week for the same weekly energy expenditure, and permit a greater number of opportunities to incorporate vigorous activities into daily living. For many (especially older) obese subjects, however, a walking or other moderate-intensity exercise program may be all they desire, and movement toward a more intense program may not be warranted. The needs and goals of the obese subject must be individually matched with the proper exercise program to achieve long-term weight management.

Programs for Reducing Body Fatness

An excessive percentage of body fat is associated with increased risk for development of hypertension, diabetes, coronary artery disease, and other chronic diseases. Recent evidence indicates that "central obesity" (fat deposited primarily in the trunk or abdominal region) is particularly problematic. In addition, obesity often carries a negative social stigma and is associated with a reduced physical working capacity. Because reduction of body fatness is a need or a goal of many exercise program participants, exercise prescriptions should be designed to aid in accomplishing this objective. The following sections present the principles that should be employed in modifying body composition.

CALORIC BALANCE

Body composition is determined by a complex set of genetic and behavioral factors. Although the contributing variables are many, the fundamental determinant of body weight and body composition is caloric balance. Caloric balance refers to the difference between caloric intake (the energy equivalent of the food ingested) and caloric expenditure (the energy equivalent of resting metabolic rate, activity, thermic effect of food). The First Law of Thermodynamics states that energy is neither created nor destroyed; therefore, body weight is lost when caloric expenditure exceeds caloric intake (negative balance), and weight is gained when the opposite situation exists. One pound of fat is equivalent to approximately 3500 kcal of energy (1 kg approximately equal to 7700 kcal). Although it is predictable that shifts in caloric balance will be accompanied by changes in body weight, the nature of the weight change varies markedly with the specific behaviors that lead to the caloric imbalance. For example, fasting and extreme caloric restriction (starvation and semistarvation diets) cause substantial losses of water and fat-free tissue. In contrast, an exercise-induced negative caloric balance attenuates the loss of fat-free mass during a weight reduction program. Moreover, adjunctive resistance training may help preserve fat-free weight. Both aerobic exercise and resistance training can contribute to the loss of body weight and fat stores and maximize the potential to maintain these changes.

RECOMMENDED WEIGHT LOSS PROGRAMS

For most persons, the optimal approach to weight loss combines a mild caloric restriction with regular endurance exercise and avoids nutritional deficiencies. A desirable weight loss program is one that meets the following criteria:

- Provides intake of not lower than 1200 kcal/day for normal adults and allows for a proper distribution of foods to meet nutritional requirements. (Note: this requirement may not be appropriate for children, older individuals, and athletes.)
- Includes foods acceptable to the dieter in terms of sociocultural background, usual habits, taste, costs, and ease in acquisition and preparation; however, these foods should be low in total fat, saturated fat, cholesterol, and sodium.
- Provides a negative caloric balance (not to exceed 500 to 1000 kcal/day), resulting in gradual weight loss without metabolic derangements, such as ketosis.
- Results in a maximal weight loss of 1 kg/week.
- Includes the use of behavior modification techniques to identify and eliminate diet habits that contribute to malnutrition.

- Includes an exercise program that promotes a daily caloric expenditure of more than 300 kcal. For many participants, this may be accomplished best with moderate-intensity, long-duration exercise, such as walking.
- Provides that new eating and physical activity habits can be continued for life to maintain the achieved lower body weight.

When the exercise component of a weight loss program is designed, the balance between intensity and duration of exercise should be manipulated to promote a high total caloric expenditure (300 to 500 kcal per day and 1000 to 2000 kcal per week for adults). Obese individuals are at an increased relative risk for orthopedic injury, and this may require that the intensity of exercise be maintained at or below the intensity recommended for improvement of cardiorespiratory endurance. Non–weight-bearing activities (and/or rotation of exercise modalities) may be necessary, and frequent modifications in frequency and duration may also be required. See Table 10-1 for exercise testing and prescription guidelines (14).

References

1. The Sixth Report of the Joint National Committee on Prevention, Detection, Evaluation, and Treatment of High Blood Pressure (JNC VI). Arch Intern Med 1997;157:2413–2446.
2. Svetkey LP, Simons-Morton D, Vollmer W, et al. Effects of dietary patterns on blood pressure. Arch Intern Med 1999;159:285–293.
3. American College of Sports Medicine. Physical activity, physical fitness, and hypertension. Position stand. Med Sci Sports Exerc 1993;25:i–x.
4. Gordon NF. Hypertension. In: Durstine JL, ed. ACSM's Exercise Management for Persons With Chronic Diseases and Disabilities. Champaign, IL: Human Kinetics, 1997:59–63.
5. Weitz JI, Byrne J, Clagett P, et al. Diagnosis and treatment of chronic arterial insufficiency of the lower extremities: a critical review. Circulation 1996;94:3026–3049.
6. Gardner AW. Peripheral arterial disease. In: Durstine JL, ed. ACSM's Exercise Management for Persons With Chronic Diseases and Disabilities. Champaign, IL: Human Kinetics, 1997:64–68.
7. Gardner AW, Poehlman ET. Exercise rehabilitation programs for the treatment of claudication pain: a meta-analysis. JAMA 1995;274:975–980.
8. Fardy PS, Webb D, Hellerstein HK. Benefits of arm exercise in cardiac rehabilitation. Physician Sportsmed 1977;5:30–41.
9. Report of the Expert Committee on the Diagnosis and Classification of Diabetes Mellitus. Diabetes Care 1997;20:1183–1197.
10. Gordon NF. The exercise prescription. In: The Health Professional's Guide to Diabetes and Exercise. Alexandria, VA: American Diabetes Association, 1995:70–82.
11. Berger M. Adjustment of insulin therapy. In: The Health Professional's Guide to Diabetes and Exercise. Alexandria, VA: American Diabetes Association, 1995:116–122.
12. Albright AL. Diabetes. In: Durstine JL, ed. ACSM's Exercise Management for Persons With Chronic Diseases and Disabilities. Champaign, IL: Human Kinetics, 1997:94–100.
13. Kuczmarski RJ, Flegal KM, Campbell SM, et al. Increasing prevalence of overweight among US adults, 1960 to 1991. JAMA 1994;272:205–211.
14. Wallace JP. Obesity. In: Durstine JL, ed. ACSM's Exercise Management for Persons With Chronic Diseases and Disabilities. Champaign, IL: Human Kinetics, 1997:106–111.

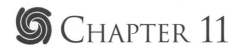 CHAPTER 11
Exercise Testing and Prescription for Children, the Elderly, and Pregnant Women

This chapter addresses recommended procedures for exercise testing and prescription for three nondiseased special populations—children, the elderly, and pregnant women. Each of these groups possesses unique physical, physiologic, and behavioral characteristics that require special consideration for exercise testing and training.

CHILDREN

Assessment of the cardiorespiratory response to exercise in children may involve fitness testing or, in those with symptoms, established disease, or suspected medical abnormalities, clinical exercise testing.

Fitness Testing

Measurement of physical fitness and health in children and adolescents is a common practice in school-based physical education. Such testing has also been used in recreational programs, public health assessments, and clinical settings. Typically a battery of simple field tests (generally 4 to 6 tests) are administered to evaluate different components of fitness and/or health (1–4). Two of the most commonly administered battery of tests are the FITNESSGRAM (1) and the President's Challenge Test (2). Each provides criterion-referenced standards for interpretation of results. Table 11-1 provides a list of common field tests of physical fitness for children, with specific reference to five components (1,2). Some communities, schools, and surveys develop their own battery of tests and standards of performance (4). Questionnaires have also been used to assess physical activity patterns of young people (5).

TABLE 11-1. Field Fitness Testing for Children*	
Fitness/Health Component	**Field Test**
Aerobic capacity	1-mile walk/run
Muscular strength and endurance	Curl-ups
	Pull-ups/push-ups
Flexibility	Sit-reach/V-sit reach
Agility	Shuttle run
Body composition	Body mass index/skinfolds

*For detailed descriptions of specific test items, the reader is referred to References 1 and 2.

Clinical Exercise Testing

Clinical laboratory exercise testing may be useful in selected pediatric groups. Primary reasons for clinical testing include evaluation of known or suspected medical abnormalities, assessment of symptoms associated with exercise, measurement of exercise capacity, promotion of self-efficacy, and individualization of an exercise program (6–8). The American College of Cardiology and American Heart Association recently published clinical selection criteria for identifying children most likely to benefit from testing based on known or suspected cardiopulmonary disorders (6), with specific reference to four categories. Contraindications to exercise testing and specific test termination criteria for young people are similar to those for adults (see Box 3-6) (3,6–8).

Interpretation of physiologic responses to exercise should be based on the age and size of the child (8–10). Peak oxygen uptake (peak $\dot{V}O_2$), when expressed in L/min, is much lower in children than in young adults. When peak $\dot{V}O_2$ is expressed relative to body weight, similar values are found in boys and young men, and higher values are observed in girls than in young adult women. Lactate production and stroke volume are lower in children than adults at matched submaximal work levels and peak effort. Most studies suggest that healthy children show less improvement in peak $\dot{V}O_2$ with aerobic training as compared with sedentary adults (9,10). Because most children do not achieve a plateau in $\dot{V}O_2$ even with exhaustive effort, attainment of a $\dot{V}O_2$ plateau does not appear to be a useful criterion for maximal effort (9).

TESTING METHODOLOGY

Exercise testing of children may be performed on either a treadmill or cycle ergometer. Often the physical abilities or disabilities of the child will dictate the modality to be used. Two disadvantages of cycle ergometry for children are that it 1) requires a greater attention span than treadmill walking because the activity is self-driven, and 2) is more likely to be limited by peripheral muscle (e.g., quadriceps) discomfort rather than central factors. The chosen protocol must be flexible enough to adapt to the child's age, fitness level, and physical stature (Table 11-2). In treadmill testing of chil-

TABLE 11-2. Protocols Suitable for Graded Exercise Testing of Children*

Modified Balke Treadmill Protocol

Subject	Speed (mph)	Initial Grade (%)	Increment (%)	Stage Duration (min)
Poorly fit	3.00	6	2	2
Sedentary	3.25	6	2	2
Active	5.00	0	2.5	2
Athlete	5.25	0	2.5	2

The McMaster Cycle Test

Height (cm)	Initial Load (watts)	Increments (watts)	Step Duration (min)
<120	12.5	12.5	2
120–139.9	12.5	25	2
140–159.9	25	25	2
≥160	25	50 (boys) 25 (girls)	2

*Adapted from Skinner J. Exercise Testing and Exercise Prescription for Special Cases. 2nd ed. Philadelphia: Lea & Febiger, 1993.

dren, adjusting grade while leaving speed constant allows the child to adapt to stage changes more readily. For cycle ergometer testing, seat height, handlebar height and position, and pedal crank length may have to be modified to accommodate children. Most children 125 cm or 50 inches tall or taller can be tested on a standard cycle ergometer. Young children are generally less cooperative than adults, often requiring special attention to achieve maximal effort. Assessment of the respiratory exchange ratio and ventilatory threshold may be helpful for test interpretation when maximal effort is not achieved. After peak effort, the workload should be decreased gradually, and the child should be allowed to recover for at least 5 minutes by walking slowly or pedaling with little or no resistance.

Exercise Prescription

Young children tend to be relatively active, although they often choose short bursts of intense energy exercise rather than sustained activities. As children move into their adolescent and young adult years, physical activity levels decline strikingly. Survey data suggest that only about 50% of American youths aged 12 to 21 years are vigorously active on a regular basis, with girls more frequently becoming less active than boys as they grow older. The increase in childhood and adolescent obesity during the last decade is attributed, in large part, to physical inactivity. Inactivity and obesity, when carried into adulthood, are associated with increased risk of developing cardiovascular disease, diabetes, and other health problems. Motivating young people to adopt a lifetime commitment to a program of regular physical activity is critically important for future health care costs and quality of life in later years (11–14).

The optimal amount and type of exercise to recommend to young children and adolescents has not been defined precisely but should be individualized based on maturity level, medical status, skill level, and prior exercise experiences. Several health agencies encourage all persons more than 6 years old to accumulate at least 30 minutes of moderate-intensity physical activity on most and preferably all days of the week (11,12). In very young children, emphasis should be directed at active play (rather than exercise), enjoyment, and creative activities that invoke sustained periods of activity. In older children, 20 to 30 minutes of vigorous exercise at least 3 times a week is encouraged for greater benefits (7,11,12). Children typically do not need a heart rate prescription to regulate intensity because they are at low cardiac risk and generally have good ability to adjust exercise according to tolerance or perceived exertion. Children should be encouraged to participate in a variety of activities that exercise all major large muscle groups and include weight-bearing activities to optimize basic skill development, weight management, aerobic fitness, and bone mineral content. In Healthy People 2000, several objectives have been established related to physical activity and fitness for children and adolescents (13). Some of the benefits obtainable from regular participation in physical activity include the following:

- Greater strength and endurance
- Enhanced bone formation
- Weight management
- Reduced anxiety and stress
- Improved self-esteem and self-efficacy
- Minimization of heart disease risk factors
- Fun and/or enjoyment
- Social interaction
- Skill development

Because physical activity experiences in childhood may be pivotal in terms of adult activity, health agencies have stepped up their efforts to encourage schools, families, and communities to promote *positive* childhood and youth physical activity experiences (11–14).

Schools are encouraged to:

- Offer daily physical education classes at each grade.
- Increase time being physically active in physical education classes.
- Discuss health benefits of physical activity.
- Eliminate or sharply decrease exemptions for physical education.

Schools and communities should:

- Provide enjoyable, lifetime physical activities.
- Meet diverse ethnic and gender activity interests.
- Promote self-efficacy and skill development.
- Provide opportunities for all skill levels.
- Not limit activities exclusively to team-oriented sports.
- Provide safe facilities outside school hours.

Parents should:

- Set a good example by being physically active.
- Offer praise, interest, and encouragement.
- Get involved in school and/or community activity programs.
- Encourage children to be active around the home.
- Provide needed transportation.

Muscular strength and endurance are important components of fitness in young people. Available evidence suggests that children can participate safely in properly designed and supervised resistance training programs (10,15). Three professional organizations have published position stands on prepubescent strength training (10). The following general guidelines and principles are offered as suggestions to those interested in developing a sound strength training program for children:

- All strength-training activities should be supervised and monitored closely by appropriately trained personnel.
- No matter how big, strong, or mature the individual appears, remember that he or she is physiologically immature.
- The primary focus, at least initially, should be directed at learning proper techniques for all exercise movements and developing an interest in resistance training.
- Proper techniques should be demonstrated first, followed by gradual application of resistance or weight.
- Proper breathing techniques (i.e., no breath-holding) should be taught.
- Stress that exercises should be performed in a manner in which the speed is controlled, avoiding ballistic (fast and jerky) movements.
- Avoid the practice of power lifting and body building.
- Perform full-range, multijoint exercises (as opposed to single-joint exercises).
- Be sure participant can understand and follow directions.

All strength training should follow approved intensity, duration, and frequency guidelines established for young people.

Intensity
- Avoid repetitive use of maximal amounts of weight in strength training programs until reaching Tanner stage 5 (adolescence) level of developmental maturity (16,17).
- Weight loads should be used that permit 8 or more repetitions to be completed per set, since heavy weights can be potentially dangerous and damaging to the developing skeletal and joint structures.
- It is not recommended that resistance exercise be performed to the point of severe muscular fatigue.
- As a training effect occurs, achieve an overload initially by increasing the number of repetitions, and then by increasing the absolute resistance.

Duration
- Perform 1 to 2 sets of 8 to 10 different exercises (with 8 to 12 repetitions per set), ensuring that all of the major muscle groups are included (in early stages of training, 1 set should be performed until the proper technique is demonstrated).
- Rest at least 1 to 2 minutes between exercises, and intersperse rest days between training days.

Frequency
- Limit strength training sessions to twice per week and encourage children and adolescents to participate in other forms of physical activity.

SAFETY CONSIDERATIONS

Because children are anatomically, physiologically, and psychologically immature, special precautions should be applied when designing exercise programs. Safety for children should always be of primary concern. Children may experience a higher incidence of overuse injuries or damage the epiphyseal growth plates if exercise is excessive or if the child encounters acute trauma. Risk of injury can be decreased significantly by ensuring appropriate matching of competition in terms of size, maturation or skill level, use of properly fitted protective equipment, liberal adaptation of rules, and proper conditioning and skill development. Whenever new activities are initiated, intensity of effort should start low and progress to higher levels according to tolerance and appropriate increments. The child's ability to tolerate temperature conditions should be evaluated carefully to avoid thermal injury (10). Children thermoregulate quite effectively in normal to moderate conditions with appropriate clothing and rehydration but have reduced ability to adapt to temperature extremes. In a hot environment, children show less heat dissipation than adults because of a lower sweat rate and evaporative heat loss and a greater heat production per kilogram of body weight. Children also acclimate to heat more slowly than adults. In a cold environment, the high surface area-to-body mass ratio of children can accelerate heat loss, increasing their risk of hypothermia. In children, exertion-related deaths are uncommon and are generally related to congenital heart defects or acquired myocarditis (12,18). Individuals with these disorders should be encouraged to remain active but refrain from vigorous or competitive athletics.

Children with certain illnesses and physical challenges merit special attention. Such children tend to be far less active than their healthy counterparts. As a result, these children may require adjustments in their exercise prescription (7,8) (Table 11-3). Special considerations in testing and training children with concomitant cardiovascular or pulmonary disorders are described elsewhere (7,8,10).

THE ELDERLY

Dynamic assessment of cardiorespiratory function and exercise prescription for older adults may require subtle differences in protocol, methodology, and dosage as compared with younger and middle-aged persons.

Exercise Testing

Because of higher rates of underlying coronary artery disease, the rationale for exercise testing within an elderly population may be even greater than that of the general adult population. Several key points deserve mention. First, knowledge of the effects of the aging process on variables measured during exercise testing is critical to the safe and effective performance of exercise testing in the elderly. A list of such changes follows (18):

Resting heart rate	↔
Maximal heart rate	↓
Maximal cardiac output	↓
Resting and exercise blood pressures	↑
Maximal oxygen uptake	↓
Residual volume	↑
Vital capacity	↓
Reaction time	↑
Muscular strength	↓
Bone mass	↓
Flexibility	↓
Fat-free body mass	↓
Percent body fat	↑
Glucose tolerance	↓
Recovery time	↑

Legend: ↔ = unchanged; ↓ = decrease; ↑ = increase.

Second, physiologic aging does not occur uniformly across the population; therefore it is not wise to define "elderly" by any specific chronologic age or set of ages. Individuals of the same age can and will differ drastically

TABLE 11-3. Exercise Prescription in the Management of Specific Pediatric Diseases*

Disease	Purposes of Program	Recommended Activities
Anorexia nervosa	Means for behavioral modification; educate regarding lean body mass versus fat	Various; emphasize those with low energy demand
Bronchial asthma	Conditioning; possible reduction of exercise-induced bronchospasm; instill confidence	Aquatic, intermittent, long warm-up
Cerebral palsy	Increase maximal aerobic power, range of motion, ambulation; control of body mass	Depends on residual ability
Cystic fibrosis	Improve mucus clearance, training of respiratory muscles	Jogging, swimming, walking, selected games
Diabetes mellitus	Help in metabolic control; control of body mass	Various; attempt equal daily energy output
Hemophilia	Prevent muscle atrophy and possible bleeding in joints	Swimming, cycling; avoid contact sports
Mental retardation	Socialization; increase self-esteem; prevent detraining	Recreational, intermittent, large variety
Muscular dystrophies	Increase muscle strength and endurance; prolong ambulatory phase	Swimming, calisthenics, wheelchair sports
Neurocirculatory disease	Increase effort tolerance; improve orthostatic response	Various; emphasize endurance-type activities
Obesity	Reduction of body mass and fat; conditioning; socialization and improved self-esteem	High in caloric expenditure but feasible to child; walking, recreational games, swimming
Rheumatoid arthritis	Prevent contractures and muscle atrophy; increase daily function	Swimming, calisthenics, cycling
Spina bifida	Strengthen upper body; control of body mass and fat; increase maximal aerobic power	Arm-shoulder resistance training, wheelchair sports (including endurance)

*Adapted from Bar-Or O. Exercise in childhood. In: Walsh RP, Shephard RJ, eds. Current Therapy in Sports Medicine, 1985–1986. Toronto: CV Mosby, 1985.

in their physiologic status and response to an exercise stimulus. Third, it is difficult to distinguish effects due to deconditioning, age-related decline, and disease. Fourth, while aging is inevitable, both the pace and potential reversibility of this process may be amenable to intervention. And finally, the possibility that an active or latent disease process may be present in the subject must always be considered. In accordance with Table 2-2, medical clearance is advised before maximal exercise testing or their participation in vigorous exercise.

Various test protocols using a variety of modalities have been used for testing the elderly population, either in their standard form or with slight modifications. Protocols are available for those who are highly deconditioned or physically limited. The following special considerations should be considered when testing the elderly (6,8):

- For those with expected low work capacities, the initial workload should be low (2 to 3 metabolic equivalents [METs]) and workload increments should be small (0.5 to 1.0 METs), e.g., Naughton protocol.
- A cycle ergometer may be preferable to a treadmill for those with poor balance, poor neuromuscular coordination, impaired vision, senile gait patterns, weight-bearing limitations, and foot problems.
- Added treadmill handrail support may be required due to reduced balance, decreased muscular strength, poor neuromuscular coordination, or fear. Handrail support or gait abnormalities, however, can reduce the accuracy of estimating peak MET capacity based on exercise duration or peak workload achieved.
- Treadmill speed may need to be adapted according to walking ability.
- For those who have difficulty adjusting to the exercise equipment, the initial stage may need to be extended, the test restarted, or the test repeated.
- Exercise-induced arrhythmias are more frequent in the elderly than in other age groups.
- Prescribed medications are common and may influence exercise electrocardiographic and hemodynamic responses.

No specific exercise test termination criteria are necessary for the elderly population beyond those previously presented (Box 5-3). However, probable attainment of a lower peak $\dot{V}O_2$ coupled with the increased prevalence of cardiovascular, metabolic, and orthopedic problems in the elderly often leads to an earlier test termination (either volitionally or due to achievement of established criteria) than with the young adult population.

Exercise Prescription

The general principles of exercise prescription (Chapter 7) apply to adults of all ages. Relative adaptations to exercise are also similar to other age groups. The percent improvement in $\dot{V}O_{2max}$ in elderly persons is comparable to that reported in younger populations. Unfortunately, physical inactivity is more common in the elderly than in any other age group and can contribute to loss of independence in advanced age (11). Particularly important components of the exercise prescription include cardiovascular fitness, resistance training, and flexibility.

CARDIOVASCULAR FITNESS

The elderly should be encouraged, whenever possible, to meet the population-wide recommendation to accumulate at least 30 minutes of moderate-intensity exercise on most and preferably all days of the week. This can be accomplished with activities such as brisk walking, gardening, yard work, housework, climbing stairs, and active recreational pursuits (see Fig. 7.1, The Activity Pyramid). For those achieving this level, additional benefits may be obtained with longer duration, moderate-intensity exercise or by substituting moderate-intensity with higher-intensity exercise. Importantly, activities performed at a given MET value represent greater relative effort in the elderly than in the young because of the decrease in peak METs with age. Before progressing to a vigorous exercise program, the elderly should consult a physician.

The optimal mode of exercise for elderly persons can be influenced by physiologic and psychosocial variables, such as work capacity, orthopedic problems, poor balance, and travel limitations:

Mode
- The exercise modality should be one that does not impose excessive orthopedic stress.
- Walking is an excellent mode of exercise for many elderly.
- Aquatic exercise and stationary cycle exercise may be especially advantageous for those with reduced ability to tolerate weight-bearing activity.
- The activity should be accessible, convenient, and enjoyable to the participant—all factors directly related to exercise adherence.
- A group setting may provide important social reinforcement to adherence.

The wide range of health and fitness levels observed among older adults may require special considerations in terms of integrating intensity, frequency, and duration into an exercise plan (11,18).

Intensity
- To minimize medical problems and promote long-term compliance, exercise intensity for inactive elderly people should start low and individually progress according to tolerance and preference.

- Many older persons suffer from a variety of medical conditions; thus, a conservative approach to increasing exercise intensity is warranted initially.
- Exercise need not be vigorous and continuous to be beneficial; a daily accumulation of 30 minutes of moderate-intensity exercise provides health benefits.
- Longer-duration or higher-aerobic intensity offers additional health and fitness benefits, although it can lead to greater risk of cardiovascular and musculoskeletal problems and lower compliance to a long-term exercise plan.
- The intensity guidelines and precautions established for younger people (see Chapter 7) for aerobic exercise training generally apply to the elderly.
- A measured peak heart rate is preferable to an age-predicted peak heart rate when prescribing aerobic exercise because of the variability in peak heart rate in persons over 65 years of age and their greater risk of underlying coronary artery disease.
- Use of percentage of peak heart rate to calculate a target heart rate range in the elderly may provide a more accurate estimate of percentage of peak $\dot{V}O_2$ than the heart rate reserve method (19).
- Elderly persons are more likely than young persons to be taking medications that can influence peak heart rate.

Duration
- Exercise duration need not be continuous to produce benefits; thus, those who have difficulty sustaining exercise for 30 minutes or who prefer shorter bouts of exercise can be advised to exercise for 10-minute periods at different times throughout the day.
- To avoid injury and ensure safety, older individuals should initially increase exercise duration rather than intensity.

Frequency
- Exercise performed at a moderate intensity should be undertaken most days of the week.
- If exercise is undertaken at a vigorous level, it should be performed at least 3 times per week, with exercise and no exercise days alternated.

RESISTANCE TRAINING

Elderly persons should be encouraged to supplement cardiorespiratory endurance activities and an active lifestyle with strength-developing exercises. Resistance training helps preserve and enhance muscular strength and endurance (muscular fitness) in older individuals, which, in turn, may help to prevent falls, improve mobility, and counteract muscle weakness and frailty (20–22). Importantly, muscular fitness may allow performance of activities of daily living with less effort and extend functional independence by living the latter years in a self-sufficient, dignified manner.

Similar to cardiorespiratory fitness, individualization of the resistance training prescription is essential and should be based on the health and/

or fitness status and specific goals of the participant. General guidelines for intensity, frequency, and duration of exercise follow:

Intensity
- Perform at least 1 set of 8 to 10 exercises that use all the major muscle groups (e.g., gluteals, quadriceps, hamstrings, pectorals, latissimus dorsi, deltoids, and abdominals).
- Each set should involve 10 to 15 repetitions that elicit a perceived exertion rating of 12 to 13 (somewhat hard).
- As a training effect occurs, achieve an overload initially by increasing the number of repetitions, and then by increasing the resistance.
- When returning from a lay-off, start with resistances of 50% or less of previous training intensity, then gradually increase the resistance.

Frequency
- Resistance training should be performed at least twice a week, with at least 48 hours of rest between sessions.

Duration
- Sessions lasting longer than 60 minutes may have a detrimental effect on exercise adherence.
- Adherence to the guidelines set forth in this chapter should permit individuals to complete total body resistance training sessions within 20 to 30 minutes.

Regardless of which specific protocol is adopted, several common sense guidelines pertaining to resistance training for older adults should be followed:

- The major goal of the resistance training program is to develop sufficient muscular fitness to enhance an individual's ability to live a physically independent lifestyle.
- The first several resistance training sessions should be closely supervised and monitored by trained personnel who are sensitive to the special needs and capabilities of the elderly.
- Begin (the first 8 weeks) with minimal resistance to allow for adaptations of the connective tissue elements.
- Teach proper training techniques for all of the exercises to be used in the program.
- Instruct older participants to maintain their normal breathing pattern while exercising.
- Stress that all exercises should be performed in a manner in which the speed is controlled (no ballistic movements should be allowed).
- Perform the exercises in a range of motion that is within a "pain-free arc" (i.e., the maximum range of motion that does not elicit pain or discomfort).

- Perform multijoint exercises (as opposed to single-joint exercises).
- Given a choice, use machines to resistance train, as opposed to free weights (machines require less skill to use, protect the back by stabilizing the user's body position, and allow the user to start with lower resistances, to increase by smaller increments, and to more easily control the exercise range of motion).
- Never permit arthritic participants to participate in strength training exercises during active periods of pain or inflammation.
- Engage in a year-round resistance training program.
- Routine activities, such as domestic work, gardening, and walking, may help to maintain muscular strength.

FLEXIBILITY

An adequate range of motion in all body joints is important to maintaining an acceptable level of musculoskeletal function, balance, and agility in older adults. Unfortunately, efforts to identify the most effective protocol for developing flexibility have been limited in comparison to the other basic components of physical fitness. What is almost universally accepted, although not documented, is the fact that maintaining adequate levels of flexibility enhances an individual's functional capabilities (e.g., bending and twisting) and reduces injury potential (e.g., risk of muscle strains, low back problems, and falls)—particularly for the aged. Exercises should be prescribed for every major joint (hip, back, shoulder, knee, upper trunk, and neck regions) in the body. A well-rounded program of stretching can counteract the usual decline in flexibility of the elderly and improve balance and agility. Yoga and tai chi movements may be helpful in this regard. Not surprisingly, it is critical that a sound stretching program be included as part of each exercise session for older adults (23):

Intensity
- Exercises should incorporate slow movement, e.g., static stretches that are sustained for 10 to 30 seconds.
- At least four repetitions per muscle group should be performed.
- The degree of stretch achieved should not cause pain, but rather mild discomfort.

Frequency
- Stretching exercises should be performed a minimum of 2 to 3 d·wk^{-1} and should be included as an integral part of the warm-up and cool-down exercises.

Duration
- The stretching phase of an exercise session should last long enough to exercise the major muscle/tendon groups.
- An entire exercise session devoted to flexibility may be appropriate for deconditioned older adults who are beginning an exercise program.

Several guidelines pertaining to stretching by older adults should be followed:

- Always precede stretching exercises with some type of warm-up activity to increase circulation and internal body temperature.
- Stretch smoothly and never bounce.
- Do not stretch a joint beyond its pain-free range of motion.
- Gradually ease into a stretch, and hold it only as long as it feels comfortable (10 to 30 seconds).

PREGNANT WOMEN

Pregnant women represent a unique clientele because of concerns that exercise could produce adverse outcomes due to 1) inadequate availability of oxygen or substrate for both maternal exercising muscle and fetus; 2) hyperthermia-induced fetal distress or birth abnormalities; and/or 3) increased uterine contraction. To date, however, human studies indicate that healthy women with uncomplicated pregnancy do not need to limit their exercise for fear of adverse effects (24,25). No consistent differences have been reported between exercisers and nonexercisers in terms of rate of spontaneous abortion or rupture, incidence of preterm labor, fetal distress or birth abnormalities, and ability to carry to term. Several physiologic adaptations occur with both pregnancy and exercise that appear to provide the physiologic reserve needed to accommodate the simultaneous needs of the fetus and maternal exercising muscle (25). Although some data suggest that strenuous exercise may lead to delivery of somewhat lighter birth weight babies, these deliveries are well within normal limits and are due in part to less baby fat.

Contraindications for exercise during pregnancy have been established by the American College of Obstetricians and Gynecologists (ACOG) and are listed in Box 11-1. For women who do not have any risk factors for adverse maternal or perinatal outcomes, the ACOG has established guide-

BOX 11-1. Contraindications for Exercising During Pregnancy*

- Pregnancy-induced hypertension
- Preterm rupture of membrane
- Preterm labor during the prior or current pregnancy
- Incompetent cervix
- Persistent second to third trimester bleeding
- Intrauterine growth retardation

*Reprinted with permission from American College of Obstetricians and Gynecologists. Exercise during pregnancy and the postpartum period (Technical Bulletin #189). Washington: American College of Obstetricians and Gynecologists, 1994.

BOX 11-2. American College of Obstetricians and Gynecologists (ACOG) Recommendations for Exercise in Pregnancy and Postpartum*

- During pregnancy, women can continue to exercise and derive health benefits even from mild to moderate exercise routines. Regular exercise (at least 3 times per week) is preferable to intermittent activity.
- Women should avoid exercise in the supine position after the first trimester. Such a position is associated with decreased cardiac output in most pregnant women. Because the remaining cardiac output will be preferentially distributed away from splanchnic beds (including the uterus) during vigorous exercise, such regimens are best avoided during pregnancy. Prolonged periods of motionless standing should also be avoided.
- Women should be aware of the decreased oxygen available for aerobic exercise during pregnancy. They should be encouraged to modify the intensity of their exercise according to maternal symptoms. Pregnant women should stop exercising when fatigued and not exercise to exhaustion. Weight-bearing exercises may under some circumstances be continued at intensities similar to those prior to pregnancy throughout pregnancy. Non–weight-bearing exercises, such as cycling or swimming, will minimize the risk of injury and facilitate the continuation of exercise during pregnancy.
- Morphologic changes in pregnancy should serve as a relative contraindication to types of exercise in which loss of balance could be detrimental to maternal or fetal well-being, especially in the third trimester. Further, any type of exercise involving the potential for even mild abdominal trauma should be avoided.
- Pregnancy requires an additional 300 kcal/day to maintain metabolic homeostasis. Thus, women who exercise during pregnancy should be particularly careful to ensure an adequate diet.
- Pregnant women who exercise in the first trimester should augment heat dissipation by ensuring adequate hydration, appropriate clothing, and optimal environmental surroundings during exercise.
- Many of the physiologic and morphologic changes of pregnancy persist 4 to 6 weeks postpartum. Thus, prepregnancy exercise routines should be resumed gradually based on a woman's physical capability.

*Reprinted with permission from American College of Obstetricians and Gynecologists. Exercise during pregnancy and the postpartum period (Technical Bulletin #189). Washington: American College of Obstetricians and Gynecologists, 1994.

lines for the safe prescription of exercise (25) (Box 11-2). When exercising, pregnant women should be aware of signs or symptoms for discontinuing exercise and seeking medical advice (Box 11-3) (26).

Although some pregnant women have undergone maximal exercise testing, it generally is not recommended except for clinical reasons. For monitoring exercise intensity, the ACOG guidelines recommend using rat-

> ## BOX 11-3. Reasons to Discontinue Exercise and Seek Medical Advice During Pregnancy*,†
>
> - Any signs of bloody discharge from the vagina
> - Any "gush" of fluid from the vagina (premature rupture of membranes)
> - Sudden swelling of the ankles, hands, or face
> - Persistent, severe headaches, and/or visual disturbance; unexplained spell of faintness or dizziness
> - Swelling, pain, and redness in the calf of one leg (phlebitis)
> - Elevation of pulse rate or blood pressure that persists after exercise
> - Excessive fatigue, palpitations, chest pain
> - Persistent contractions (>6–8/h) that may suggest onset of premature labor
> - Unexplained abdominal pain
> - Insufficient weight gain (<1.0 kg/mo during last two trimesters)

*Adapted from Wolfe LA, Hall P, Webb KA, et al. Prescription of aerobic exercise during pregnancy. Sports Med 1989;8:273–301.

†Participants and the exercise instructor should know these signs and symptoms, and the participant should consult the physician monitoring her pregnancy if any are encountered. Women who develop preeclampsia, eclampsia, severe anemia, phlebitis, significant infection, signs of fetal intrauterine growth retardation, or other significant medical problems should discontinue participation in the exercise program.

ing of perceived effort rather than heart rate due to chronotropic alterations during pregnancy that make standard training heart rate formulas less appropriate.

The ACOG guidelines differentiate between women who exercise and become pregnant and women who start exercising during pregnancy (25). The ACOG guidelines recommend that women who currently participate in a regular exercise program can continue their training program during pregnancy, without major modifications. However, many women choose to modify intensity, duration, and/or frequency during the course of pregnancy due to overall comfort level and specific symptoms. Those who plan to begin an exercise program after becoming pregnant are advised to seek physician approval and begin exercising with low-intensity, low- (or non-) impact activities, such as walking and swimming. Although exercise may not be appropriate for every pregnant woman, most pregnant women—especially with physician authorization—can gain maternal health benefits while subjecting the developing fetus to minimal risk. Commonly cited potential benefits of a properly designed prenatal exercise program include the following:

- Improved aerobic and muscular fitness
- Facilitation of recovery from labor

- Enhanced maternal psychologic well-being that may help counter feelings of stress, anxiety, and/or depression frequently experienced during pregnancy
- Establishment of permanent healthy lifestyle habits
- More rapid return to prepregnancy weight, strength, and flexibility levels
- Fewer obstetric interventions
- Shorter active phase of labor and less pain
- Less weight gain
- Improved digestion and reduced constipation
- Greater energy reserve
- Reduced "postpartum belly"
- Reduced back pain during pregnancy

References

1. FITNESSGRAM. The Test Administration Manual. Dallas: Institute for Aerobics Research, 1994.
2. President's Council on Physical Fitness and Sports. The presidential physical fitness award program. Washington: 1997.
3. Bar-Or O. Exercise in childhood. In: Walsh RP, Shephard RJ, eds. Current Therapy in Sports Medicine, 1985–1986. Toronto: CV Mosby, 1985.
4. Ross JG. Evaluating fitness and activity assessments from the National Children and Youth Fitness Studies I and II. In: Assessing Physical Fitness and Physical Activity in Population-based Surveys. Rockville, MD: US Department of Health and Human Services, Publication (PHS) DHHS 89–1253, 1989.
5. Pereira MA, FitzGerald SJ, Gregg EW, et al. A collection of physical activity questionnaires for health-related research. Med Sci Sports Exer 1997;29(suppl):S170–189;S201–205.
6. Gibbons RJ, Balady GJ, Beasley JW, et al. ACC/AHA guidelines for exercise testing. A report of the American College of Cardiology/American Heart Association Task Force on Practice Guidelines (Committee on Exercise Testing). J Am Coll Cardiol 1997;30:260–315.
7. Tomassoni TL. Introduction: the role of exercise in the diagnosis and management of chronic disease in children and youth. Med Sci Sports Exerc 1996;28:403–405.
8. Skinner J. Exercise Testing and Exercise Prescription for Special Cases. 2nd ed. Philadelphia: Lea & Febiger, 1993.
9. Armstrong N, Welsman JR. Assessment and interpretation of aerobic fitness in children and adolescents. Exerc Sport Sci Rev 1994;22:435–476.
10. Rowland TW. Exercise and Children's Health. Champaign, IL: Human Kinetics, 1990.
11. US Department of Health and Human Services. Physical activity and health: a report of the Surgeon General. Atlanta, GA: US Department of Health and Human Services, Centers for Disease Control and Prevention, National Center for Chronic Disease Prevention and Health Promotion, 1996.
12. Pate RR, Pratt M, Blair SN, et al. Physical activity and public health. A recommendation from the Centers for Disease Control and Prevention and the American College of Sports Medicine. JAMA 1995;273:402–407.
13. Public Health Service. Healthy People 2000: National Health Promotion and Disease Prevention Objectives. Washington: US Government Printing Office, DHHS Publication (PHS) 91-50212, 1991.
14. US Department of Health and Human Services. Guidelines for school and community programs to promote lifelong physical activity among young people. Morb Mort Weekly Rep 1997;46:1–36.
15. Freedson PS, Ward A, Rippe JM. Resistance training for youth. In: Grana WA, Lombardo JA, Sharkey BJ, et al., eds. Advances in Sports Medicine and Fitness. Vol. 3. Chicago: Yearbook Medical Publishers, 1990.
16. Tanner JM. Growth at Adolescence. 2nd ed. Oxford: Blackwell Scientific Publications Ltd., 1982.
17. Joffe A. Adolescent medicine. In: Oski FA, DeAngelis CD, Feighin RD, et al., eds. Principles and Practice of Pediatrics. 2nd ed. Philadelphia: Lippincott, 1994:763–775.

18. Fletcher GF, Balady G, Froelicher VF, et al. Exercise standards. A statement for healthcare professionals from the American Heart Association. Circulation 1995;91:580–615.
19. Kohrt WM, Spina RJ, Holloszy JO, et al. Prescribing exercise intensity for older women. J Am Geriatr Soc 1998;46:129–133.
20. Fiatarone MA, O'Neill EF, Ryan ND, et al. Exercise training and nutritional supplementation for physical frailty in very elderly people. N Engl J Med 1994;330:1769–1775.
21. Taunton JE, Martin AD, Rhodes EC, et al. Exercise for the older woman; choosing the right prescription. Br J Sports Med 1997;31:5–10.
22. Ades PA, Ballor DL, Ashikaga T, et al. Weight training improves walking endurance in healthy elderly persons. Ann Intern Med 1996;124:568–572.
23. Pollock ML, Gaesser GA, Butcher JD, et al. The recommended quantity and quality of exercise for developing and maintaining cardiorespiratory and muscular fitness, and flexibility in healthy adults. Med Sci Sports Exerc 1998;30:975–991.
24. Clapp III JF. The effect of continuing regular endurance exercise on the physiologic adaptations to pregnancy outcome. Am J Sports Med 1996;24:S28–S29.
25. American College of Obstetricians and Gynecologists. Exercise during pregnancy and the postpartum period (Technical Bulletin #189). Washington: American College of Obstetricians and Gynecologists, 1994.
26. Wolfe LA, Hall P, Webb KA, et al. Prescription of aerobic exercise during pregnancy. Sports Med 1989;8:273–301.

SECTION IV

Special Considerations

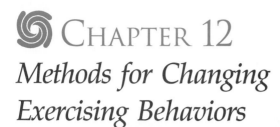 Chapter 12
Methods for Changing Exercising Behaviors

Improving compliance to exercise and other behaviors known to decrease death and disability from cardiovascular disease is an important and complex subject. The term compliance can have subjective, even paternalistic, connotations when used to describe nonadherence to recommended medical therapeutics. As health care professionals, it is important to acknowledge that although behavior change may seem important and necessary, the process for the client or patient involves complex emotional and physical changes. For instance, a person with hypertension may not experience any negative symptoms from this condition. However, taking medications known to lessen stroke and heart attack from hypertension may result in side effects such as fatigue or constipation. "Compliance" in this situation may be problematic unless specific educational strategies are implemented. Fitness and rehabilitation professionals face the challenge of working with clients and their families, as well as the community, to develop methods of changing negative health-related behaviors. To achieve positive changes in health-related behaviors, a clear understanding of adult learning processes and the psychological influences on learning and behavior change are important. This chapter addresses the challenge of exercise compliance, concepts of adult learning, and psychological components of successful behavior change, and suggests practical strategies to improve behavioral change outcomes.

Exercise Compliance

Fitness and cardiac exercise programs have typically reported dropout rates ranging from 9 to 87%, highlighting the compliance problem among those who voluntarily enter physical conditioning programs (1,2). Dropout rates are generally highest in the first 3 months, increasing to approximately 50% within 1 year (Fig. 12-1). Although widely differing definitions of "exercise dropout" in these studies may have contributed to the variability in results,

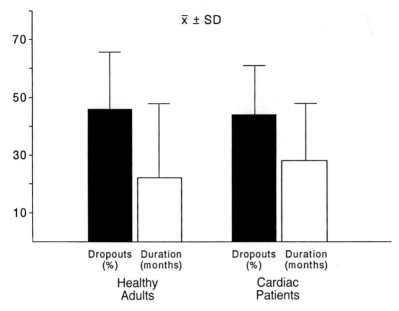

FIGURE 12-1. Relationship between the dropout rate (percent) and the duration of exercise training (months) in 7 studies with a total of 734 healthy adults and 14 studies with a total of 3887 cardiac patients.

it appears that exercise is not unlike other health-related behaviors (e.g., medication compliance, smoking cessation, weight reduction) in that typically half or less of those who initiate the behavior will continue, irrespective of initial health status or type of program.

To understand why people sometimes lack the motivation for regular physical activity, one must first acknowledge a simple yet important fact: exercise is voluntary and time-consuming. Therefore, it may extend the day or compete with other valued interests and responsibilities of daily life. The traditional approach to the exercise compliance problem has involved attempting to persuade dropouts to become reinvolved. An alternative approach, however, involves the identification and subsequent monitoring of "dropout prone" individuals, with an aim toward preventing recidivism.

Principal factors related to long-term exercise noncompliance include cigarette smoking, blue collar employment, inactive leisure time, and inactive occupation. The noncompliance rate appears to increase progressively, from 59% in the presence of smoking alone, the single most discriminating variable, to 95% with all four variables (3,4). Additional characteristics of the early exercise dropout are shown in Box 12-1, with specific reference to personal, program, and related factors. Nevertheless, psychosocial variables, including perception of the program, personal convenience factors, and family lifestyle components appear to present the major impediment to exercise compliance, accounting for almost half of all dropouts in rehabilitation programs (2,5). A brief questionnaire designed to assess "self-

BOX 12-1. Variables Predicting the Exercise Dropout*

Personal Factors
  Smoker
  Inactive leisure time
  Inactive occupation
  Blue collar worker
  Type A personality
  Increased physical strength
  Extroverted
  Poor credit rating
  Overweight and/or low ponderal index
  Poor self-motivation
  Depressed
  Hypochondriacal
  Anxious
  Introverted
  Low ego strength
Program Factors
  Inconvenient time and/or location
  Excessive cost
  High-intensity exercise
  Lack of exercise variety, e.g., running only
  Exercising alone
  Lack of positive feedback or reinforcement
  Inflexible exercise goals
  Low enjoyment ratings for running programs
  Poor exercise leadership
Other Factors
  Lack of spouse support
  Inclement weather
  Excessive job travel
  Injury
  Job change and/or move

*Adapted from Franklin BA. Program factors that influence exercise adherence: practical adherence skills for clinical staff. In: Dishman R, ed. Exercise Adherence: Its Impact on Public Health. Champaign, IL: Human Kinetics, 1988:237–258.

motivation" can be used, along with measures of intention and self-efficacy, to predict male and female dropout-prone behavior (Fig. 12-2) (6,7).

ADULT LEARNING

Learning and changing behavior involves a clear understanding of multiple factors that influence learning potential. Individual, social, environmental, and medical factors collectively influence learning and behavior (8). Cultural beliefs and practices exert strong influences on health-related behaviors.

A	B	C	D	E	
5	4	3	2	1	1. I get discouraged easily.
5	4	3	2	1	2. I don't work any harder than I have to.
1	2	3	4	5	3. I seldom if ever let myself down.
5	4	3	2	1	4. I'm just not the goal-setting type.
1	2	3	4	5	5. I'm good at keeping promises, especially the ones I make myself.
5	4	3	2	1	6. I don't impose much structure on my activities.
1	2	3	4	5	7. I have a very hard-driving, aggressive personality.

Directions: Circle the number beneath the letter corresponding to the alternative that best describes how characteristic the statement is when applied to you. The alternatives are:

        A. *extremely* uncharacteristic of me.
        B. *somewhat* uncharacteristic of me.
        C. neither characteristic nor uncharacteristic of me.
        D. *somewhat* characteristic of me.
        E. *extremely* characteristic of me.

Scoring: Add together the seven numbers you circled. A score ≤24 suggests dropout-prone behavior. The lower the self-motivation score, the greater the likelihood toward exercise noncompliance. If the score suggests dropout proneness, it should be viewed as an incentive to remain active, rather than a self-fulfilling prophecy to quit exercising.

FIGURE 12-2. Self-motivation assessment scale to determine likelihood of exercise compliance. (Copyright ©1978 by Dishman RK, Ickes W, Morgan WP. Self-motivation and adherence to habitual physical activity. J Appl Social Psychol 1980;10:115–132. From Falls HB, Baylor AM, Dishman RK. Essentials of fitness. Appendix A–13. Philadelphia: Saunders College, 1980. Reproduced by permission of the copyright holders.)

Asking persons whose diets are culturally and socially defined to eat a "healthy" low-fat diet can be confusing and unsuccessful. Assessment of baseline knowledge about a disease as well as beliefs regarding treatment outcomes sets the stage for a successful educational program. If a person does not believe that a behavior change will result in beneficial outcomes, behavior change is not likely to occur. For example, believing that taking a cholesterol-lowering medication will result in liver damage usually indicates that a patient will have difficulty complying with this intervention.

    Adults learn largely based on their beliefs, culture, prior experiences, and knowledge. Generally accepted principles of learning indicate that adults:

- Are self-directed.
- Participate in decision-making.
- Base learning on past experiences.
- Use problem-solving as a basis for learning.
- Learn only when they are "ready" to learn, for example, when they are physically and emotionally stable and are aware that there is a need to learn (9,10).

Psychological Components of Successful Behavior Change

Successful behavior change is based upon an understanding of certain psychological theories. Behavior modification, social cognitive theory, and stages of motivational readiness (also known as the transtheoretical model) are fundamental to guiding our behavioral interventions.

Behavior modification theory has added greatly to our ability to effect long-term behavior change. Cardiac rehabilitation programs began to use behavior modification theory in the 1970s (11). This theory involves the patient actively in the change process. This is achieved by clients and/or patients doing the following:

- Setting short- and long-term, realistic, and measurable goals
- Determining their "confidence" that they can achieve each goal
- Signing a contract with a clear description of the desirable goal and means to achieve the goal
- Receiving feedback on their success and revising the plan as appropriate
- Receiving lifestyle physical activity counseling, including specific cognitive and behavioral counseling strategies (e.g., diaries, prompts) to increase the adoption and maintenance of physical activity in daily living (12–14)
- Developing social support systems to provide encouragement and help during difficult times (15–17)

Social cognitive theory provides great insight into the interrelationships between beliefs, understanding, environment, and behavior. Beliefs are seen as the fundamental driving force behind behavior. The perceived ability to achieve successful behavior change can be measured by assessing "self-efficacy." Clients or patients who have a low "self-efficacy" are less likely to be successful at behavior change (18,19). As a result, these individuals are often seen as "noncompliant." Assessing "self-efficacy" and beliefs regarding behavior change sets the stage for successful long-term change (18,19). Methods of assessing "self-efficacy" include having clients or patients rate their confidence that they can make a behavior change on a scale from 0 to 100%. The lower the rating, the less likely it is that an individual will be able to make and sustain long-term change. Ratings less than 70% are associated with a lower chance of successful change. With a low self-efficacy rating, education needs to be directed at discovering the beliefs and/or barriers to change. For instance, a patient may have a low rating of self-efficacy to stop smoking if the spouse or partner continues to smoke. In this case, efforts to address smoking cessation with a partner may increase confidence and chances for long-term successful change.

Readiness for change theory has received wide acceptance and use by health care practitioners. This theory addresses the individual's ability to make permanent change based upon their emotional and intellectual "readi-

---

BOX 12-2. Stages of "Readiness to Change" Model*

1. Precontemplation—patients express lack of interest in making change. Moving patients through this stage involves utilization of multiple resources to stress the importance of the desired change. This can be achieved through written materials, educational classes, physician and family persuasion and other means.
2. Contemplation—patients are "thinking" about making a desired change. This stage can be influenced by helping patients define the risks and benefits of making or not making the desired change (e.g., starting an exercise program).
3. Preparation—patients are doing some physical activity but not meeting the recommended criteria, i.e., 30 minutes of moderate-intensity physical activity for ≥5 days/week or 3 to 5 days/week of vigorous-intensity activity for ≥20 minutes.
4. Action—patients are meeting the above-referenced (preparation) criteria on a consistent basis but they have not maintained the behavior for 6 months.
5. Maintenance—patients have been in action for 6 months or more.

*Modified for physical activity interventions (see references 12,13).

ness to change" (20). Clients or patients can be evaluated as to the stage of readiness they express before being given the challenge to change a behavior. The stages, as modified for physical activity interventions, are defined as precontemplation, contemplation, preparation, action, and maintenance. Box 12-2 describes each of these stages (12,13,17,21,22). Individuals should also be counseled to deal with hypokinetic lapses or relapses, and to recognize that these behaviors are not necessarily tantamount to failure.

STRATEGIES TO IMPROVE BEHAVIORAL CHANGE OUTCOMES

Using self-efficacy measures and integrating the stages of change into educational strategies can greatly influence behavioral and lifestyle outcomes. In addition, providing written and visual materials as well as experimental educational tools (e.g., yoga classes for relaxation) can influence and support behavioral change. Written plans and documentation of progress should be integrated into the patient record.

Use of behavior modification strategies, such as setting goals, making agreements or contracts, providing frequent feedback, scheduling appropriate rewards, assessing and integrating social support, and providing prompts, are critical in modulating health behavior change (15). Box 12-3 further defines these strategies, with specific reference to techniques to initiate and maintain exercise behaviors (23).

We must be careful not to define our beliefs and practices as the "gold standard" of behavior. Labeling patients as "noncompliant" because they

BOX 12-3. Behavioral Management Strategies for Initiating and Maintaining Exercise Adherence*

Techniques	Practical Applications/Recommendations
Initiation of Exercise	
Preparation	The exercise professional should establish realistic expectations among new participants. Overly pessimistic or optimistic expectations should be corrected.
Shaping	This strategy is analogous to the physiologic principle of progression. Begin the exercise program at a dosage (intensity, frequency, duration) that is comfortable for the participant, and increase the volume slowly until the optimal level is attained.
Goal-setting	Goals should be individualized and based upon the participant's physiologic and psychosocial status. Goals can be set for both supervised and unsupervised exercise. Short-term goals that are specific, yet flexible, are more effective than longer-term goals.
Reinforcement	Participants should be queried as to what reinforcers (rewards) would work for them. One of the most effective rewards may be praise from program staff that is specific to each individual. Certificates, patches, and attendance charts can also be used as reinforcers.
Stimulus control	Environmental cues or stimuli (e.g., written notes, watch alarms) may be used to remind participants to maintain their exercise commitment. Having a routine time and place for exercise establishes powerful stimulus control.
Contracting	A behavioral contract has been shown to enhance the commitment to exercise. Signing the contract formalizes the agreement and makes it more significant.
Cognitive strategies	Participants should be oriented to the advantages and disadvantages of exercise. Individuals who select their own flexible goals generally demonstrate better adherence as compared with those whose goals are rigidly set by exercise professionals.
Maintenance of Exercise	
Generalization training	Specific steps should be taken to "generalize" the exercise habit from the gymnasium or home setting to other environments (e.g., walk breaks at work, using stairs, gardening, parking the car away from stores).

BOX 12-3. (continued)

Techniques	Practical Applications/Recommendations
Social support	The support of family, friends, and coworkers should be sought from the beginning. Finding a compatible exercise partner often serves to enhance exercise adherence.
Self-management	Participants should be encouraged to be their own behavior therapists. They should practice self-reinforcement by focusing on increased self-esteem, enjoyment of the exercise itself, and the anticipated health and fitness benefits.
Relapse prevention training	Exercise professionals should prepare participants for situations that may produce a relapse and ways of coping with them so that a complete relapse is avoided. Relapses should be viewed as inevitable challenges, rather than failures.

*Adapted from Martin JE, Dubbert PM. Behavioral management strategies for improving health and fitness. J Cardiac Rehabil 1984;4:200–208.

do not participate in behaviors that we believe are beneficial to their health is not necessarily the optimal approach to understanding and facilitating healthy behavior change. A more successful approach is to assess an individual's educational level, resources to facilitate change, readiness to learn, and personal beliefs. Such individually tailored education and counseling are more likely to result in long-term change. In addition, health care professionals should live the life they prescribe. In doing this, their actions as "role models" can positively influence the behaviors of those they counsel and educate.

Methods of behavior change are often effective in altering many health-related behaviors, but their use does not guarantee success. The techniques presented here should be integrated into the exercise program in a way that is appropriate to the population, the setting, and the expertise of the staff. An effective program would selectively incorporate several of these techniques into a focused multifactorial program; however, it is not necessary to use all of them (12,13). The techniques are only introduced in this chapter; additional readings, relevant training, or consultation from an expert in behavior change should be used to complement this information. The ACSM's Resource Manual for Guidelines for Exercise Testing and Prescription contains several chapters that address health counseling skills (24), principles of health behavior change (15), and initiation, adoption, and maintenance strategies to promote physical activity (25,26). Other texts are available that provide an in-depth, yet practical approach to behavior change methodology (27).

Practical Recommendations to Enhance Exercise Adherence

In addition to educating people about exercise, it is necessary to motivate them to act and maintain a personal fitness program (28). Unfortunately, exercise testing and exercise prescription are often overemphasized in relation to the behavioral components of the program. As a result, negative forces often outweigh the positive forces contributing to sustained participant interest and adherence. Such imbalance (Fig. 12-3) leads to a decline in adherence while program effectiveness diminishes. Research and empiric experience suggest that the following program modifications and motivational strategies may enhance participant interest, enthusiasm, and long-term adherence.

RECRUIT PHYSICIAN SUPPORT OF THE EXERCISE PROGRAM
According to a recent clinical study, the single most important factor determining patient's participation in exercise was receiving a strong recommendation from their primary care physician (29). Simple physician counseling has also been shown to be highly effective in motivating patients to make other significant lifestyle changes (e.g., smoking cessation).

MINIMIZE INJURIES AND/OR COMPLICATIONS WITH A MODERATE EXERCISE PRESCRIPTION
Oftentimes, novice exercisers become discouraged due to muscular soreness or injury from increasing the activity dosage too abruptly. Excessive intensity ($\geq 85\%$ $\dot{V}O_{2max}$), frequency (≥ 5 $d \cdot wk^{-1}$), or duration of training

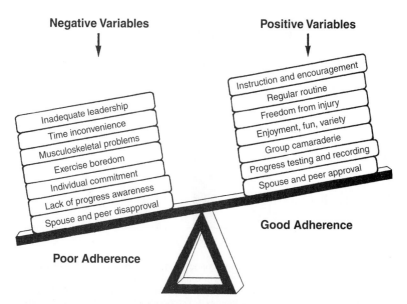

FIGURE 12-3. Variables affecting adherence to a physical conditioning program. Negative variables often outweigh positive variables, resulting in poor adherence.

(≥45 min·session⁻¹) offer the participant little additional gain in aerobic fitness, yet the incidence of orthopedic injury increases substantially (Fig. 12-4) (30,31). Attention to warm-up, proper walking or running shoes, and training on appropriate terrain (i.e., avoiding hard and uneven surfaces) should aid in decreasing attrition due to injury. Participants should be counseled to discontinue exercise and seek medical advice if they experience excessive muscle soreness, orthopedic injury, or premonitory signs or symptoms, including abnormal heart rhythms (palpitations), chest pain or pressure, or dizziness.

ADVOCATE EXERCISING WITH OTHERS

Poorer long-term adherence has been reported in programs in which an individual exercises alone compared with those that incorporated group dynamics (32). Commitments made as part of a group tend to be stronger than those made independently (33). The social support provided by others may offer the incentive to continue even during periods of sagging interest.

EMPHASIZE VARIETY AND ENJOYMENT IN THE EXERCISE PROGRAM

The type of physical activity program has also been shown to influence long-term exercise adherence. Calisthenics, when relied on too heavily in an exercise program, readily become monotonous and boring, leading

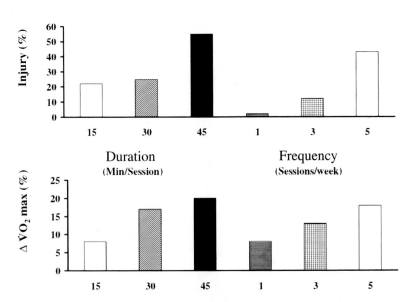

FIGURE 12-4. Relationship between frequency and duration of exercise training, improvement in $\dot{V}O_{2max}$, and the incidence of orthopedic injury. Above an exercise duration of 30 min/session, or a frequency of 3 sessions/week, additional improvement in $\dot{V}O_{2max}$ is small, yet the injury rate increases disproportionately. (Adapted from Pollock ML, Gettman L, Milesis C, et al. Effects of frequency and duration of training on attrition and incidence of injury. Med Sci Sports 1977;9:31–36.)

to poor exercise adherence. The most successful physical conditioning regimens are those that are pleasurable and offer the greatest diversification.

PROVIDE POSITIVE REINFORCEMENT THROUGH PERIODIC TESTING

Exercise testing, body fatness assessment, and serum lipid profiling may be done at the start of the exercise program and at regular intervals thereafter to assess the individual's response to the conditioning stimulus. Favorable changes in these measures can serve as powerful motivators that produce renewed interest and dedication.

RECRUIT SUPPORT OF THE PROGRAM AMONG FAMILY AND FRIENDS

Lack of social support is frequently found to be a precursor to exercise noncompliance. Accordingly, attention should be focused not only on the participant, but also on family and friends. Spouse support and approval appears to play a key role in this regard. The importance of this influence became evident in one study that showed that the husband's adherence to the exercise program was directly related to the wife's attitude toward it (33). Of those men whose spouses had a positive attitude toward the exercise program, 80% demonstrated good-to-excellent adherence, and only 20% exhibited fair-to-poor adherence. In contrast, when the spouse was neutral or negative, 40% showed good-to-excellent adherence and 60% demonstrated fair-to-poor adherence (Fig. 12-5).

INCLUDE AN OPTIONAL RECREATIONAL GAME TO THE CONDITIONING PROGRAM FORMAT

The standard warm-up, endurance phase, and cool-down used in most exercise programs offer little in terms of fun or variety. A recreational game may be included as an option to this format. Game modifications that serve to minimize skill and competition and maximize participant success are particularly important in preventive and rehabilitative exercise programs. Through such modifications the leader is better able to emphasize the primary goal of the activity: enjoyment of the game for its own sake (34).

ESTABLISH REGULARITY OF WORKOUTS

If individuals start their workouts at the same time each day, they will accept them as part of their routine schedule, and exercise will become habitual. Availability of morning and evening sessions should serve to further increase the compatibility of an exercise commitment with the varied schedules of participants.

USE PROGRESS CHARTS TO RECORD EXERCISE ACHIEVEMENTS

The importance of immediate, positive feedback on reinforcement of health-related behaviors is well documented. A progress chart that allows participants to document daily and cumulative exercise achievements (e.g., mileage) can facilitate this objective. One example is the computerized exercise session progress report system developed at a preventive medicine

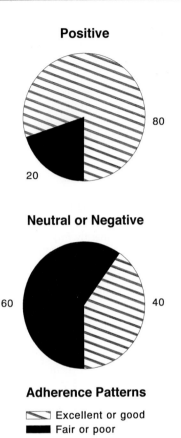

FIGURE 12-5. Relation of wives' attitudes to husband's adherence to an exercise training program. Adapted from Heinzelman F, Bagley RW. Response to physical activity programs and their effects on health behavior. Public Health Rep 1970;85:905–911.

center in Dallas, Texas. The system provides exercisers with an updated record of the number of "aerobic points" they have earned, the miles they have run, and related training accomplishments. A practical alternative, however, is a progress chart that allows the participant to record his or her daily workout mileage. If the chart is strategically placed near the running track or locker room, it becomes a matter of pride to motivate individuals to "increase" their exercise totals.

RECOGNIZE PARTICIPANT ACCOMPLISHMENTS THROUGH A SYSTEM OF REWARDS

Peer recognition is another powerful motivator. Recognition of lifestyle, health, or exercise achievements can be made in the form of inexpensive trophies, plaques, ribbons, certificates, or "iron-on" insignias. To this end, an annual awards ceremony or banquet is recommended.

PROVIDE QUALIFIED, ENTHUSIASTIC EXERCISE PROFESSIONALS

Although numerous variables affect exercise adherence, perhaps the single most important is the exercise leader (35,36). Exercise staff should be well-trained, compassionate, sensitive, empathetic, tactful, innovative, and enthusiastic. Box 12-4 lists recommended behavioral strategies of the good exercise professional. Workshop and certification offerings by the American College of Sports Medicine (ACSM) serve to promote "quality control" and knowledge and proficiency standards for program personnel.

POPULATION-SPECIFIC BARRIERS TO PHYSICAL ACTIVITY

Women, older adults, and obese individuals are faced with several unique barriers to exercise participation, which may account for their lower initial enrollment, poorer attendance, and higher drop-out rates. The role of caregiver is typically the woman's—maintaining the home and caring for children, an older spouse, or a family member. Women are also less likely to drive to an exercise facility. Some women may be uncomfortable participating in a male-dominated physical conditioning program. Several factors may restrict physical activity with patients of increasing age: poor health, fear of injury, and inaccessibility to fitness facilities. Among obese individuals, unique barriers include previous negative experiences with exercise (feelings of inadequacy, limited physical skills) and the physiologic and psychosocial burden of their excess weight. Nevertheless, these obstacles can oftentimes be overcome with careful program design, including interventions to improve self-efficacy (37). The role of the health care provider is to facilitate the decision to participate in regular exercise and other health-related habits, to support these lifestyle changes over time, and to provide training to prevent relapse to the former undesirable behavior.

PROGRAM MODELS: GROUP VERSUS HOME-BASED EXERCISE THERAPY

Considerable data are available regarding the safety, efficacy, and cost-effectiveness of traditional supervised group exercise. Such programs may be more appropriate for persons with concomitant neurologic, cardiovascular, orthopedic, or pulmonary conditions. Others may require the social reinforcement of group dynamics to maintain their exercise adherence. Furthermore, supervised programs facilitate education regarding both exercise and lifestyle changes for coronary risk reduction, provide variety and recreational opportunities, and offer staff reassurance and the potential for enhanced safety and surveillance (38). Moreover, it appears that patients who remain active in a formal cardiac rehabilitation program for an extended length (more than 1 year) continue to maintain or improve their body composition, functional capacity, and blood lipids, in contrast to those

BOX 12-4. Behavioral Strategies of the Good Exercise Professional

1. Show a sincere interest in the participant. Learn why participants have gotten involved in your program and what they hope to achieve.
2. Be enthusiastic in your instruction and guidance.
3. Develop a personal association and relationship with each participant: learn clients' names and greet them by shaking hands.
4. Consider the various reasons why adults exercise (i.e., health, recreation, weight loss, social, personal appearance) and allow for individual differences.
5. Remove or reduce as many initial barriers to participation as possible. If cost, distance, child care, or other factors make it difficult for clients to attend, assist them to overcome these obstacles whenever possible.
6. Initiate participant follow-up (e.g., postcards or telephone calls) when several unexplained absences occur in succession. Novice exercisers should be advised that an inevitable slip in attendance does not imply failure.
7. Practice what you preach. Participate in the exercise sessions yourself.
8. Honor special days (e.g., birthdays) or exercise accomplishments with extrinsic rewards such as T-shirts, ribbons, or certificates.
9. Attend personally to orthopedic and musculoskeletal problems. Provide alternatives to floor exercise.
10. Counsel participants on proper foot apparel and exercise clothing.
11. Avoid constant references to complicated medical or physiologic terminology. Concentrate on a few selected terms to provide a little education at a time.
12. Arrange for occasional visits by personal physicians.
13. Provide a constant flow of newspaper or magazine articles to the participants on topics related to physical activity and other relevant information.
14. Encourage an occasional visitor or participant to lead activity.
15. Have a designated area for participant counseling with an appropriate decor.
16. Give clear and concise information. Listen, summarize, and clarify to ensure that your communications have been correctly understood.
17. Introduce "first-time" exercisers on the gymnasium floor or in the locker room. This orientation will encourage a sense of belonging to the group.
18. Reinforce participants by complimenting them on their appearance as they are exercising. Your conversation during exercise may also serve as a distracter from any unpleasant sensations that they may be experiencing.
19. Use goal setting as a motivational tool. Build on areas of participant perceived interest, "How would he or she like to be different?"
20. Show your optimism. This creates a positive self-fulfilling prophesy where the participant succeeds largely because of your belief that he or she can persevere.

who exit after only 3 months (39). However, such programs are associated with inconvenient hours, increased cost, and extended travel time. In one study, patients undergoing gymnasium-based exercise training spent more time in their cars going to and from the program than their counterparts in a home-training comparison group spent on their cycle ergometers (40).

For many participants, medically directed home exercise may be a reasonable alternative to promote weight management, enhance psychologic status, and improve functional capacity, especially if a training partner can be recruited. Advantages of home-training programs include lesser cost, increased practicability, convenience, and the potential to promote independence and self-responsibility for health and fitness needs (40). Home-based fitness programs also can be as effective as group interventions for improving functional capacity and modifying coronary risk factors (e.g., smoking, hyperlipidemia) (41,42). Drawbacks, however, include the limited means of teaching clients (patients) necessary principles and proscriptions for exercise, the lack of opportunity to counsel and encourage lifestyle changes, and the absence of direct medical surveillance, emergency care, and peer support. Several program modifications have been used to overcome these limitations successfully, including regular telephone contact between staff and participants, mail (e.g., completion of activity logs), fax, video recording, the Internet, and transtelephonic ECG monitoring of those at increased risk of future cardiac events (40,42).

In summary, contemporary models must be developed to ensure that apparently healthy adults and patients with heart disease can more easily participate in comprehensive, exercise-based programs of primary and secondary prevention. The challenge for those developing these models is to incorporate techniques to facilitate optimal adherence and overcome many of the current limitations of home or group programs, while maximizing their benefits.

OTHER TARGETS FOR HEALTH BEHAVIOR CHANGE

Fitness and exercise-based rehabilitation program personnel are often asked questions about additional ways to implement healthier lifestyles. Although these individuals should not be expected to be experts in all areas, it is appropriate that they serve as a resource person to direct the participant to accurate information and additional services. Upon intake to the program, it may be worthwhile for staff to assess related lifestyle habits and risk factors, such as dietary patterns (including consumption of high-fat, high calorie foods), smoking status, body composition, lipids and lipoproteins, and psychosocial well-being. Based on initial screening tests, participants should be counseled regarding the value of a complementary risk reduction program, and realistic goals should be defined and mutually agreed upon. A listing of qualified local professionals and services related to each of these areas should be developed, with specific reference to smoking cessation, weight reduction, dietary modification, and stress management.

Smoking Cessation

Because cigarette smoking represents the primary preventable cause of death and disability in the United States today, every health professional has an obligation to strongly urge cigarette smokers to quit. Unfortunately, there is little or no evidence of a reduction in cigarette smoking resulting from exercise training as a sole intervention (38). Nevertheless, exercise program staff can play an important role in this regard. After establishing rapport with clients and/or patients, program staff should direct those who want to quit to well-designed education, counseling, and behavioral interventions (including relapse prevention) targeted at smoking cessation. Such programs generally produce quit rates of 15 to 25% in the general population of smokers (43). Quit rates increase substantially for persons with smoking-related cardiorespiratory diseases, with up to 70% of patients quitting 1 year after acute myocardial infarction (using biochemical verification of smoking status) when provided with an intensive nurse-managed program (42). In contrast, self-quit rates have been estimated to be less than 3% in the general population of smokers (44).

The following "steps" are suggested in helping people stop smoking, as delineated in the guidelines put forth by the Agency for Health Care Policy and Research (45):

Step 1: Identify smokers at every encounter.
Step 2: Advise smokers to quit.
Step 3: Ask smokers if they are willing to make a quit attempt.
Step 4: Aid smokers in quitting.
Step 5: Arrange for follow-up.

When counseling smokers about a quit attempt (step 4), it is important to provide interventions and strategies to effectively address challenges of withdrawal symptoms, psychologic cravings, relapse, weight gain, and high-risk social environments. Additional resources for smoking cessation materials and clinics include the American Heart Association (AHA), American Lung Association, and the American Cancer Society. A comprehensive review on what health care professionals can do to favorably impact smoking prevalence can be found in *ACSM's Resource Manual for Guidelines for Exercise Testing and Prescription* (43).

Weight Management

People who are overweight or obese—a growing health problem that affects millions of Americans—are at increased risk of complications from hypertension, lipid disorders, type 2 diabetes, coronary heart disease, stroke, gallbladder disease, osteoarthritis, sleep apnea and other respiratory problems, and certain cancers. In response to the emerging body of scientific data about the link between excess adiposity and coronary heart disease, the AHA reclassified obesity as a major, modifiable risk factor for heart disease (46).

Recently, the federal government issued clinical practice guidelines on the identification, evaluation, and treatment of an increasing number of both men and women who are overweight or obese (47). According to the guidelines, assessment of obesity involves evaluation of two simple measures, height and weight, to calculate body mass index (BMI), defined as weight in kilograms divided by height in meters squared (kg/m^2). Because BMI describes body weight relative to height, it is strongly correlated with total body fat content in adults. A BMI between 25 and 29.9 is considered overweight; obesity is signified by a BMI of 30 or more.

The guidelines note that from 1960 to 1994, the prevalence of obesity in adults (BMI of ≥ 30) increased from less than 13% to nearly 23% of the U.S. population, with most of the increase occurring in recent years. Although the causes of obesity are complex and include genetic, hormonal, and other medical conditions, most people who are excessively fat exercise too little relative to their caloric intake. According to the *Physical Activity and Health* report by the Surgeon General (48), low levels of physical activity, resulting in fewer calories used than consumed, contribute to the high prevalence of obesity in the United States. Nevertheless, inactivity is only half of the energy balance equation; total calories also count. Despite a modest decrease in the percentage of calories consumed as fat, surveys indicate that Americans are consuming more calories overall (46).

According to the guidelines, the most successful strategies for weight loss include calorie reduction, increased physical activity, and behavior therapy designed to improve eating and exercise habits. Specific behavioral recommendations may include keeping a food diary; eating only fruit for snacks; reducing fried foods; using a smaller plate; parking the car farther away from stores when shopping; eliminating home extension phones; and reducing television viewing time. The initial objective should be to reduce body weight by about 10% from baseline, with a goal of 1 to 2 lb per week over a 6-month treatment period (49). With success, and if warranted, further weight loss can be initiated. *A continued physical activity program appears to be the best predictor of long-term weight loss and its subsequent maintenance.* Finally, physicians should have their patients on a combined program of caloric restriction and exercise for at least 6 months before embarking on drug therapy. Additional information on weight management can be found in the *ACSM's Resource Manual for Guidelines for Exercise Testing and Prescription* (50).

Dietary Modification

The typical American diet is high in calories, fat (particularly saturated fat), cholesterol, and sodium, and low in fiber. This dietary profile contributes to a number of chronic diseases, including obesity, diabetes, coronary heart disease, and hypertension. Accordingly, the goals of dietary modification often are to reduce or maintain body weight and fat stores, decrease elevated plasma total and low-density lipoprotein cholesterol, and lower blood pressure.

The process of changing eating behaviors is complex and includes assessing the individual's motivation and readiness for change, analyzing eating patterns using a food diary, establishing realistic goals, providing instructions on food preparation and eating out, and altering the eating environment (51). A well-trained exercise professional may be able to provide assistance in achieving these objectives, but consultation with a registered dietitian should also be encouraged, especially for those with specialized needs. Additional information on nutrition can be found in *ACSM's Resource Manual for Guidelines for Exercise Testing and Prescription* (51).

Stress Management

Although "being stressed" is typically equated to "being anxious," it also is associated with a variety of emotional correlates, including anger, alarm, lack of control, vulnerability, and depression (52). Exercise may help to alleviate feelings of distress and mild depression in some people; however, as a sole intervention, it does not consistently improve measures of anxiety and depression after an acute cardiac event (53). However, training in behavioral modification, stress management, and relaxation techniques, with or without concomitant exercise therapy, has been shown to be effective in lowering levels of self-reported emotional stress and in modifying Type-A behavior (38).

Stress management techniques aimed at attenuating physiologic responses like heart rate and blood pressure, inducing an improved sense of well-being, modifying behavior patterns (e.g., responding rather than reacting), enhancing coping mechanisms, and promoting positive thinking have become increasingly popular. Effective programs to facilitate these objectives may include methods to avoid stressful situations, adjustment and/or adaptation techniques to cope more appropriately with stressors, and using relaxation or biofeedback to neutralize physiologic reactions to stress (54). The best specific stress management techniques remain elusive, and no single intervention has been universally accepted. Most people can be trained easily in relaxation therapy, but other stress management techniques may require more intensive instruction by a behavioral therapist. Additional information on stress management can be found in *ACSM's Resource Manual for Guidelines for Exercise Testing and Prescription* (52).

Although a variety of techniques are commonly promulgated for relaxation training, including yoga, self-hypnosis, progressive muscular relaxation, breathing exercises, and biofeedback, there is no convincing evidence that one form of therapy is more effective than another (55). Group stress management programs are offered by many hospitals, universities, health promotion programs, and private practitioners. However, participants with emotional disorders should be referred for more intensive counseling to a licensed psychiatrist, psychologist, or social worker. Preliminary screening with a variety of psychosocial inventories, including the SF-36 (56), Beck Depression Inventory (57), or Spielberger State-Trait Anxiety Inventory (58), can be helpful in this regard.

References

1. Franklin BA. Program factors that influence exercise adherence: practical adherence skills for clinical staff. In: Dishman R, ed. Exercise Adherence: Its Impact on Public Health. Champaign, IL: Human Kinetics, 1988:237–258.
2. Oldridge NB. Compliance with exercise rehabilitation. In: Dishman R, ed. Exercise Adherence: Its Impact on Public Health. Champaign, IL: Human Kinetics, 1988:283–304.
3. Oldridge NB, Donner AP, Buck CW, et al. Predictors of dropout from cardiac rehabilitation. Ontario Exercise Heart Collaborative Study. Am J Cardiol 1983;51:70–74.
4. Oldridge NB, Jones NL. Preventive use of exercise rehabilitation after myocardial infarction. Acta Med Scand (Suppl) 1986;711:123–129.
5. Oldridge NB, Wicks JR, Hanley C, et al. Noncompliance in an exercise rehabilitation program for men who have suffered a myocardial infarction. Can Med Assoc J 1978;118:361–364.
6. Dishman RK, Ickes W, Morgan WP. Self-motivation and adherence to habitual physical activity. J Appl Social Psychol 1980;10:115–132.
7. Falls HB, Baylor AM, Dishman RK. Essentials of fitness. Appendix A–13. Philadelphia: Saunders College, 1980.
8. Bartlett EE. Behavioral diagnosis: a practical approach to patient education. Patient Couns Health Educ 1982;4(1):29–35.
9. Comoss PM. Education of the coronary patient and family: Principles and practice. In: Wenger NK, Hellerstein HK, eds. Rehabilitation of the Coronary Patient. 3rd ed. New York: Churchill Livingston, 1992:439–460.
10. Cupples SA. Inpatient cardiac rehabilitation: patient education implementation and documentation. J Cardiopulm Rehabil 1995;15:412–417.
11. Nash J. Taking charge of your weight and well being. Palo Alto, CA: Bull Publishing, 1986.
12. Dunn AL, Marcus BH, Kampert JB, et al. Reduction in cardiovascular disease risk factors: 6-month results from Project Active. Prev Med 1997;26:883–892.
13. Dunn AL, Marcus BH, Kampert JB, et al. Comparison of lifestyle and structured interventions to increase physical activity and cardiorespiratory fitness. JAMA 1999;281:327–334.
14. Andersen RE, Wadden TA, Bartlett SJ, et al. Effects of lifestyle activity vs structured aerobic exercise in obese women. JAMA 1999;281:335–340.
15. Taylor CB, Miller NH. Principles of health behavior change. In: Roitman J, Southard D, eds. ACSM's Resource Manual for Guidelines for Exercise Testing and Prescription. 3rd ed. Baltimore: William & Wilkins, 1998:542–547.
16. Miller NH, Taylor CB. Lifestyle Management for Patients with Coronary Heart Disease. Champaign, IL: Human Kinetics, 1995.
17. Miller NH, Hill M, Kottke T, et al. The multilevel compliance challenge: recommendations for a call to action. A statement for healthcare professionals. Circulation 1997;95:1085–1090.
18. Bandura A. Self-efficacy. In: Social Foundations of Thought and Action. Englewood Cliffs, NJ: Prentice Hall, 1986:390–453.
19. Bandura A. Social Learning Theory. Englewood Cliffs, NJ: Prentice Hall, 1977.
20. Prochaska J, DiClemente C. Transtheoretical therapy, toward a more integrative model of change. Psych Theory Res Prac 1982;19:276–288.
21. Prochaska JO, DiClemente CC. Common processes of change in smoking, weight control and psychological distress. In: Schiffman S, Wills TA, eds. Coping and Substance Use. San Diego: Academic Press, 1985:345–363.
22. Marlatt GA, Gordon JR, eds. Relapse Prevention: Maintenance Strategies in the Treatment of Addictive Behaviors. New York: Guilford Press, 1985.
23. Martin JE, Dubbert PM. Behavioral management strategies for improving health and fitness. J Cardiac Rehabil 1984;4:200–208.
24. Southard DR, Southard BH. Health counseling skills. In: Roitman J, Southard DR, eds. ACSM's Resource Manual for Guidelines for Exercise Testing and Prescription. 3rd ed. Baltimore: Williams and Wilkins, 1998:523–526.
25. King AC, Kiernan M. Physical activity promotion: antecedents. In: Roitman J, Southard DR, eds. ACSM's Resource Manual for Guidelines for Exercise Testing and Prescription. 3rd ed. Baltimore: Williams and Wilkins, 1998:559–563.
26. King AC, Martin JE. Physical activity promotion: adoption and maintenance. In: Roitman J, Southard DR, eds. ACSM's Resource Manual for Guidelines for Exercise Testing and Prescription. 3rd ed. Baltimore: Williams and Wilkins, 1998:564–569.
27. Kanfer FH, Goldstein AP, eds. Helping People Change: A Textbook of Methods. 3rd ed. New York: Pergamon, 1988.
28. Wilmore JH. Individual exercise prescription. Am J Cardiol 1974;33:757–759.
29. Ades PA, Waldmann ML, McCann WJ, et al. Predictors of cardiac rehabilitation participation in older coronary patients. Arch Intern Med 1992;152:1033–1035.

30. Kilbom A, Hartley L, Saltin B, et al. Physical training in sedentary middle-aged and older men. I. Medical evaluation. Scand J Clin Lab Invest 1969;24:315–322.
31. Pollock ML, Gettman L, Milesis C, et al. Effects of frequency and duration of training on attrition and incidence of injury. Med Sci Sports 1977;9:31–36.
32. Massie JF, Shephard RJ. Physiological and psychological effects of training—a comparison of individual and gymnasium programs, with a characterization of the exercise 'drop-out.' Med Sci Sports 1971;3:110–117.
33. Heinzelman F, Bagley RW. Response to physical activity programs and their effects on health behavior. Public Health Rep 1970;85:905–911.
34. Franklin BA, Stoedefalke KG. Games-as-aerobics: activities for cardiac rehabilitation programs. In: Fardy PS, Franklin BA, Porcari JP, et al., eds. Training Techniques in Cardiac Rehabilitation. Champaign, IL: Human Kinetics, 1998:106–136.
35. Oldridge NB. What to look for in an exercise class leader. Phys Sportsmed 1977;5:85–88.
36. Oldridge NB. Qualities of an exercise leader. In: Blair SN, Painter P, Pate RR, et al., eds. ACSM's Resource Manual for Guidelines for Graded Exercise Testing and Exercise Prescription. Philadelphia: Lea and Febiger, 1988:239–243.
37. Blair SN, Horton E, Leon AS, et al. Physical activity, nutrition, and chronic disease. Med Sci Sports Exerc 1996;28:335–349.
38. Wenger NK, Froelicher ES, Smith LK, et al. Cardiac rehabilitation guideline No. 17. Rockville, MD: US Department of Health and Human Services, Public Health Service, Agency for Health Care Policy and Research and the National Heart, Lung, and Blood Institute. AHCPR publication No. 96-0672, October 1995.
39. Brubaker PH, Warner JG Jr, Rejeski WJ, et al. Comparison of standard- and extended-length participation in cardiac rehabilitation on body composition, functional capacity, and blood lipids. Am J Cardiol 1996;78:769–773.
40. DeBusk RF, Haskell WL, Miller NH, et al. Medically directed at-home rehabilitation soon after clinically uncomplicated myocardial infarction: a new model for patient care. Am J Cardiol 1985;55:251–257.
41. Haskell WL, Alderman EL, Fair JM, et al. Effects of intensive multiple risk factor reduction on coronary atherosclerosis and clinical cardiac events in men and women with coronary artery disease. The Stanford Coronary Risk Intervention Project (SCRIP). Circulation 1994;89:975–990.
42. DeBusk RF, Miller NH, Superko HR, et al. A case-management system for coronary risk factor modification after acute myocardial infarction. Ann Intern Med 1994;120:721–729.
43. Miller NH, Smith PM. Smoking cessation. In: Roitman J, Williams M, eds. ACSM's Resource Manual for Guidelines for Exercise Testing and Prescription. 3rd ed. Baltimore: Williams & Wilkins, 1998:36–42.
44. Cohen S, Lichtenstein E, Prochaska JO, et al. Debunking myths about self-quitting. Evidence from 10 prospective studies of persons who attempt to quit smoking by themselves. Am Psychol 1989;44:1355–1365.
45. Fiore MC, Wetter DW, Bailey WC, et al. Smoking cessation clinical practice guideline. Rockville, MD: Agency for Health Care Policy and Research, Public Health Service, US Departttment of Health and Human Services, 1996.
46. Eckel RH, Krauss RM. American Heart Association Call to Action: obesity as a major risk factor for coronary heart disease. Circulation 1998;97:2099–2100.
47. Pi-Sunyer FX, Becker DM, Bouchard C, et al. Clinical guidelines on the identification, evaluation, and treatment of overweight and obesity in adults. National Institutes of Health, National Heart, Lung and Blood Institute, 1998.
48. US Department of Health and Human Services. Physical activity and health: a report of the Surgeon General. Atlanta, GA: US Department of Health and Human Services, Centers for Disease Control and Prevention, National Center for Chronic Disease Prevention and Health Promotion, 1996.
49. Expert panel on the identification, evaluation, and treatment of overweight and obesity in adults. Executive summary of the clinical guidelines on the identification, evaluation, and treatment of overweight and obesity in adults. Arch Intern Med 1998;158:1855–1867.
50. Grilo CM, Brownell KD. Interventions for weight management. In: Roitman J, Southard DR, eds. ACSM's Resource Manual for Guidelines for Exercise Testing and Prescription. 3rd ed. Baltimore: Williams & Wilkins, 1998:570–577.
51. Steen SN, Butterfield G. Diet and nutrition. In: Roitman J, Williams M, eds. ACSM's Resource Manual for Guidelines for Exercise Testing and Prescription. 3rd ed. Baltimore: Williams & Wilkins, 1998:27–35.
52. Sotile WM. Stress management. In: Roitman J, Southard DR, eds. ACSM's Resource Manual for Guidelines for Exercise Testing and Prescription. 3rd ed. Baltimore: Williams & Wilkins, 1998:548–553.
53. Blumenthal JA, Emery CF, Rejeski WJ. The effects of exercise training on psychosocial functioning after myocardial infarction. J Cardiopulm Rehabil 1988;8:183–193.

54. Schwartz MS. Biofeedback: A Practitioner's Guide. New York: Guilford Press, 1987.
55. Sotile WM. Psychosocial Interventions for Cardiopulmonary Patients: A Guide for Health Professionals. Champaign, IL: Human Kinetics, 1996.
56. Ware J, Sherbourne C. The MOST 36-item short-form health survey (SF-36), I: conceptual framework and item selection. Med Care 1992;30:473–481.
57. Beck A, Weissman A, Lester D, et al. The measurement of pessimism: the hopeless scale. J Consult Clin Psychol 1974;42:861–865.
58. Spielberger C, Gorsuch R, Luschene R. Manual for the State Trait Anxiety Inventory. Palo Alto, CA: Consulting Psychologists Press, 1970.

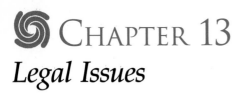

CHAPTER 13
Legal Issues

This chapter presents basic information about how the legal system affects health/fitness and clinical exercise professionals. Key elements of the tort system are reviewed, including the ways that written or oral contracts dictate certain provider obligations (duties) owed to a client and how standards of care, performance failures, and proximate cause contribute to or are involved in negligence and malpractice actions. Information is provided about liability and risk management issues that are important to consider with informed consent, delivery of exercise services, and the conduct and credentialing of exercise personnel. The scope of this chapter, however, permits only a cursory treatment of this subject. Interested readers who want more comprehensive information and analysis of new litigation issues involving exercise, should consult other sources (1–3).

Legal issues affect virtually every dimension of the work that exercise professionals and program managers complete in the course of delivering service to clients. To appreciate the many sources of legal vulnerability, consider all the points of provider interaction with clients in the context of exercise and other services, where insult or injury may occur, and how they might be perceived by clients as attributable to some professional failure. These areas may include preactivity health screening, exercise tests, health-fitness counseling, exercise prescription, and the comprehensive delivery of physical activity programs. Such matters may also involve written operating manuals, policies, procedures, and practices within an exercise program and how these collectively dictate the standard of service (care) delivered to clients. In addition, the way that programs write and use marketing materials to portray the competence of staff and sophistication of programs may also be of significant legal importance. These include the contract and informed consent process, how consultations about clients are conducted with health care providers, and how service fulfillment is documented. Finally, the physical settings where activity programs are carried out, how equipment is used and maintained, how exercise personnel are trained and credentialed, and what steps are employed to instruct, monitor, and supervise the exercising client are all of concern. Each and every one of these dimensions of service might be a focus of legal challenge should a legal claim and suit arise from a personal injury to a client.

Fortunately, a limited number of legal principles have broad application

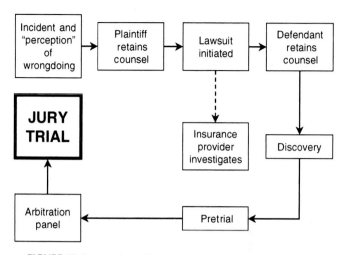

FIGURE 13-1. Hypothetical example of a personal injury lawsuit.

to the work of exercise professionals, even though it is important to recognize that the laws do vary considerably from one state to the next. These principles and their implications for delivery of service need to be well understood so that exercise programs may keep the risks of legal problems to a minimum. So-called "risk management" efforts justify themselves because they offer some degree of protection for professionals and programs against the imposition of damages in the event of legal claim and suit. A risk management orientation, moreover, adds further value to a program because it assigns priorities to client satisfaction, documents client outcomes, and aims to reduce injuries.

Personal injury lawsuits are expensive and psychologically traumatic for defendants and plaintiffs alike. From start to finish, such lawsuits involve many steps and require several months, if not years, before finally coming to resolution through jury trial (Fig. 13-1). Thus, every exercise professional needs to know certain basics of the legal system in the United States, how it affects his or her work, and how to minimize these legal risks.

CONTRACTS, INFORMED CONSENT, AND TORTS

Legal claims against exercise professionals often center on alleged violations of contract or tort law. These two broad legal areas, along with written and statutory laws, define and govern most legal relationships between individuals, including those affecting exercise professionals and their clients.

Contract Law

The law of contracts defines undertakings that may be specified among individuals. A legal contract is defined simply as a promise or performance bargained for and given in exchange for another promise or performance, all of which is supported by something of value, which within the legal system is referred to as "consideration." In the exercise setting, professionals may provide something of value by giving clients information about their health/fitness status and recommendations on exercise training. They also may perform certain procedures for clients, including health screenings, exercise tests, exercise prescriptions, activity counseling, and exercise monitoring. They may do these services in exchange for payment or reimbursement, for the acquisition of research data, or for some other consideration that has value to the exercise professional. If the client's expectations as defined within this relationship are not fulfilled, a lawsuit for breach of contract *may* be instituted. Such potential suits allege nonfulfillment of certain promises or a breach of alleged warranties that the law sometimes imposes on many contractual relationships. Contract law also has implications for an exercise professional's business relations with parties other than clients, e.g., equipment companies, independent service contractors, and employees.

Informed Consent

Breach of contract-type claims or suits predicated on tort law principles that are lodged or filed against exercise professionals may arise from failure to obtain adequate informed consent from clients. Although there are a variety of potential deficiencies associated with the informed consent process that may lead to claim and suit, these often involve negligence actions. Legally, to perform a specific procedure, the *client* first must give the provider an *informed* consent. The intention is to ensure that the client enters into the procedure after a full disclosure of all relevant facts, knowledge of the material risks, information about any alternative procedures that are available and might satisfy certain of the objectives, and any benefits associated with that activity for which informed consent is sought. Informed consent can be written or the law may imply it, depending on how the 2 parties to the procedure conducted themselves. The written approach certainly is preferable to any oral or implied form, should questions later arise (see Chapter 3 for sample forms [2,4,5]). If the informed consent is written and includes the professional's notations on important questions received (from the client) and answers given (by the professional), this may be helpful if legal questions arise later. Such notations tend to support the requirement that client comprehension was part of the process that led him/her to agree to affix their signature to the informed consent and thereby agree to the procedure. To give valid informed consent, the individual must meet the following criteria:

1. Be of lawful age
2. Not be mentally incapacitated
3. Know and fully comprehend the importance and relevance of the material risks
4. Give consent voluntarily and not under any mistake of fact or duress

Suits arising from the informed consent process frequently occur when an injured party claims that a professional was negligent in the explanation of the procedure, including the risks, and that the participant would not, but for the negligence of the professional, have undergone the procedure. These cases are often decided upon the testimony of expert witnesses who determine whether the professional engaged in substandard conduct in securing the informed consent. These informed-consent cases can involve claims related to contract laws, warranties, negligence, and malpractice. Suits arising from alleged deficiencies in the informed consent process related to testing, exercise prescription, or physical activity have become more commonplace (3). The law is moving toward a requirement for an ever-broadening disclosure of risk to participants. Some courts have even gone so far as to require the disclosure of all possible risks, as opposed to those which are simply material. Such requirements impose unusual burdens and raise substantial medico-legal concerns.

Another important element of the informed consent process relates at least tangentially to confidentiality and disclosure of any personal and sensitive information that may be gathered from the client in the course of evaluating health status or delivering health-exercise services. Provision should be made in the informed consent or preferably through other documentation to secure the client's written authorization to disclose specific test results and exercise progress reports to health care professionals who have a "need to know," e.g., a primary-care physician and/or to those the client wants such information to be provided to. Written authorization should also be secured from clients in situations when there is an intent to use their data in reporting group statistics for program evaluation or research purposes—even when such information is presented in ways not identifiable with the client. Many states and the federal government have promulgated privacy statutes that may affect the release of personally identifiable material regarding a program participant. The application of these laws to a program and its rights to release information depend on a variety of factors that should be decided on the basis of advice from local legal counsel.

Torts

A tort is defined simply as a type of civil wrong. Noncontractual civil wrongs are resolved judicially through the tort system by an adversarial process in which competing interests are judged and damages for determined wrongs are awarded to the injured party. Most claims of tort that affect exercise professionals are based on allegations of either negligence or malpractice, causing personal injury or death. Negligence actions are a form of tort resolved within the tort system.

NEGLIGENCE AND/OR MALPRACTICE

Negligence may be defined as a failure to conform one's conduct to a generally accepted standard or duty. A cause of action in negligence is established by proof of a breach of that duty which proximately results in harm and damage to the injured party (Fig. 13-2). Thus, establishment of negligence requires that a number of conditions be satisfied. Among the various requirements, it first must be established that some harm or injury actually occurred. Secondly, it must be determined that this injury was specifically attributable to (*proximately caused*) the particular action of an exercise professional (*commission*) or his or her failure to act (*omission*) in accordance with *due care* when the action was performed. When negligence claims arise, the matter of whether an exercise professional provided due care is an issue of critical importance. Once a duty is established, the nature and scope of the expected performance usually is determined by reference to current standards and guidelines published by peer professional associations.

Malpractice is a special type of negligence action involving claims against certain professionals who usually have *public authority to practice (arising from specific state statutes)*—for alleged breaches of professional duties and responsibilities toward patients or other persons to whom they owed a particular standard of care or duty. By statute or case law, some states include nurses, physical therapists, dentists, psychologists, and other health professionals in this group. Very recently, Louisiana became the first state to pass legislation to license and regulate exercise practitioners who work under the authority of physicians with patients in cardiopulmonary rehabilitation treatment programs (6). The Louisiana State Board of Medical Examiners is charged with regulating this new group of licensed professionals. There are specific provisions in the Louisiana act that may affect practitioners in a variety of ways. Some of these ways cannot easily be predicted, but the more obvious possibilities include a somewhat higher level of autonomy in practice, changes in the availability and provision of liability insurance, increased costs of liability insurance, and exposure to claims of malpractice.

In negligence or malpractice actions, proof of the standard of care and breach thereof is established through expert witness testimony supplied at time of trial (Fig. 13-3). In years past, expert witness testimony tended to result in the expression of individualized opinions about what constitutes the standard of care under some specific set of facts that apply to a particular legal case. Frequently, however, such testimonial expressions provided inconsistent and often biased views about the so-called standard of care. Uncertainties sometimes resulted from such cases, and this often created a sense of professional anxiety and confusion about the actual standard of care that should be exercised in the field. In at least a partial response to this oft-perceived problem, many professional associations developed and published practice standards or guidelines to delineate clear benchmarks

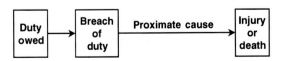

FIGURE 13-2. Legal basis for negligent tort actions.

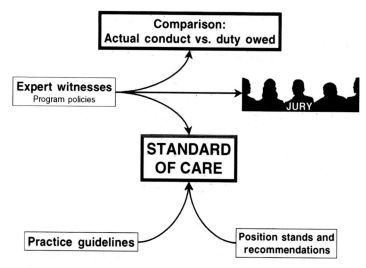

FIGURE 13-3. How standards influence questions of professional conduct in court.

of expected care available to professionals to use in their delivery of service. A great number of such statements have been published over the last 10 years. Some of these statements when compared to others are duplicitous and inconsistent. Wherever feasible, standard-setting organizations should therefore collaborate in their efforts to create or update their practice guidelines. Fortunately, this type of collaboration is increasing among prominent organizations concerned within public health and exercise (7). The result is the development of practice guidelines that are more uniform in scope, detail, and language. In court, such uniform standards may lessen the potential effect of wide-ranging opinions from expert witnesses on the outcome of personal injury cases, since such witnesses may differ considerably in their view of the applicable standard.

Defenses to Negligence and/or Malpractice Actions

If properly given, informed consents can sometimes be used as legal defenses to claims based on either contract or tort principles. In such cases, defense counsel may seek to characterize an informed consent type document as *an assumption of the risks by the plaintiff.* Assumption of the risks of the procedure, however, is often difficult to establish without an explicit written statement or clear conduct that demonstrates such an assumption. In addition, an assumption of the risks never relieves the exercise professional of the duty to perform in a competent and professional manner. In some jurisdictions, it may be advisable or even necessary to obtain consent, an expressed assumption of risk, or even a prospective waiver or release from a participant and/or the participant's spouse, and perhaps, in a limited number of states, to make it binding on any children or the participant's executor, administrators, and heirs.

Informed consents often are confused with so-called *releases*. Releases are statements sometimes written into consent-type documents that contain *exculpatory* language, i.e., wording that professes to relieve the provider from any legal responsibility in the event of a participant's injury or death due to any error or omission or even negligence. These releases also are sometimes referred to as *prospective waivers* of responsibility or liability and in some states may be disfavored (7). In medical settings, the use of such releases, with certain limited exceptions, has been declared invalid as being against public policy. In nonmedical settings, however, particularly with certain activities that may carry a high risk of injury, such as auto racing, sky diving, rafting dangerous rapids, and even as to exercise or fitness activities, the use of such releases may be valid in some jurisdictions. In these and all other circumstances that involve composition and use of consent, release, and waiver-type documents, and in the adoption of risk management tools for a particular setting, it is imperative that exercise professionals consult local legal counsel and risk management professionals to determine the legal validity and appropriateness of such documents.

Other defenses to claims of negligence or malpractice may also be available. In some states, for example, proof of a client's negligence, referred to in law as *contributory negligence*, can preclude any recovery of damages from a defendant (exercise professional). In many states, however, this rule has been modified by adoption of a so-called system of *comparative negligence*. In jurisdictions where comparative negligence is applicable, the negligence of the injured party is compared with the negligence of all defendants in the case. Then, if the negligence of the injured party is found to be less than that of all defendants in the case (or in some states in any case), the plaintiff is allowed to recover. However, the amount of recovery is reduced by the sum of the injured party's own negligence.

Liability Insurance

Liability insurance is an effective mechanism for exercise professionals to protect themselves against financial loss in the event of claim and suit. Such insurance policies provide an insurance-paid defense for any covered claims and suits, as well as *indemnification* from any judgment or settlement that is not excluded from the terms of coverage up to the limits of the applicable coverage.

STANDARDS OF CARE

Standards of care express the ways and means by which services should be delivered to clients so as to give reasonable assurance that the desired outcomes will be achieved in a safe manner. In most professions, such standards are developed and periodically revised by consensus among professionals or national associations of providers. These documents address what are considered to be the benchmark methods, procedures, and processes that are applied in almost all settings, regardless of location, resources, and/or training of the provider. In reality, the national standard of practice at any point in time typically is influenced by a variety of sources, including published statements from professional associations, government policies, and state and national government regulations. In recent years, the promulgation of standards has increased dramatically in medicine and related health care fields, as well as in the fitness profession. This circumstance mandates that professionals stay abreast of new pronouncements and regulations dealing with these issues.

Without knowledge of the most relevant and current standard-type documents and incorporation of their tenants into the professional's operating protocols and records of service fulfillment, the individual practitioner becomes more vulnerable to damage and loss in the event of legal challenges arising from personal injury lawsuits. The reason for this derives from the critical role that *standards of care* play in the legal arena. To clarify, consider that, in law, proof of negligence consequent to an injury of a client often depends on whether it can be established that there was a clear causal connection between the injury to the client and what the professional did or failed to do. To establish what should or shouldn't have been done in a given case, the court relies heavily on interpretations from these standard-type documents (provided through expert witnesses). The use of these standards in certain cases dealing with exercise testing and exercise leadership already has occurred (8).

Several organizations have published documents that influence the legal standard of care in the health/fitness and exercise rehabilitation fields. It is beyond the scope of this chapter to list or discuss all of these in detail. The sources listed below represent recent updates from a select group of national organizations that have particular importance for health-related exercise programs. This is by no means a comprehensive list:

- The American College of Sports Medicine (*ACSM's Guidelines for Exercise Testing and Prescription*) (4)
- The American Heart Association (9–13)
- The American Association of Cardiovascular and Pulmonary Rehabilitation (5,14,15)
- The Agency for Health Care Policy and Research (16)
- The American College of Cardiology (9)
- The Association for Fitness in Business (17)

Documents from these organizations and others, including the Aerobics and Fitness Association of America (AFAA), International Health, Racquet & Sportsclub Association (IHRSA), and American Council on Exercise (ACE), vary in scope and applicability to different situations. Professionals should carefully consider the purposes and methods of their services, uses of technologies, medically related protocols, and their clientele before deciding which standards and guidelines are most applicable. Deficiencies or disparities in the published standards and guidelines have importance for safety and legal exposure. In such cases, professionals should adopt the most stringent set of standards and then couple this adoption of such statements with operational approaches that are as conservative as possible (without compromising their ability to meet client goals and needs). In final decisions in this area, as with others mentioned in this chapter, practitioners should seek the advice of their local legal counsel or other advisors.

Policies, Protocols, Forms, and Fulfillment

Policies and procedures that are correlated to relevant national standards provide yet another important step in managing legal risks for exercise programs. Likewise, program forms and checklists created for such protocols as preactivity health/fitness screening of clients, exercise testing, exercise monitoring, and client orientation/instruction represent tangible links to national standards as a function of their design and relationship to a program's operating manual. Finally, the thoroughness and consistency by which staff members record information on these forms and also act on such information is of critical importance to the defense of legal challenges. Consistent and accurate record keeping, done contemporaneously with delivery of service, provides powerful verification of fulfillment in accordance with the standard that a program has adopted. Of course, such recordings can be most damaging in a liability case should these provide evidence of negligence and proximate cause in connection with harm to a client. Exercise professionals should design and use recording forms and protocol checklists routinely to assure standardization in every area where injury and/or legal risks are considered significant. These might include, but are not limited to, dated checklists of equipment and supplies reviewed for exercise emergency situations, checklists for instructing new clients in exercise routines or explaining specific cautions for avoidance of injury, and inspection checklists for routine examination of equipment and facilities.

FACILITY AND EQUIPMENT ISSUES

Issues related to facilities and equipment are often involved in litigation related to exercise. Although some cases pertaining to equipment arise due to claims of improper design or manufacture, a good number of these also deal with improper provider assembly, maintenance or repair, or failures to properly provide instruction, warning, or supervision to clients. Many programs face such claims without adequate preparation and without having met the appropriate standard of care in reference to the equipment used in their facilities. All these potential equipment liability areas deserve close and ongoing attention so that claims and suits might be minimized.

The ACSM recently led a multiorganizational project to develop health/fitness facility standards and guidelines. Although the goal was to promote quality of physical activity programs and consumer service, publication of the document added considerable definition to the standard of care for design and operation of all health-fitness facilities (4,18). The first edition was published in 1992 and included 650 standards and guidelines. It was organized into 22 chapters covering a wide range of facility, equipment, and operational domains. However, significant concerns were voiced almost immediately after publication from a number of sectors in the industry. The greatest among these were concerns related to the costs of compliance associated with adhering to the 397 "standards" items and the increased legal vulnerability that might be engendered by facilities that failed to adhere to these standards (18).

The second edition of this work attempted to consolidate material, simplify format, and reexamine the industry concerns. Now, only six benchmarks are categorized as "standards" (i.e., mandatory performance expectations), while approximately 500 guidelines are offered more as recommendations for enhancing quality in programs. The six standards are safety-related benchmarks related to emergency response, preactivity screening, competency levels of physical activity supervisors, warning-type signage, and conditions necessitating supervision of youth. All health/fitness professionals should carefully review this publication because its standards and guidelines undoubtedly will have significant influence on deciding the standard of care in legal claim and suit. The same is true, of course, for those practicing in rehabilitative exercise (4,5,14) and health promotion (17) relative to facility and equipment standards and guidelines that are applicable to their settings.

LEGAL CONCERNS AND THE ROLES OF LICENSED AND NONLICENSED EXERCISE PROFESSIONALS

Providing exercise services with some degree of independence while collaborating with licensed providers can potentially create legally precarious circumstances for the exercise professional. A prime example relates to the question of who is legally authorized and who is proscribed from providing emergency cardiac care in community or clinic settings for exercising cardiac patients. There is no doubt that the emergency response standard for this situation is clear and universal (see Appendix B and related publications [5,10]) in calling for a defibrillator, crash ("code") cart with artificial airways, suction pump, and emergency drugs. Furthermore, the standard is clear that such settings should include an on-site provider who is able to administer advanced cardiac life support (ACLS) as delineated by the AHA (10). The provider of emergency services, however, must understand that he or she cannot assume such duties unless the physician in charge has given written *standing orders* to that effect *and* the individual has legal authority under state statutes to accept such standing orders. This almost is never the case for the nonlicensed exercise professional, with or without current successful training in an ACLS program of the AHA.

The health care reform movement has compounded these challenges because of the increasing trend to staff health care services with paraprofessionals to reduce costs. In fact, various states have undertaken efforts to expand nursing practice and other medical practice laws beyond mere observation, reporting, and recording of patient signs/symptoms. Various physician assistant or similar paraprofessional laws allow more nonphysicians to have expanded treatment authority when dealing with patients. Despite these developments, however, some nonphysicians who perform services that might be characterized as "medical" or are otherwise reserved in law for certain statutorily defined and controlled allied health professions need to understand their special legal risks. In such situations, the nonlicensed provider runs the risk of engaging in unauthorized practices that could lead to both criminal and civil sanctions. Many states have defined the practice of medicine broadly so that nonlicensed persons engaged in exercise testing and prescription activities could, under some circumstances, fall within the limits of such statutes. Without the presence or assistance of a physician or other licensed allied health professional for certain aspects of these exercise services, claims as to the unauthorized practice of medicine could be put forth.

Under some of these state statutes, such practices are often classified as crimes, usually misdemeanors, punishable by imprisonment for less than 1 year, a fine, or both. In addition, a person found to have engaged in the unauthorized practice of medicine or some other allied health profession faces (after the fact) the legal expectation to provide an elevated standard of care in the event of participant injury or death. Under this rule, the exercise professional's actions would be compared to an assumed standard of care of a physician or other allied health professional acting under the same or similar circumstances. In the event that the professional's actions do not meet this standard (which the nonphysician or allied health professional cannot meet because of inadequacies of knowledge, skill, authorization, and experience), liability may result.

Exercise professionals often are placed in collaborative roles with licensed health care providers in the setting of clinical exercise testing and delivery of rehabilitative exercise services. This has prompted the ACSM and others (9,15) to clarify roles and responsibilities for these collaborative situations between physicians and nonlicensed exercise professionals. The most comprehensive effort in this area to date is reflected by the competency certifications of the ACSM (see Appendix F for knowledge, skills, and abilities that define the ACSM certification programs). The latter is complemented by the AACVPR Core Competency position statement for Cardiac Rehabilitation Specialists (15). Another development in this area occurred when the Louisiana legislature passed the previously mentioned bill to license clinical exercise physiologists, or CEPs (6). This particular act authorizes exercise professionals with specified qualifications to provide care to patients who are enrolled in cardiopulmonary rehabilitation programs, so long as they do so in Louisiana while under the direction, approval, and supervision of a licensed physician. This law is so new that it is not yet possible to assess its implications for differentiation of practice patterns among CEPs. However, it may well evolve into a variety of new collaborative arrangements for CEPs and physicians that were unanticipated by the practice act.

In 2000, the ACSM plans to implement a national Registry for Clinical Exercise Physiologists$_{SM}$, i.e., the RCEP (19). This plan, promulgated by the ACSM Board of Trustees in 1996, will recognize professionals who have achieved a master's degree in exercise physiology, have significant clinical experience, and have passed a comprehensive written examination. The intent is to provide a credential that will advance patient care in an ever-broadening range of chronic diseases and conditions where emerging scientific and clinical evidence indicates that the exercise provides therapeutic effects, functional benefits, or both. The scope of clients to be served by the RCEP will be considerable and will include, but is not limited to, those with cardiovascular, pulmonary, metabolic, immunologic, inflammatory, orthopedic, and neuromuscular diseases and conditions. The RCEP's scope of competencies will encompass exercise evaluation, exercise prescription, exercise supervision, exercise education, and exercise outcome evaluation. The RCEP's clients will be restricted to those who are referred by and are under the continuing care of a licensed physician. This credential is expected to increase access to quality exercise services for patients, with the added assurance that the outcomes will promote fitness development, health-related quality of life, and independent living. Of equal importance, this new ACSM credential will, by design, include certain steps that will help reshape related academic programs in higher education across the United States and facilitate career opportunities nationally for exercise clinicians. The fact that the RCEP is expected to work with patients under conditions of significant autonomy, yet do so only on the basis of physician referral, will pose some special liability concerns, as well as those concerns related to practice areas reserved by various state laws to licensed health care professionals. Therefore, RCEPs will need individualized legal counsel in their jurisdictions, special liability insurance coverage, and rigorous standards of practice so that they may appropriately manage their legal risks.

Summary

As more and more middle-aged and older adults with varied co-morbidities engage in professionally directed exercise programs, the number of untoward events during these activities will escalate. These injuries will result in a rising number of negligence-type claims that will ultimately find resolution in court. The probabilities of such actions are low, particularly for individuals and organizations that operate programs in a manner commensurate with rigorous standards and guidelines. Awareness of the main areas of legal vulnerability and adoption of legally sensitive practices may help to reduce risks of litigation. Simultaneously, this should result in more efficacious and satisfying programs for clients. Ultimately, the most effective shield against claims of negligence may be development of professional competency by individual practitioners and a daily pattern of adhering to the most relevant and rigorous published guidelines. Professionals would be well advised to keep up to date as information on new standards and litigation in this rapidly changing field becomes available (3).

References

1. Herbert D, Herbert W. Legal considerations. In: Roitman JL, ed. ACSM's Resource Manual

for Guidelines for Exercise Testing and Training. 3rd ed. Baltimore: Williams & Wilkins, 1998:610–615.

2. Herbert DL, Herbert WG. Legal Aspects of Preventive, Rehabilitative and Recreational Exercise Programs. 3rd ed. Canton, OH: PRC Publishing, Inc., 1993.

3. The Exercise Standards and Malpractice Reporter (Published six times per year; Canton, OH: PRC Publishing, Inc., 44718-3629).

4. American College of Sports Medicine. ACSM's Health/Fitness Facility Standards and Guidelines. 2nd ed. Champaign, IL: Human Kinetics, 1997.

5. American Association for Cardiovascular and Pulmonary Rehabilitation. Guidelines for Cardiac Rehabilitation and Secondary Prevention Programs. 3rd ed. Champaign, IL: Human Kinetics Publications, 1999.

6. Herbert WG. Licensure of clinical exercise physiologists: impressions concerning the new law in Louisiana. The Exercise Standards and Malpractice Reporter 1995;9:65, 68–70.

7. Cotten DJ, Cotten MB. Legal Aspects of Waivers in Sports, Recreation and Fitness Activities. Canton, OH: PRC Publishing, Inc., 1997.

8. Tart vs. McGann. US District Court, Southern District of New York, Case No. 81-CIV-IL-3899 (ELP 1981). *Cited* in 697 F. 2d 75 (2d Cir. 1982).

9. American College of Cardiology/American Heart Association. Guidelines for exercise testing. J Am Coll Cardiol 1997;30:260–315 and Circulation 1997;96:345–354.

10. American Heart Association. Guidelines for cardiopulmonary resuscitation and emergency cardiac care. JAMA 1992;268:2171–2183.

11. Fletcher GF, Blair SN, Blumenthal J, et al. The AHA medical/scientific statement on exercise. Circulation 1992;86:340–344.

12. Balady GJ, Fletcher BJ, Froelicher ES, et al. The AHA medical/scientific statement on cardiac rehabilitation programs. Circulation 1994;90:1602–1610.

13. Fletcher GF, Balady G, Froelicher VF, et al. The AHA medical/scientific statement on exercise standards. Circulation 1995;91:580–615.

14. American Association for Cardiovascular and Pulmonary Rehabilitation. Guidelines for Pulmonary Rehabilitation Programs. 2nd ed. Champaign, IL: Human Kinetics, 1998.

15. AACVPR core competencies for cardiac rehabilitation specialists. J Cardiopulm Rehabil 1994;14:87–92.

16. Agency for Health Care Policy and Research. Cardiac rehabilitation. Clinical practice guideline No. 17. Rockville, MD: US Department of Health and Human Services, Publication No. 96-0672, 1995.

17. Association for Fitness in Business. Guidelines for Employee Health Promotion Programs. Champaign, IL: Human Kinetics, 1992.

18. Herbert DL. Preparing to meet new industry standards for health and fitness facilities: where do we go from here? The Exercise Standards and Malpractice Reporter 1993;7:40–43.

19. American College of Sports Medicine. *(http://www.acsm.org).*

SECTION V

Appendices

Appendix A
Common Medications

 TABLE A-1. Generic and Brand Names of Common Drugs by Class

Generic Name	Brand Name*
β-Blockers	
Acebutolol	Sectral
Atenolol	Tenormin
Betaxolol	Kerlone
Bisoprolol	Zebeta
Carteolol	Cartrol
Esmolol	Brevibloc
Metoprolol	Lopressor, Toprol
Nadolol	Corgard
Penbutolol	Levatol
Pindolol	Visken
Propranolol	Inderal
Sotalol	Betapace
Timolol	Blocadren
β-Blockers in Combinations With	
Diuretics	Inderide, Lopressor Hydrochlorothiazide (HCTZ), Tenoretic, Timolide, Ziac, Corzide
α- and β-Adrenergic Blocking Agents	
Carvedilol	Coreg
Labetalol	Normodyne, Trandate
α₁-Adrenergic Blocking Agents	
Doxazosin	Cardura
Prazosin	Minipress
Terazosin	Hytrin

TABLE A-1. *(continued)*

Generic Name	Brand Name*
Antiadrenergic Agents Without Selective Receptor Blockade	
Clonidine	Catapres
Guanabenz	Wyntensin
Guanadrel	Hylorel
Guanethidine	Ismelin
Guanfacine	Tenex
Methyldopa	Aldomet
Reserpine	Serpasil
Nitrates and Nitroglycerin	
Amyl nitrite	Amyl nitrite
Isosorbide mononitrate	Ismo, Monoket, Imdur
Isosorbide dinitrate	Isordil, Sorbitrate, Dilatrate
Nitroglycerin, sublingual	Nitrostat
Nitroglycerin, translingual	Nitrolingual
Nitroglycerin, transmucosal	Nitrogard
Nitroglycerin, sustained release	Nitrong, Nitrocine, Nitroglyn, Nitro-Bid
Nitroglycerin, transdermal	Minitran, Nitro-Dur, Transderm-Nitro, Deponit, Nitrodisc, Nitro-Derm
Nitroglycerin, topical	Nitro-Bid, Nitrol
Calcium Channel Blockers	
Amlodipine	Norvasc
Bepridil	Vascor
Diltiazem	Cardizem, Dilacor, Tiazac
Felodipine	Plendil
Isradipine	DynaCirc
Nicardipine	Cardene
Nifedipine	Adalat, Procardia
Nimodipine	Nimotop
Nisoldipine	Sular
Verapamil	Calan, Isoptin, Covera, Verelan
Cardiac Glycosides	
Digitoxin	Crystodigin
Digoxin	Lanoxin
Peripheral Vasodilators (Nonadrenergic)	
Hydralazine	Apresoline
Minoxidil	Loniten
Isoxsuprine	Vasodilan
Papaverine	Pavabid

TABLE A-1. (*continued*)

Generic Name	Brand Name*

Angiotensin-Converting Enzyme (ACE) Inhibitors
Benazepril	Lotensin
Captopril	Capoten
Enalapril	Vasotec
Fosinopril	Monopril
Lisinopril	Zestril, Prinivil
Moexipril	Univasc
Perindopril erbumine	Aceon
Quinapril	Accupril
Ramipril	Altace
Trandolapril	Mavik

ACE Inhibitors + Diuretics
Captopril and HCTZ	Capozide
Enalapril maleate and HCTZ	Vaseretic
Lisinopril and HCTZ	Prinzide, Zestoretic
Moexipril and HCTZ	Uniretic

Angiotensin II Receptor Antagonists
Irbesartan	Avapro
Losartan	Cozaar
Valsartan	Diovan

Diuretics
Thiazides
Hydrochlorothiazide (HCTZ)	Esidrix

"Loop"
Bumetanide	Bumex
Ethacrynic acid	Edecrin
Furosemide	Lasix

Potassium-sparing
Amiloride	Midamor
Spironolactone	Aldactone
Triamterene	Dyrenium

Combinations
Triamterene and HCTZ	Dyazide, Maxzide
Amiloride and HCTZ	Moduretic

Others
Metolazone	Zaroxolyn

Antiarrhythmic Agents
Class I
IA
Disopyramide	Norpace
Moricizine	Ethmozine
Procainamide	Pronestyl, Procan SR
Quinidine	Quinora, Quinidex, Quinaglute, Quinalan, Cardioquin

TABLE A-1. (*continued*)

Generic Name	Brand Name*
Antiarrhythmic Agents	
Class I	
IB	
Lidocaine	Xylocaine, Xylocard
Mexiletine	Mexitil
Phenytoin	Dilantin
Tocainide	Tonocard
IC	
Flecainide	Tambocor
Propafenone	Rythmol
Class II	
β-Blockers	
Class III	
Amiodarone	Cordarone
Bretylium	Bretylol
Sotalol	Betapace
Class IV	
Calcium channel blockers	
Antihyperlipidemic Agents	
Atorvastatin	Lipitor
Cerivastatin	Baycol
Cholestyramine	Questran, Cholybar, Prevalite
Clofibrate	Atromid
Colestipol	Colestid
Fluvastatin	Lescol
Gemfibrozil	Lopid
Lovastatin	Mevacor
Nicotinic acid (niacin)	Nicobid, Nicolar, Slo-Niacin, Niaspan
Pravastatin	Pravachol
Simvastatin	Zocor
Sympathomimetic Agents	
Albuterol	Proventil, Ventolin
Ephedrine	Primatene
Epinephrine	Adrenalin
Isoetharine	Bronkosol
Metaproterenol	Alupent
Terbutaline	Brethine
Others	
Clopidogrel	Plavix
Dipyridamole	Persantine
Pentoxifylline	Trental
Warfarin	Coumadin

*Represent selected brands; these are not necessarily all-inclusive.

TABLE A-2. Effects of Medications on Heart Rate, Blood Pressure, the Electrocardiogram (ECG), and Exercise Capacity

Medications	Heart Rate	Blood Pressure	ECG	Exercise Capacity
I. β-Blockers (including carvedilol, labetalol)	↓*(R and E)	↓ (R and E)	↓ HR*(R) ↓ ischemia†(E)	↑ in patients with angina; ↓ or ↔ in patients without angina
II. Nitrates	↑ (R) ↑ or ↔ (E)	↓ (R) ↓ or ↔ (E)	↑ HR (R) ↑ or ↔ HR (E) ↓ ischemia†(E)	↑ in patients with angina; ↔ in patients without angina; ↑ or ↔ in patients with congestive heart failure (CHF)
III. Calcium channel blockers				
Amlodipine Felodipine Isradipine Nicardipine Nifedipine Nimodipine Nisoldipine	↑ or ↔ (R and E)	↓ (R and E)	↑ or ↔ HR (R and E) ↓ ischemia†(E)	↑ in patients with angina; ↔ in patients without angina
Bepridil Diltiazem Verapamil	↓ (R and E)	↓ (R and E)	↓ HR (R and E) ↓ ischemia†(E)	

TABLE A-2. (continued)

Medications	Heart Rate	Blood Pressure	ECG	Exercise Capacity
IV. Digitalis	↓ in patients with atrial fibrillation and possibly CHF Not significantly altered in patients with sinus rhythm	↔ (R and E)	May produce nonspecific ST-T wave changes (R) May produce ST segment depression (E)	Improved only in patients with atrial fibrillation or in patients with CHF
V. Diuretics	↔ (R and E)	↔ or ↓ (R and E)	↔ or PVCs (R) May cause PVCs and "false positive" test results if hypokalemia occurs May cause PVCs if hypomagnesemia occurs (E)	↔, except possibly in patients with CHF
VI. Vasodilators, nonadrenergic	↑ or ↔ (R and E)	↓ (R and E)	↑ or ↔ HR (R and E)	↔, except ↑ or ↔ in patients with CHF
ACE inhibitors	↔ (R and E)	↓ (R and E)	↔ (R and E)	↔, except ↑ or ↔ in patients with CHF
α-Adrenergic blockers	↔ (R and E)	↓ (R and E)	↔ (R and E)	↔
Antiadrenergic agents without selective blockade	↓ or ↔ HR (R and E)	↓ (R and E)	↓ or ↔ HR (R and E)	↔

All antiarrhythmic agents may cause new or worsened arrhythmias (proarrhythmic effect)

VII. Antiarrhythmic agents				
Class I				
Quinidine Disopyramide	↑ or ↔ (R and E)	↓ or ↔ (R) ↔ (E)	↑ or ↔ HR (R) May prolong QRS and QT intervals (R) Quinidine may result in "false negative" test results (E)	↕
Procainamide	↔ (R and E)	↔ (R and E)	May prolong QRS and QT intervals (R) May result in "false positive" test results (E)	↕
Phenytoin Tocainide Mexiletine	↔ (R and E)	↔ (R and E)		↕
Flecainide Moricizine	↔ (R and E)	↔ (R and E)	May prolong QRS and QT intervals (R) ↔ (E)	↕
Propafenone	↓ (R) or ↔ (E)	↔ (R and E)	↓ HR (R) ↓ or ↔ HR (E)	↕
Class II β-Blockers (see I.)				
Class III Amiodarone	↓ (R and E)	↔ (R and E)	↓ HR (R) ↔ (E)	↕
Class IV Calcium channel blockers (see III.)				

TABLE A-2. (continued)

Medications	Heart Rate	Blood Pressure	ECG	Exercise Capacity
VIII. Bronchodilators	↔ (R and E)	↔ (R and E)	↔ (R and E)	Bronchodilators ↑ exercise capacity in patients limited by bronchospasm
Anticholinergic agents Methylxanthines	↑ or ↔ (R and E)	↔	↑ or ↔ HR May produce PVCs (R and E)	
Sympathomimetic agents	↑ or ↔ (R and E)	↑, ↔, or ↓ (R and E)	↑ or ↔ HR (R and E)	↔
Cromolyn sodium	↔ (R and E)	↔ (R and E)	↔ (R and E)	↔
Corticosteroids	↔ (R and E)	↔ (R and E)	↔ (R and E)	↔
IX. Antihyperlipidemic agents		Clofibrate may provoke arrhythmias, angina in patients with prior myocardial infarction Nicotinic acid may ↓ BP All other antihyperlipidemic agents have no effect on HR, BP, and ECG		↔
X. Psychotropic medications Minor tranquilizers	May ↓ HR and BP by controlling anxiety; no other effects			
Antidepressants	↑ or ↔ (R and E)	↓ or ↔ (R and E)	Variable (R) May result in "false positive" test results (E)	
Major tranquilizers	↑ or ↔ (R and E)	↓ or ↔ (R and E)	Variable (R) May result in "false positive" or "false negative" test results (E)	
Lithium	↔ (R and E)	↔ (R and E)	May result in T wave changes and arrhythmias (R and E)	

Medication			
XI. Nicotine	↑ or ↔ (R and E)	↑ (R and E)	↑ or ↔ HR May provoke ischemia, arrhythmias (R and E)	↔, except ↓ or ↔ in patients with angina
XII. Antihistamines	↔ (R and E)	↔ (R and E)	↔ (R and E)	↔
XIII. Cold medications with sympathomimetic agents	Effects similar to those described in sympathomimetic agents, although magnitude of effects is usually smaller			↔
XIV. Thyroid medications Only levothyroxine	↑ (R and E)	↑ (R and E)	↑ HR May provoke arrhythmias ↑ ischemia (R and E)	↔, unless angina worsened
XV. Alcohol	↔ (R and E)	Chronic use may have role in ↑ BP (R and E)	May provoke arrhythmias (R and E)	↔
XVI. Hypoglycemic agents Insulin and oral agents	↔ (R and E)	↔ (R and E)	↔ (R and E)	↔
XVII. Dipyridamole	↔ (R and E)	↔ (R and E)	↔ (R and E)	↔
XVIII. Anticoagulants	↔ (R and E)	↔ (R and E)	↔ (R and E)	↔
XIX. Antigout medications	↔ (R and E)	↔ (R and E)	↔ (R and E)	↔
XX. Antiplatelet medications	↔ (R and E)	↔ (R and E)	↔ (R and E)	↔

TABLE A-2. (*continued*)

Medications	Heart Rate	Blood Pressure	ECG	Exercise Capacity
XXI. Pentoxifylline	↔ (R and E)	↔ (R and E)	↔ (R and E)	↑ or ↔ in patients limited by intermittent claudication
XXII. Caffeine	Variable effects depending upon previous use Variable effects on exercise capacity May provoke arrhythmias			
XXIII. Anorexiants/diet pills	↑ or ↔ (R and E)	↑ or ↔ (R and E)	↑ or ↔ HR (R and E)	

Key: ↑ = increase; ↔ = no effect; ↓ = decrease; R = rest; E = exercise; HR = heart rate; PVCs = premature ventricular contractions.

*β-Blockers with ISA lower resting HR only slightly.

†May prevent or delay myocardial ischemia (see text).

APPENDIX B
Emergency Management

The following key points are essential components of all emergency medical plans:

- All personnel involved with exercise testing and supervision should be trained in basic cardiopulmonary resuscitation (CPR) and preferably advanced cardiac life support (ACLS).
- There should be at least one, and preferably two, licensed and trained ACLS personnel and a physician immediately available at all times when maximal sign- or symptom-limited exercise testing is performed.
- Telephone numbers for emergency assistance should be posted clearly on all telephones. Emergency communication devices must be readily available and working properly.
- Emergency plans should be established and posted. Regular rehearsal of emergency plans and scenarios should be conducted and documented.
- Regular drills should be conducted at least quarterly for all personnel.
  —A specific person or persons should be assigned to the regular maintenance of the emergency equipment and to the regular surveillance of all pharmacologic substances.
  —Records should be kept documenting function of emergency equipment such as defibrillator, oxygen supply and suction. In addition, expiration dates for pharmacologic agents and other supportive supplies (e.g., intravenous equipment and intravenous fluids) should be kept.
  —Hospital emergency departments (or code teams) and other sources of support such as paramedics (if exercise testing is performed outside of a hospital setting) should be advised as to the exercise testing laboratory location as well as the usual times of operation.

If a problem occurs during exercise testing, the nearest physician or other licensed and trained ACLS provider (paramedic or code team) available should be summoned immediately. The physician should decide whether to call for evacuation to the nearest hospital if testing is not carried out in the hospital. If a physician is not available and any question exists as to the status of the patient, then emergency transportation to the closest hospital should be summoned immediately.

Equipment and drugs that should be available in any area where maximal exercise testing is performed are listed in Table B-1. Only those personnel authorized by law to use certain equipment (e.g., defibrillators, syringes, needles) and dispense drugs can lawfully do so. It is mandatory that such personnel be immediately available during maximal exercise testing of persons with known coronary artery disease.

Tables B-2 through B-4 provide sample plans for nonemergency situations (Table B-2) and emergency situations (B-3 and B-4). These plans are provided only as examples, and specific plans must be tailored to individual program needs and local standards.

 TABLE B-1. Emergency Equipment and Drugs

Equipment

Portable, battery-operated defibrillator-monitor with hardcopy printout or memory, cardioversion capability, direct-current capability in case of battery failure (equipment must have battery low-light indicator). Defibrillator should be able to perform hard wire monitoring in case of exercise testing monitor failure

Sphygmomanometer including aneroid cuff and stethoscope

Airway supplies including oral, nasopharyngeal, and/or intubation equipment (only in situations where licensed and trained personnel are available for use)

Oxygen, available by nasal cannula and mask

AMBU bag with pressure release valve

Suction equipment

Intravenous fluids and stand

Intravenous access equipment in varying sizes including butterfly IV supplies

Syringes and needles in multiple sizes

Tourniquets

Adhesive tape, alcohol wipes, gauze pads

Emergency documentation forms (incident/accident form or code charting form)

TABLE B-1. (*continued*)

Drugs (IV Form Unless Otherwise Indicated)

Aspirin, adult strength/oral
American Heart Association ACLS, 1997 (1)
    Pharmacology I (agents used for full cardiac arrest including the antiar-
      rhythmics)
        Oxygen*
        Epinephrine*
        Atropine*
        Glucose tablets
      Antiarrhythmics
        Lidocaine*
        Procainamide*
        Bretylium*
        Verapamil and Diltiazem*
        Adenosine*
    Pharmacology II (agents used to treat acute myocardial infarction and
      its complications, including inotropic vasoactive agents and antihy-
      pertensive vasodilators)
      Inotropic vasoactive agents
        Epinephrine
        Norepinephrine
        Dopamine
        Dobutamine
        Isoproterenol
        Milrinone
        Digitalis
        Vasodilators/antihypertensives
        Sodium nitroprusside
        Nitroglycerin
        β-Adrenergic blockers
          Propranolol
          Metoprolol
          Atenolol
          Esmolol
        Diuretics
          Furosemide
      Thrombolytic agents
        Ansioylated plasminogen activator complex
        Streptokinase
        Tissue plasminogen activator

IV, intravenous.

*Agents used in cardiac arrest algorithms.

TABLE B-2. Plan for Nonemergency Situations

Level: Basic	Intermediate	High
At a field, pool, or park without emergency equipment	At a gymnasium or outside facility with basic equipment plus defibrillator and possibly a small "start-up" kit with drugs	Hospital or hospital adjunct with all the equipment of intermediate level plus a "code cart" containing emergency drugs and equipment for IV drug administration, intubation, drawing arterial blood gas samples, and suctioning. Victim may be inpatient or outpatient

Level: Basic	Intermediate	High
First Rescuer	First Rescuer	First Rescuer

1. Instruct victim to stop activity
2. Remain with victim until symptoms subside
  a. If symptoms worsen, use basic first aid
  b. If symptoms do not subside, bring victim to ER or physician's office for evaluation
3. Advise victim to seek medical advice before further activity
4. Document event
	Same as Basic level No. 1–4
	Add:
	5. Take vital signs
	6. Monitor and record ECG rhythm
	7. Bring record of vital signs and ECG rhythm strip to ER/physician's office if symptoms do not subside and visit is necessary
		Inpatient facility
		Same as Intermediate level No. 1–6
		Add:
		7. Call for medical personnel on duty
		8. Notify primary physician
		9. Request new consult from physician to resume exercise if more than three consecutive exercise sessions are interrupted for same complaint

Level: Basic	Intermediate	High
Second Rescuer	**Second Rescuer**	**Second Rescuer**
1. Assist first rescuer, drive victim to ER or physician's office, if necessary	Same as Basic level No. 1 Add: 2. Bring blood pressure cuff and ECG monitor to site 3. Assist with taking and monitoring vital signs	Same as Intermediate level No. 1–3

ECG, electrocardiogram; ER, emergency room (center); IV, intravenous.

TABLE B-3. Plan for Potentially Life-Threatening Situations

Level: Basic	Intermediate	High
At a field, pool, or park without emergency equipment	At a gymnasium or outside facility with basic equipment plus defibrillator and possibly a small "start-up" kit with drugs	Hospital or hospital adjunct with all the equipment of intermediate level plus a "code cart" containing emergency drugs and equipment for oxygen, intravenous drug administration, intubation, drawing arterial blood gas samples, and suctioning Victim may be inpatient or outpatient

Level: Basic	Intermediate	High
First Rescuer	**First Rescuer**	**First Rescuer**

1. Establish responsiveness
  a. Responsive:
    Instruct victim to sit
    Activate EMS
    Direct second rescuer to call EMS
    Stay with victim until EMS team arrives
    Note time of incident
    Apply pressure to any bleeding
    Note if victim takes any medication (i.e., nitroglycerin)
    Take pulse
  b. Unresponsive:
    Place victim supine
    Open airway
    Activate EMS
    Check respiration. If absent, follow directions in Table B-4
    Maintain open airway
    Check pulse. If absent follow directions in Table B-4
	Same as Basic level No. 1 and 2
	Add:
	3. Apply monitor to victim and record rhythm. Monitor continuously
	4. Take vital signs every 1 to 5 minutes
	5. Document vital signs and rhythm. Note time, and victim signs and symptoms
		Same as Intermediate level No. 1–5
		Also may adapt/add:
		1. Call nurse on ward
		2. Call nurse if physician is off ward
		3. Notify primary physician as soon as possible

Direct second rescuer to call EMS
Stay with victim; continue to monitor respiration and pulse

2. Other considerations
   a. If bleeding, compress area to decrease/stop bleeding
   b. Suspected neck fracture: open airway with a jaw-thrust maneuver; do not hyperextend neck
   c. If seizing; prevent injury by removing harmful objects; place something under head if possible

   Turn victim on side, once seizure activity stops, to help drain secretions

Level: Basic	Intermediate	High
Second Rescuer	**Second Rescuer**	**Second Rescuer**

1. Call EMS
2. Wait to direct emergency team to scene
3. Return to scene to assist
	Same as Basic level No. 1–3
	Add:
	4. Bring all emergency equipment and
	  a. Place victim on monitor
	  b. Run ECG rhythm strips
	  c. Take vital signs
		Same as Intermediate level No. 1–4

Level: Basic	Intermediate	High
Third Rescuer	**Third Rescuer**	**Third Rescuer**
1. Direct emergency team to scene or 2. Assist first rescuer	Same as Basic level	Same as Basic level

ECG, electrocardiogram; EMS, emergency medical services.

TABLE B-4. Plan for Life-Threatening Situations

Level: Basic	Intermediate	High
At a field, pool, or park without emergency equipment	At a gymnasium or outside facility with basic equipment plus defibrillator and possibly a small "start-up" kit with drugs	Hospital or hospital adjunct with all the equipment of intermediate level plus a "code cart" containing emergency drugs and equipment for intravenous drug administration, intubation, oxygenation, drawing arterial blood gas samples, and suctioning. Victim may be inpatient or outpatient

Level: Basic	Intermediate	High
First Rescuer	First Rescuer	First Rescuer
1. Position victim (pull from pool if necessary) and place supine, determine unresponsiveness 2. Call for help (911 or local EMS number) 3. Open airway; look, listen, and feel for the air 4. Give 2 ventilations if no respirations 5. Check pulse (carotid artery) 6. Administer 15:2 compression/ventilation if no pulse 7. Continue ventilation if no respiration	Step No. 1–7 for Basic level	Step No. 1–7 for Basic level

Level: Basic	Intermediate	High
Second Rescuer	**Second Rescuer**	**Second Rescuer**

1. Locate nearest phone and call EMS
2. Return to scene and help with 2-person CPR, or
3. Remain at designated area and direct emergency team to location
	Step No. 1–3 of Basic level
	Add:
	4. Return to scene, bringing defibrillator: take "quick look" at rhythm
	Document rhythm (do not defibrillate unless certified to do so and this activity is part of your clinical privileges for the facility in which the work is being completed)
	5. Place monitor leads on patient and monitor rhythm during CPR
	6. Bring emergency drug kit if available
	  a. Open oxygen equipment and use AMBU bag with oxygen at 10 L/min, i.e., 100% (2) (if trained to do so)
	  b. Open drug kit and prepare intravenous line and drug administration (must only be done by trained, licensed professionals)
	  c. Keep equipment at scene for use by emergency personnel
		Step No. 1–6 of Intermediate level

Level: Basic	Intermediate	High
Third Rescuer	**Third Rescuer**	**Third Rescuer**
1. Assist with 2-person CPR or 2. Help direct emergency team to site 3. Help clear area	Same as Basic level	Same as Basic level

EMS, emergency medical services.

References

1. Advanced cardiac life support. Greenville, TX: American Heart Association, 1997–1999.
2. Basic life support for health care providers. Greenville, TX: American Heart Association, 1994.

APPENDIX C
Electrocardiogram (ECG) Interpretation

The tables in this appendix provide a quick reference source for ECG recording and interpretation. Each of these tables should be used as part of the overall clinical picture when making diagnostic decisions about an individual.

 TABLE C-1. Precordial (Chest Lead) Electrode Placement

Lead	Electrode Placement
V_1	4th intercostal space just to the right of the sternal border
V_2	4th intercostal space just to the left of the sternal border
V_3	At the midpoint of a straight line between V_2 and V_4
V_4	On the midclavicular line in the 5th intercostal space
V_5	On the anterior axillary line and horizontal to V_4
V_6	On the midaxillary line and horizontal to V_4 and V_5

 TABLE C-2. ECG Interpretation Steps

1. Check for correct calibration (1 mV = 10 mm) and paper speed (25 mm/sec)
2. Calculate the heart rate and determine the heart rhythm
3. Measure intervals (PR, QRS, QT)
4. Determine the mean QRS axis and mean T wave axis in the limb leads
5. Look for morphologic abnormalities of the P wave, QRS complex, ST segments, T waves and U waves (e.g., chamber enlargement, conduction delays, infarction, repolarization changes)
6. Interpret the present ECG
7. Compare the present ECG with previous available ECGs
8. Conclusion, clinical correlation, and recommendations

TABLE C-3. Resting 12-lead ECG: Normal Limits

Parameter	Normal Limits	Abnormal If:	Possible Interpretation(s)*
Heart rate	60–100 beats·min⁻¹	<60 >100	Bradycardia Tachycardia
PR interval	0.12–0.20 sec	<0.12 sec >0.20 sec	Preexcitation (i.e., WPW, LGL) First-degree AV block
QRS duration	Up to 0.10 sec	If ≥0.11 sec	Conduction abnormality (i.e., incomplete or complete BBB, WPW, aberrant conduction)
QT interval	Rate dependent: Normal QT = KV/RR where K = 0.37 for men and children and 0.40 for women	QTc long QTc short	Drug effects, electrolyte abnormalities, ischemia Digitalis effect, hypercalcemia
QRS axis	−30° to +110°	<−30° >+110° Indeterminate	Left axis deviation (i.e., chamber enlargement, hemiblock, infarction) Right axis deviation (i.e., RVH, pulmonary disease, infarction) All limb leads transitional

T axis	Generally same direction as QRS axis	The T axis (vector) is typically deviated away from the area of "mischief" (i.e., ischemia, BBB, hypertrophy)	Chamber enlargement, ischemia, drug effects, electrolyte disturbances
ST segments	Generally at isoelectric line (PR segment) or within 1 mm. The ST may be elevated up to 3 mm in leads V_1–V_4.	Elevation of ST segment	Injury, ischemia, pericarditis, electrolyte abnormality, normal variant
		Depression of ST segment	Injury, ischemia, electrolyte abnormality, drug effects, normal variant.
Q waves	<0.04 sec and <25% of R wave amplitude (exceptions lead III & V_1)	>0.04 sec and/or >25% of R wave amplitude except lead III (the lead of exceptions) and V_1	Infarction or pseudoinfarction (as from chamber enlargement, conduction abnormalities, WPW, COPD, cardiomyopathy)
Transition zone	Usually between V_2 and V_4	Before V_2 After V_4	Counterclockwise rotation Clockwise rotation

bpm, beats per minute; WPW, Wolff-Parkinson-White syndrome; LGL, Lown-Ganong-Levine syndrome; QTc, QT corrected for heart rate; COPD, chronic obstructive pulmonary disease.

*If supported by other electrocardiograms (ECGs) and related clinical criteria.

TABLE C-4. Normal QT Interval* as a Function of Heart Rate[†]

	Age (y)							
	18–29		30–39		40–49		50–60	
Heart Rate	L	U	L	U	L	U	L	U
115–84	0.30	0.37	0.30	0.37	0.31	0.37	0.31	0.37
83–72	0.32	0.39	0.33	0.39	0.33	0.40	0.33	0.40
71–63	0.34	0.41	0.35	0.41	0.35	0.41	0.35	0.42
62–56	0.36	0.42	0.36	0.43	0.37	0.43	0.37	0.43
55–45	0.39	0.45	0.39	0.45	0.39	0.46	0.39	0.46

*A good rule of thumb for the QT interval is that at normal heart rates between 60 and 100 beats·min[−1], the T wave should be completely finished being inscribed before you get half way between the previous and subsequent R waves. In other words, if you bisect the RR interval, the T wave should end before you get to that bisecting line.

[†]Adapted from Simonson E, Cady LD, Woodbury M. The normal QT interval. Am Heart J 1962;63:747, by permission of CV Mosby. Reproduced from Chou TC. Electrocardiography in Clinical Practice. Philadelphia: WB Saunders, 1996:16.

L, lower limit in seconds; U, upper limit in seconds.

TABLE C-5. Localization of Transmural Infarcts*

Typical ECG Leads	Infarct Location
V_1–V_3	Anteroseptal
V_3–V_4	Localized anterior
V_4–V_6, I, aVL	Anterolateral
V_1–V_6	Extensive anterior
I, aVL	High lateral
II, III, aVF	Inferior
V_1–V_2	True posterior (R/S >1)
V_1, V_{3R}, V_{4R}	Right ventricular

*Based on abnormal Q waves except for true posterior myocardial infarction, which is reflected by abnormal R waves.

TABLE C-6. Supraventricular versus Ventricular Ectopic Beats*

Parameter		Supraventricular (Normal Conduction)	Supraventricular (Aberrant Conduction)	Ventricular
QRS complex	Duration	Up to 0.10 sec	≥0.11 sec	≥0.11 sec
	Configuration	Normal	Widened QRS usually with unchanged initial vector	Widened QRS often with abnormal initial vector. QRS usually not preceded by a P wave.
			P wave precedes QRS.	
P wave		Present or absent but with relationship to QRS.	Present or absent but with relationship to QRS.	Present or absent but without relationship to QRS.
Rhythm		Usually less than compensatory pause.	Usually less than compensatory pause.	Usually compensatory pause.

*Numerous ECG criteria exist to try to distinguish premature ventricular contractions (PVCs) from aberrant conduction. Standard ECG texts review these. A major clinical problem is the patient with a wide QRS tachycardia. Such tachycardias can be ventricular or supraventricular with aberrant conduction. A good rule of thumb is that any wide QRS tachycardia in a patient with heart disease or a history of heart failure is likely to be ventricular tachycardia, especially if AV dissociation is identified.

TABLE C-7. Atrioventricular (AV) Block

Interpretation	P Wave Relationship to QRS	PR Interval	R-R Interval
1° AV block	1 : 1	>0.20 sec	Regular or follows P-P interval
2° AV block: Mobitz I (Wenckebach)	>1 : 1	Progressively lengthens until a P-wave fails to conduct	Progressively shortens; pause less than two other cycles
2° AV block: Mobitz II	>1 : 1	Constant but with sudden dropping of QRS	Regular except for pause, which usually equals two other cycles
3° AV block	None	Variable but P-P interval constant	Usually regular (escape rhythm)

TABLE C-8. Atrioventricular (AV) Dissociation*

Type of AV Dissociation	Electrophysiology	Example	Significance	Comment
AV dissociation due to complete AV block	AV block	Sinus rhythm with complete AV block	Pathologic	Unrelated P wave and QRS complexes. PP interval is shorter than RR interval
AV dissociation by default causing interference	Slowing of the primary or dominant pacemaker with escape of a subsidiary pacemaker	Sinus bradycardia with junctional escape rhythm	Physiologic	Unrelated P wave and QRS complexes. PP interval is longer than RR interval
AV dissociation by usurpation	Acceleration of a subsidiary pacemaker usurping control of the ventricles	Sinus rhythm with either AV junctional or ventricular tachycardia	Physiologic	Unrelated P wave and QRS complexes. PP interval is longer than RR interval
Combination	AV block and interference	Atrial fibrillation with accelerated AV junctional pacemaker and block below this pacemaker	Pathologic	Unrelated P wave and QRS complexes

*What is meant by "AV dissociation"? When the atria and ventricles beat independently, their contractions are "dissociated" and AV dissociation exists. Thus, P waves and QRS complexes in the ECG are unrelated. AV dissociation may be complete or incomplete, transient or permanent. The causes of AV dissociation are "block" and "interference," and both may be present in the same ECG. "Block" is associated with a pathologic state of refractoriness, preventing the primary pacemaker's impulse from reaching the lower chamber. An example of this is sinus rhythm with complete AV block. "Interference" results from slowing of the primary pacemaker or acceleration of a subsidiary pacemaker. The lower chamber's impulse "interferes" with conduction by producing physiologic refractoriness, and AV dissociation results. An example of this is sinus rhythm with AV junctional or ventricular tachycardia and no retrograde conduction into the atria. A clear distinction must be made between block and interference. This table describes the four types of AV dissociation.

Appendix D
Metabolic Calculations

A fundamental aspect of exercise testing and prescription is the ability to measure or estimate energy expenditure during exercise. Because exercise, like all metabolic events, produces heat, the rate of heat produced is directly proportional to the energy expended.

Calorimetry

Because *direct calorimetry*—the measurement of heat production—is difficult to assess in exercising humans, the rate of energy expenditure during exercise is typically measured by *indirect calorimetry*—by measuring the rate of oxygen uptake ($\dot{V}O_2$) of the exercising individual. In this notation, the V stands for volume, the O_2 for oxygen, and the dot above the V denotes a rate, that is, a volume of oxygen per unit of time. For $\dot{V}O_2$ to accurately reflect energy expenditure, the exercise must be primarily aerobic. The $\dot{V}O_2$ will underestimate energy expenditure when the contribution from anaerobic metabolism is large.

$\dot{V}O_2$ provides much useful information for exercise professionals:

- Under steady-state conditions, $\dot{V}O_2$ provides a measure of the energy cost of exercise.
- The rate of oxygen uptake during maximal exercise ($\dot{V}O_{2max}$) indicates the capacity for oxygen transport and utilization.
- $\dot{V}O_{2max}$ also serves as the criterion measure of cardiorespiratory fitness.
- In combination with the measured rate of carbon dioxide output ($\dot{V}CO_2$), $\dot{V}O_2$ provides general information about the fuels being used for exercise.

Various expressions of O_2 uptake are used depending on the purpose for its measurement:

- The **absolute** rate of oxygen uptake is typically given by the units liters per minute ($L \cdot min^{-1}$). In this form, $\dot{V}O_2$ can be converted to a rate of energy expenditure, given that the consumption of 1 L of O_2 results in the liberation of approximately 5 kcal (i.e., 20.9 kJ) of energy.
- The **relative** rate of oxygen uptake is typically given by the units, milliliters per kg of body mass per minute ($mL \cdot kg^{-1} \cdot min^{-1}$). This form is used to compare the $\dot{V}O_2$ of individuals who vary in body size. In some instances, one may express $\dot{V}O_2$ relative to kg of fat-free mass, to square meters of surface area, or to other indices of body size.
- The **gross** rate of oxygen uptake is the total consumption rate under any circumstances, whether expressed in absolute or relative units.
- The **net** rate of oxygen uptake is the consumption rate above resting oxygen uptake, as in the increased oxygen cost incurred when exercising. **Net $\dot{V}O_2$** is used to describe the caloric cost of exercise; **gross $\dot{V}O_2$** includes the caloric costs of rest and exercise.

MEASUREMENT OF $\dot{V}O_2$

The actual measurement of $\dot{V}O_2$ is typically performed in laboratory or clinical settings using a procedure called *open-circuit spirometry*. In open-circuit spirometry, the subject inspires room air and expires into a gas collection system, which measures the volume of air and the fractions of O_2 and CO_2 in the expired air. Typically, an integrated metabolic cart with a computer interface calculates the O_2 consumption ($\dot{V}O_2$) and CO_2 production ($\dot{V}CO_2$) rates.

Respiratory Exchange Ratio and Respiratory Quotient

Both respiratory exchange ratio (RER) and respiratory quotient (RQ) are calculated as $\dot{V}CO_2/\dot{V}O_2$ and are unitless variables. Although these two calculated variables are sometimes used synonymously, there is one important distinction between them. Respiratory exchange ratio is a ventilatory measurement and reflects gas exchange between the lungs and the pulmonary blood. Respiratory quotient is a measurement based solely on cellular respiration and is equivalent to RER only under steady-state conditions. RQ provides information about substrate utilization at the cellular level, equaling 1.0 for carbohydrate oxidation, 0.7 for fat oxidation, and approximately 0.8 for protein oxidation. RQ therefore always falls between 0.7 and 1.0. RER, however, exceeds 1.0 during heavy non–steady-state or maximal exercise due to hyperventilation (which increases CO_2 release by the lungs) and buffering of lactic acid in the blood (which provides a nonmetabolic source of CO_2). The energy expenditure associated with a given level of oxygen uptake varies slightly with RQ (about 4.69 kcal per L of O_2 at an RQ of 0.7, and 5.05 at an RQ of 1). When RQ is not known, the value 5 $kcal \cdot L^{-1}$ is used.

ESTIMATION OF ENERGY EXPENDITURE— METABOLIC CALCULATIONS

When it is not possible or feasible to measure $\dot{V}O_2$ directly, reasonable estimates can still be made during steady-state exercise. Regression equations have been derived from laboratory data relating mechanical measures of work rate to their metabolic equivalents. These equations are appropriate for general clinical and laboratory usage when standard ergometric devices are available but spirometry is not. They also estimate or predict energy expenditure (and thus weight loss) for some nonergometric exercise modalities (e.g., indoor or outdoor walking or running). Alternatively, these equations may be used during exercise prescription to determine the exercise intensity associated with a desired level of energy expenditure for any of these ergometric or nonergometric activities. Several cautionary notes about the use of metabolic calculations are in order:

- The measured $\dot{V}O_2$ at a given work rate is highly reproducible for a given individual; however, the intersubject variability in measured $\dot{V}O_2$ may have a standard error of estimate (SEE) as high as 7%. Since the equations are often used to predict $\dot{V}O_2$, it is important to remember that the variance of a predicted value is much larger than the SEE (i.e., the prediction interval is greater than the confidence interval).
- As noted previously, these equations are appropriate only for steady-state submaximal aerobic exercise. Failure to achieve a steady state results in an overestimation of $\dot{V}O_2$.
- Although the accuracy of these equations is unaffected by most environmental influences (heat and cold), variables that change the mechanical efficiency (e.g., gait abnormalities; wind, snow, or sand) result in a loss of accuracy.
- Inherent assumptions for the use of the equations presuppose that ergometers are calibrated properly and used appropriately, e.g., no rail-holding during treadmill exercise.

Despite these caveats, proper and judicious use of metabolic calculations provides a valuable tool for the exercise professional.

Derivation of Metabolic Equations

Table D-1 presents the metabolic equations for the gross or total oxygen cost of walking, running, leg ergometry, arm ergometry, and stepping in metric units. To obtain the net oxygen cost, just subtract 3.5 mL·kg^{-1}·min^{-1}. The following paragraphs explain the derivation of each equation. The equations associated with each section yield the gross oxygen cost in mL·kg^{-1}·min^{-1}.

TABLE D-1. Metabolic Equations for Gross $\dot{V}O_2$ in Metric Units*

Walking
$$\dot{V}O_2 = (0.1 \cdot S) + (1.8 \cdot S \cdot G) + 3.5$$
Treadmill and Outdoor Running
$$\dot{V}O_2 = (0.2 \cdot S) + (0.9 \cdot S \cdot G) + 3.5$$
Leg Ergometry
$$\dot{V}O_2 = (10.8 \cdot W \cdot M^{-1}) + 7$$
Arm Ergometry
$$\dot{V}O_2 = (18 \cdot W \cdot M^{-1}) + 3.5$$
Stepping
$$\dot{V}O_2 = (0.2 \cdot f) + (1.33 \cdot 1.8 \cdot H \cdot f) + 3.5$$

*Where $\dot{V}O_2$ is gross oxygen consumption in $mL \cdot kg^{-1} \cdot min^{-1}$; S is speed in $m \cdot min^{-1}$; M is body mass in kg; G is the percent grade expressed as a fraction; W is power in watts; f is stepping frequency in min^{-1}; H is step height in meters.

Note: These equations are presented in conventional units following each mode of exercise, simplifying the calculations.

WALKING AND RUNNING

During walking, approximately 0.1 mL O_2 is needed for transporting each kg of body mass per meter (m) of horizontal distance covered, i.e., 0.1 $mL \cdot kg^{-1} \cdot m^{-1}$ (1). The oxygen demand of running is twice as great, i.e., 0.2 $mL \cdot kg^{-1} \cdot m^{-1}$ (2,3). The oxygen demand of raising one's body mass against gravity at sea level is approximately 1.8 mL per kg of body mass for each m of vertical distance (1.8 $mL \cdot kg^{-1} \cdot m^{-1}$) (4–6). The vertical distance is the product of the distance along the surface and the sine of the angle the surface makes with the horizontal. Typically, the tangent (i.e., fractional grade) is substituted for the sine, and this introduces only a small error for grades less than 20%. The oxygen cost of vertical ascent in treadmill running is half that of walking, or 0.9 $mL \cdot kg^{-1} \cdot m^{-1}$ (3), and over-ground inclined running has the same oxygen cost as treadmill grade running (7). Running on a level surface is more costly than walking due to the greater vertical displacement that occurs between each step. Some of the vertical displacement of horizontal running is applied to the vertical ascent during grade running, reducing the coefficient for that factor. The resting oxygen uptake, 3.5 $mL \cdot kg^{-1} \cdot min^{-1}$, is added to give the gross cost.

Walking Appropriate for speeds of 50 to 100 $m \cdot min^{-1}$ (1.9 to 3.7 mph)

$$\dot{V}O_2 = 0.1 \text{ (speed)} + 1.8 \text{ (speed) (fractional grade)} + 3.5$$

Running Appropriate for speeds over 134 $m \cdot min^{-1}$ (5.0 mph) or for speeds as low as 80 $m \cdot min^{-1}$ (3 mph) if the individual is truly jogging/running

$$\dot{V}O_2 = 0.2 \text{ (speed)} + 0.9 \text{ (speed) (fractional grade)} + 3.5$$

where $\dot{V}O_2$ is in $mL \cdot kg^{-1} \cdot min^{-1}$ and speed is in $m \cdot min^{-1}$ (1 mph = 26.8 $m \cdot min^{-1}$).

LEG AND ARM ERGOMETRY

Determine the power output during leg or arm ergometry from the following:

- Power = R·D·f, where
  Power is in watts
  R is the resistance setting in Newtons
  D is the distance in meters (m) the flywheel travels for 1 pedal revolution
  f is the pedaling frequency (s^{-1})
- It is common to calculate the power in $kg \cdot m \cdot min^{-1}$ as follows:
  Power = (kg setting) (D) (pedaling cadence in rpm)
- One watt is approximately equal to 6 $kg \cdot m \cdot min^{-1}$ (more precisely, 6.12)
- The distance, D, for some commonly used ergometers is:
  — 6 m for Monark (Monark Exercise AB, Vanberg, Sweden) leg ergometers
  — 3 m for Tunturi (Turku, Finland) and BodyGuard ergometers
  — 2.4 m for Monark arm ergometers

Performing cycle ergometry with the legs entails an oxygen demand associated with unloaded cycling (i.e., the movement of the legs), a cost that is directly proportional to the external load, and resting oxygen uptake. At 50 to 60 rpm, the oxygen cost of unloaded cycling is approximately 3.5 $mL \cdot kg^{-1} \cdot min^{-1}$ above rest (8–10). The cost of cycling against the external load is approximately 1.8 $mL \cdot kg^{-1} \cdot m^{-1}$, as in the vertical component of walking (5), and resting oxygen uptake is 3.5 $mL \cdot kg^{-1} \cdot min^{-1}$.

The arms are such a small mass that performing cycle ergometry with them does not require the inclusion of a special term for unloaded cycling. However, the arms are less efficient than the legs in cycling, most likely due to the recruitment of accessory muscles needed to stabilize the torso, and the oxygen cost is approximately 3 $mL \cdot kg^{-1} \cdot m^{-1}$ (11–13). The resting oxygen uptake of 3.5 $mL \cdot kg^{-1} \cdot min^{-1}$ is added to obtain the gross cost.

Leg Cycling Appropriate for power outputs between 50 and 200 W (300 and 1200 $kg \cdot m \cdot min^{-1}$)

$$\dot{V}O_2 = 1.8 \text{ (work rate)} \cdot M^{-1} + 7$$

Arm Cycling Appropriate for power outputs between 25 and 125 W (150 and 750 $kg \cdot m \cdot min^{-1}$)

$$\dot{V}O_2 = 3 \text{ (work rate)} \cdot M^{-1} + 3.5$$

where $\dot{V}O_2$ is in $mL \cdot kg^{-1} \cdot min^{-1}$, work rate is in $kg \cdot m \cdot min^{-1}$, and M is the subject's body mass in kg.

STEPPING ERGOMETRY

Stepping is traditionally performed in a four-part process of lifting one leg onto a box or other fixed object, then pushing with this leg to raise the body and place the other leg on the box, then stepping down with the first and then second leg. The oxygen cost of stepping has a horizontal component and a vertical component because one moves forward and backward horizontally, not just up and down. The oxygen demand of the horizontal movement is approximately 0.2 mL O_2 per four-cycle step per kg of body mass. As noted previously, the O_2 demand of vertical ascent is 1.8 mL·kg^{-1}·m^{-1}, and approximately one-third of this must be added to account for the O_2 cost of stepping down (6). The resting oxygen uptake is added to obtain the total oxygen cost.

Stepping   Appropriate for stepping rates between 12 and 30 steps·min^{-1}, and step heights between 0.04 and 0.40 m (1.6 to 15.7 in)

$$\dot{V}O_2 = 0.2 \text{ (stepping rate)} + 1.33 \cdot 1.8 \text{ (step height) (stepping rate)} + 3.5$$

where $\dot{V}O_2$ is in mL·kg^{-1}·min^{-1}, stepping rate is in steps·min^{-1}, and step height is in m (1 inch = 0.0254 m).

Tables of MET values based on the formulas for walking, running, cycling, and stepping are provided later in this appendix.

ESTIMATING $\dot{V}O_{2max}$

$\dot{V}O_{2max}$ can be estimated from the final grade and speed (treadmill), power output (leg or arm ergometer), or step rate and height (stepping) achieved in a conventional graded exercise test using the above equations. However, because a steady state is not achieved in the final stage of a maximal graded exercise test, these equations may overestimate $\dot{V}O_{2max}$. Other prediction equations are available to estimate $\dot{V}O_{2max}$. One such generalized equation in common use, based on the Bruce protocol, is as follows (14):

$$\dot{V}O_{2max}(\text{mL·kg}^{-1}\text{·min}^{-1}) = 14.8 - 1.379 \text{ (time in min)} \\ + 0.451 \text{ (time}^2) - 0.012 \text{ (time}^3) \\ \text{SEE} = 3.35 \text{ mL·kg}^{-1}\text{·min}^{-1}$$

It is typically desirable to test patients without the use of handrail support. However, with some patient and elderly populations this may not be possible. A validated equation has been published for use when treadmill walking is done with handrail support using the Bruce protocol (15):

$$\dot{V}O_{2max}(\text{mL·kg}^{-1}\text{·min}^{-1}) = 2.282 \text{ (time in min)} + 8.545 \\ \text{SEE} = 4.92 \text{ mL·kg}^{-1}\text{·min}^{-1}$$

Ramp treadmill protocols were discussed in Chapter 5, and published prediction equations can be used to estimate $\dot{V}O_{2max}$ based on data collected during ramp style exercise tests. One such equation is based on an *individualized* ramp protocol (16):

$$\dot{V}O_{2max}(mL \cdot kg^{-1} \cdot min^{-1}) = 0.72x + 3.67$$
$$SEE = 4.4\ mL \cdot kg^{-1} \cdot min^{-1}$$

where x equals predicted $\dot{V}O_2$ based on peak speed/grade using ACSM walking equation.

Another validated equation for use with the *standardized* Bruce Ramp treadmill protocol (17) is as follows:

$$\dot{V}O_{2max}(mL \cdot kg^{-1} \cdot min^{-1}) = 3.9\ (\text{time in minutes}) - 7.0$$
$$SEE = 3.4\ mL \cdot kg^{-1} \cdot min^{-1}$$

For cycle ergometry, the following equations have been published, based on the final power completed in a 15 W per min protocol (18):

Males:

$$\dot{V}O_{2max}(mL \cdot min^{-1})* = 10.51\ (\text{power in W}) + 6.35\ (\text{body mass in kg})$$
$$- 10.49\ (\text{age in y}) + 519.3$$
$$SEE = 212\ mL \cdot min^{-1}$$

Females:

$$\dot{V}O_{2max}(mL \cdot min^{-1})* = 9.39\ (\text{power in W}) + 7.7\ (\text{body mass in kg})$$
$$- 5.88\ (\text{age in y}) + 136.7$$
$$SEE = 147\ mL \cdot min^{-1}$$

*Divide by kg to obtain the value in $mL \cdot kg^{-1} \cdot min^{-1}$.

FIELD TEST EQUATIONS

When large numbers of individuals are being tested, or when the use of standard ergometry is not possible, field tests are commonly used to predict $\dot{V}O_{2max}$. These tests involve endurance walks or runs over level terrain designed to either 1) cover a fixed distance (such as 1 or 1.5 miles) with time as the criterion measure or 2) measure the distance covered in a fixed period of time (such as 12 or 15 minutes). Some tests incorporate other predictor

TABLE D-2. Common Field Test Equations to Estimate $\dot{V}O_{2max}$

1. Rockport Walking Test (1-mile walk) (19)
   - $\dot{V}O_{2max}(mL\cdot kg^{-1}\cdot min^{-1}) = 132.853 - 0.1692$ (body mass in kg) $- 0.3877$ (age in y) $+ 6.315$ (gender) $- 3.2649$ (time in min) $- 0.1565$ (HR); gender $= 0$ for female, 1 for male; heart rate (HR) is taken at end of walk
     $SEE = 5.0$ mL·kg^{-1}·min^{-1}
2. 1.5-mile Run Test*
   - $\dot{V}O_{2max}$ (mL·kg^{-1}·min^{-1}) $= 3.5 + 483/$(time in min)

*This formula is a transposition of the running metabolic equation for gross $\dot{V}O_2$.

variables, such as age, gender, or body weight. Field test equations for the 1-mile walk and the 1.5-mile run are given in Table D-2.

USING THE METABOLIC CALCULATIONS

Use of metabolic calculations is relatively simple and straightforward for the experienced professional, but it is often a source of confusion for the novice user. Although an advanced knowledge of mathematics is not necessary, the ability to solve for an unknown variable in a simple algebraic expression is essential.

The equations presented in Table D-1 may be used to estimate the gross $\dot{V}O_2$ of various forms of exercise when the workload on the exercise

TABLE D-3. Approximate Energy Requirements in METs for Horizontal and Grade Walking

	mi·h^{-1}	1.7	2.0	2.5	3.0	3.4	3.75
% Grade	m·min^{-1}	45.6	53.6	67.0	80.4	91.2	100.5
0		2.3	2.5	2.9	3.3	3.6	3.9
2.5		2.9	3.2	3.8	4.3	4.8	5.2
5.0		3.5	3.9	4.6	5.4	5.9	6.5
7.5		4.1	4.6	5.5	6.4	7.1	7.8
10.0		4.6	5.3	6.3	7.4	8.3	9.1
12.5		5.2	6.0	7.2	8.5	9.5	10.4
15.0		5.8	6.6	8.1	9.5	10.6	11.7
17.5		6.4	7.3	8.9	10.5	11.8	12.9
20.0		7.0	8.0	9.8	11.6	13.0	14.2
22.5		7.6	8.7	10.6	12.6	14.2	15.5
25.0		8.2	9.4	11.5	13.6	15.3	16.8

TABLE D-4. Approximate Energy Requirements in METs for Horizontal and Uphill Jogging/Running

mi·h⁻¹	5	6	7	7.5	8	9	10
% Grade m·min⁻¹	134	161	188	201	214	241	268
0	8.6	10.2	11.7	12.5	13.3	14.8	16.3
2.5	9.5	11.2	12.9	13.8	14.7	16.3	18.0
5.0	10.3	12.3	14.1	15.1	16.1	17.9	19.7
7.5	11.2	13.3	15.3	16.4	17.4	19.4	
10.0	12.0	14.3	16.5	17.7	18.8		
12.5	12.9	15.4	17.7	19.0			
15.0	13.8	16.4	18.9				

apparatus and, in the case of cycle ergometry, the client's body mass are known. The equations yield $\dot{V}O_2$ in relative units, i.e., mL·kg⁻¹·min⁻¹. To determine net $\dot{V}O_2$, i.e., the $\dot{V}O_2$ above resting level caused by the exercise, simply subtract 3.5 mL·kg⁻¹·min⁻¹ from the gross value.

If the caloric cost of exercise is desired, the $\dot{V}O_2$ must first be expressed in net terms. This is then converted to L·min⁻¹ by multiplying the $\dot{V}O_2$ in mL·kg⁻¹·min⁻¹ by body mass (kg) and dividing by 1000 (i.e., 1000 mL per L). $\dot{V}O_2$ expressed in L·min⁻¹ is multiplied by 5 kcal·L⁻¹ to obtain caloric expenditure. As described in Chapter 7, caloric expenditure can be calculated from METs as follows: kcal·min⁻¹ = (METs × 3.5 × body weight in kg)/200.

The metabolic equations also may be used to estimate a target work rate at a desired level of oxygen uptake or energy expenditure. Once this level is expressed in mL·kg⁻¹·min⁻¹, the equation is solved for the unknown

 TABLE D-5. Approximate Energy Expenditure in METs During Leg Cycle Ergometry

Body Wt.		Power Output (kg·m·min⁻¹ and Watts)						
kg	lb	300 50	450 75	600 100	750 125	900 150	1050 175	1200 (kg·m·min⁻¹) 200 (Watts)
50	110	5.1	6.6	8.2	9.7	11.3	12.8	14.3
60	132	4.6	5.9	7.1	8.4	9.7	11.0	12.3
70	154	4.2	5.3	6.4	7.5	8.6	9.7	10.8
80	176	3.9	4.9	5.9	6.8	7.8	8.8	9.7
90	198	3.7	4.6	5.4	6.3	7.1	8.0	8.9
100	220	3.5	4.3	5.1	5.9	6.6	7.4	8.2

TABLE D-6. Approximate Energy Expenditure in METs
During Arm Ergometry

Body Wt.		Power Output (kg·m·min⁻¹ and Watts)					
kg	lb	150	300	450	600	750	900 (*kg·m·min⁻¹*)
		25	50	75	100	125	150 (*Watts*)
50	110	3.6	6.1	8.7	11.3	13.9	16.4
60	132	3.1	5.3	7.4	9.6	11.7	13.9
70	154	2.8	4.7	6.5	8.3	10.2	12.0
80	176	2.6	4.2	5.8	7.4	9.0	10.6
90	198	2.4	3.9	5.3	6.7	8.1	9.6
100	220	2.3	3.6	4.9	6.1	7.4	8.7

variable on the workload side of the equation. In the case of treadmill exercise, there are two unknown variables, speed and fractional grade. It is best to select an appropriate speed based on the ability and comfort of the client, and then solve for the fractional grade.

Step 1: If a target energy expenditure or oxygen uptake is known, express this $\dot{V}O_2$ in mL·kg⁻¹·min⁻¹.

Common Conversions:
— (caloric expenditure in kcal·min⁻¹)/5 = $\dot{V}O_2$ in L·min⁻¹
— ($\dot{V}O_2$ in L·min⁻¹) (1000)/(body mass in kg) = $\dot{V}O_2$ in mL·kg⁻¹·min⁻¹
— mph × 26.8 = m·min⁻¹
— 60 ÷ min/mile = mph
— caloric content of 1 lb adipose tissue = 3500 kcal
— METs × 3.5 mL·kg⁻¹·min⁻¹ = $\dot{V}O_2$ in mL·kg⁻¹·min⁻¹
— (weight in lb)/2.2 = mass in kg
— (power in W) × 6 = workload in kg·m·min⁻¹

Step 2: Select the appropriate metabolic equation and solve for the unknown.

Sample Metabolic Calculations

A 30-year-old man has a resting heart rate of 60 beats·min⁻¹, a maximal heart rate of 190 beats·min⁻¹, weighs 180 lb, and has a $\dot{V}O_{2max}$ of 48 mL·kg⁻¹·min⁻¹. He wishes to begin an exercise program in which he can 1) walk on a treadmill at 3.5 mph (a comfortable speed for him) or 2) cycle on a Monark ergometer. You decide to begin his exercise prescription at an exercise intensity of 70% $\dot{V}O_{2max}$.

TABLE D-7. Approximate Energy Expenditure in METs During Stair Stepping

Step Height		Stepping Rate per Minute					
in	m	20	22	24	26	28	30
4	0.102	3.5	3.8	4.0	4.3	4.5	4.8
6	0.152	4.2	4.6	4.9	5.2	5.5	5.8
8	0.203	4.9	5.3	5.7	6.1	6.5	6.9
10	0.254	5.6	6.1	6.5	7.0	7.5	7.9
12	0.305	6.3	6.8	7.4	7.9	8.4	9.0
14	0.356	7.0	7.6	8.2	8.8	9.4	10.0
16	0.406	7.7	8.4	9.0	9.7	10.4	11.1
18	0.457	8.4	9.1	9.9	10.6	11.4	12.1

Q: *What is his target $\dot{V}O_2$?*

A: Target $\dot{V}O_2$ = (exercise intensity) $\times$ ($\dot{V}O_{2max}$)
= 0.70×48
= 33.6 mL·kg^{-1}·min^{-1}

Q: *How steep should the treadmill grade be if he is walking at 3.5 mph?*
3.5 mph $\times$ 26.8 = 93.8 m·min^{-1}

A: $\dot{V}O_2$ = 0.1 (speed) + 1.8 (speed) (frac. grade) + 3.5 mL·kg^{-1}·min^{-1}
33.6 = 0.1 (93.8) + 1.8 (93.8) (frac. grade) + 3.5
30.1 = 0.1 (93.8) + 1.8 (93.8) (frac. grade)
30.1 = 9.38 + 168.8 (frac. grade)
20.7 = 168.8 (frac. grade)
0.123 = frac. grade = 12.3% grade

Q: *What is his target work rate on the Monark bike?*

A: First determine his body mass:
180 lb/2.2 = 81.8 kg
$\dot{V}O_2$ = 7.0 + 1.8 (work rate)/(body mass)
33.6 = 7.0 + 1.8 (work rate)/81.8
26.6 = 1.8 (work rate)/81.8
2176 = 1.8 (work rate)
1209 kg·m·min^{-1} = work rate

Q: *If he is comfortable pedaling at 60 rpm on a Monark cycle, what resistance setting should be used?*

A: Work rate = (resistance setting) (D) (pedal cadence)
1209 = (resistance setting) (6) (60)
1209 = (resistance setting) 360
3.36 kg = resistance setting

Q: **What will be his net caloric expenditure during 30 minutes of exercise?**

A: Net $\dot{V}O_2$ = 33.6 − 3.5 = 30.1 mL·kg^{-1}·min^{-1}
   ($\dot{V}O_2$ in mL·kg^{-1}·min^{-1}) (body mass)/1000 = $\dot{V}O_2$ in L·min^{-1}
   (30.1) (81.8)/1000 = 2.46 L·min^{-1}
   2.46 L·min^{-1} × 5 = 12.3 kcal·min^{-1}
   12.3 kcal·min^{-1} × 30 min = 369 kcal

Q: **What is an appropriate target heart rate according to the heart rate reserve method?**

A: HR_{max} = 190 beats·min^{-1}
   Target HR = (exercise intensity) (HR_{max} − HR_{rest}) + HR_{rest}
   = (0.70) (190 − 60) + 60
   = (0.70) (130) + 60
   = 91 + 60
   = 151 beats·min^{-1} (or, approximately 25 beats in a 10-second pulse count)

Practice Metabolic Calculations (With Answers)

1. A man weighing 176 lb runs at a pace of 9 minutes per mile outdoors, on level ground. What is his estimated gross $\dot{V}O_2$?

2. To match this exercise intensity (from #1 above) on a Tunturi cycle ergometer, what setting would you use at a pedaling rate of 60 rpm?

3. If this same man exercised at this intensity 5 times per week for 30 minutes each session, how long would it take him to lose 12 lb (assuming all calories expended in this exercise are in excess of food intake)? Hint: Use the net $\dot{V}O_2$ to calculate the exercise energy expenditure.

4. For a desired training intensity of 75% $\dot{V}O_{2max}$, at what heart rate should a 45-year-old woman exercise? Her resting heart rate is 70 beats·min^{-1}.

5. A 198-lb cardiac patient wishes to use an arm ergometer for part of his rehabilitation program. He works at a power output of 300 kg·m·min^{-1} for 15 minutes, then at 450 kg·m·min^{-1} for 15 minutes. What is his average *net* $\dot{V}O_2$ (in mL·kg^{-1}·min^{-1}) over this session?

6. If an individual reduces his or her dietary intake by 1750 kcal per week, how much weight (in lb) would he or she lose in 6 months (26 weeks)?

7. If an 18-year-old girl steps up and down on a 12-inch step at a rate of 20 steps (complete up and down cycles) per minute, what would her gross $\dot{V}O_2$ be (in mL·kg^{-1}·min^{-1})?

8. A 71-year-old man weighing 180 lb walks on a motor-driven treadmill at 3.5 mph and a 15% grade. What is his gross MET level?

Answers

1. 39.2 mL·kg^{-1}·min^{-1}
2. 7.9 kg (or kp)
3. About 20 weeks
4. About 150 beats·min^{-1}
5. 12.5 mL·kg^{-1}·min^{-1}
6. 13 lb
7. 21.9 mL·kg^{-1}·min^{-1}
8. 10.9 METs

References

1. Dill DB. Oxygen cost of horizontal and grade walking and running on the treadmill. J Appl Physiol 1965;20:19–22.
2. Balke B. A simplified field test for assessment of physical fitness. Civil Aeromedical Research Institute Report 63-66. Oklahoma City: Civil Aeromedical Research Institute.
3. Margaria R, Cerretelli P, Aghemo P, et al. Energy cost of running. J Appl Physiol 1963; 18:367–370.
4. Balke B, Ware RW. An experimental study of "physical fitness" of Air Force personnel. US Armed Forces Med J 1959;10:675–688.
5. Nagle FJ, Balke B, Baptista G, et al. Compatibility of progressive treadmill, bicycle, and step tests based on oxygen uptake responses. Med Sci Sports 1971;3:149–154.
6. Nagle FJ, Balke B, Naughton JP. Gradational step tests for assessing work capacity. J Appl Physiol 1965;20:745–748.
7. Bassett DR Jr, Giese MD, Nagle FJ, et al. Aerobic requirements of overground versus treadmill running. Med Sci Sports Exerc 1985;17:477–481.
8. Lang PB, Latin RW, Berg KE, et al. The accuracy of the ACSM cycle ergometry equation. Med Sci Sports Exerc 1992;24:272–276.
9. Latin RW, Berg KE. The accuracy of the ACSM and a new cycle ergometry equation for young women. Med Sci Sports Exerc 1994;26:642–646.
10. Londeree BR, Moffitt-Gerstenberger J, Padfield JA, et al. Oxygen consumption of cycle ergometry is nonlinearly related to work rate and pedal rate. Med Sci Sports Exerc 1997;29:775–780.
11. Franklin BA. Exercise testing, training, and arm ergometry. Sports Med 1985;2:100–119.
12. Stenberg J, Åstrand PO, Ekblom B, et al. Hemodynamic response to work with different muscle groups, sitting and supine. J Appl Physiol 1967;22:61–70.
13. Bevegard S, Freyschuss U, Strandell T. Circulatory adaptation to arm and leg exercise in supine and sitting position. J Appl Physiol 1966;21:37–46.
14. Foster C, Jackson AS, Pollock ML, et al. Generalized equations for predicting functional capacity from treadmill performance. Am Heart J 1984;107:1229–1234.
15. McConnell TR, Clark BA. Prediction of maximal oxygen consumption during handrail-supported treadmill exercise. J Cardiopulm Rehabil 1987;7:324–331.
16. Myers J, Buchanan N, Smith D, et al. Individualized ramp treadmill: observations on a new protocol. Chest 1992;101:236S–241S.
17. Kaminsky LA, Whaley MH. Evaluation of a new standardized ramp protocol: the BSU/Bruce ramp protocol. J Cardiopulm Rehabil 1998;18:438–444.
18. Storer TW, Davis JA, Caiozzo VJ. Accurate prediction of $\dot{V}O_{2max}$ in cycle ergometry. Med Sci Sports Exerc 1990;22:704–712.
19. Kline GM, Porcari JP, Hintermeister R, et al. Estimation of $\dot{V}O_{2max}$ from a 1-mile track walk, gender, age, and body weight. Med Sci Sports Exerc 1987;19:253–259.

APPENDIX E
Environmental Considerations

Ambient environmental conditions can exacerbate the physiologic strain of exercise. Environmental factors of greatest concern for people engaged in recreational, fitness, or competitive athletic activity (and the clinicians and trainers advising them) are weather and altitude.

HEAT AND HUMIDITY

Heat can have life- and health-threatening effects on people who are exercising. Exercise results in the production of large amounts of body heat that must be dissipated; if not, body temperature increases, eventually reaching dangerous levels. High ambient temperature and humidity impede the body's normal mechanisms for dissipating body heat. Unfortunately, no single standard defines safe upper limits for temperature and humidity during exercise. However, the American College of Sports Medicine (ACSM) has a position stand with recommendations concerning heat stress and distance running (1). Furthermore, guidelines promulgated to manage heat stress effects in industrial and military settings also can be applied to exercise environments (2,3). These guidelines can help to prevent excessive elevations in body temperature during physical exertion and mitigate the deleterious effects of dehydration.

When the environment's heat stress potential is assessed, factors influencing the body's thermal balance must include air temperature, humidity, air movement (i.e., windspeed) and, when outdoors, solar radiation from sunlight. One index integrating the effects of all these factors into a single value quantifying heat stress is the wet-bulb globe temperature, or WBGT. The WBGT combines three measurements: dry-bulb air temperature (T_b); natural wet-bulb temperature ($T_{wb(n)}$) measured by placing a wetted wick over the thermometer bulb exposed to natural air movement; and globe temperature (T_g), that is, the temperature measured inside a 15-cm diameter copper globe painted flat black. The WBGT is determined easily using inexpensive portable meters, or it can be calculated from weather-services data. WBGT is calculated as follows:

$$\text{WBGT} = 0.7\, T_{wb(n)} + 0.2\, T_g + 0.1\, T_b \text{ (outdoors)}$$
$$\text{or}$$
$$\text{WBGT} = 0.7\, T_{wb(n)} + 0.3\, T_g \text{ (indoors)}$$

Guidelines for controlling heat stress often base recommendations on the WBGT. The first such use of WBGT was in the mid 1950s at military bases, where WBGT limits for physical activities during hot weather were established. Subsequently, other organizations promulgated similar WGBT guidelines for monitoring and/or quantifying heat stress and preventing heat injury during work and recreation (1–3). Use of WBGT-based guidelines has successfully reduced the incidence of heat illness during hot-weather physical activity (4). However, limitations concerning the use of WBGT should be appreciated. The WBGT was derived empirically rather than rationally from physiologic principles governing human body heat balance and thermoregulation. With high humidity, the WBGT tends to underestimate the risk of heat illness (4). Furthermore, WBGT does not account for factors such as clothing, exercise intensity, age, fitness, acclimatization, and health status, all of which influence the body's thermal balance and modify the physiologic strain imposed by a given environmental stress.

When recommending heat-illness prevention guidelines for exercise programs, fitness professionals and clinicians can use WBGT standards established by the National Institute for Occupational Safety and Health (NIOSH) (2) for the workplace as a convenient starting point. The NIOSH standard provides recommended heat-stress alert limits, which are WBGT levels at which the risk of heat injury is increased, but exercise can still be undertaken provided that actions to alleviate the heat stress are employed. These actions include limiting the maximum duration of continuous exercise completed and incorporating required rest breaks before another exercise period is initiated. Table E-1 provides recommended exercise-rest intervals derived from NIOSH standards for moderate and vigorous exercise under worsening heat stress weather conditions. Other strategies to alleviate heat stress include the following:

- Choose clothing affording no barrier to heat loss and sweat evaporation
- Reschedule exercise for a cooler time of day
- Relocate to shady, breezier site or indoors with fans and air conditioning
- Slow exercise or add rest breaks to maintain the same target heart rate (THR) as normally prescribed

Heat acclimatization increases heat tolerance, both in terms of a decreased risk for heat illness while exercising and an improved capacity or

TABLE E-1. Guidelines for Safe Exercise Duration–Rest Periods for Healthy Unacclimatized Persons*

WBGT (°F)	Moderate Exercise Work/Rest	Vigorous Exercise Work/Rest
70–72.9	NL	45/15 min
73–76.9	40/20 min	30/30 min
77–79.9	30/30 min	20/40 min
80–81.9	20/40 min	10/50 min
82–83.9	10/50 min	None
84–86	None	None

*Adapted from NIOSH recommendations.

NL, no limit to work time per hour.

Times indicate recommended maximum duration of intermittent exercise followed by the rest period for cool-down before beginning another exercise bout.

Rest means minimal physical activity (sitting or standing), in shade if possible.

endurance for exercise in the heat. With heat acclimatization, lower heart rates and body temperatures are elicited at a given exercise intensity, sweating rate increases, and the sweat becomes more dilute. Thus, heat dissipation is facilitated, and the physiologic strain of exercise in the heat is diminished. The best method of inducing heat acclimation is to exercise in the heat, progressively increasing the duration and/or intensity of exercise each day. Individuals whose exercise prescription specifies a THR should maintain the same exercise heart rate in the heat. This approach reduces the risk of heat illness while allowing acclimatization to develop. For example, in hot or humid weather, a reduced speed or resistance will achieve the THR, even though the work of the heart (myocardial oxygen uptake) remains unchanged. As acclimatization occurs, a progressively higher exercise intensity will be tolerated and required to elicit the THR. The first exercise session in the heat may last as little as 10 to 15 minutes for safety reasons, but exercise duration can be increased gradually to its usual length. Most healthy people become fully acclimatized to the heat in 10 to 14 days, although illness or alcohol consumption may slow this process.

The other key for preventing heat illness and optimizing performance in persons who exercise in hot and/or humid conditions is to maintain proper hydration. Profuse sweating during exercise-heat stress can lead to dehydration unless adequate replacement fluids are consumed. Even mild dehydration impairs temperature regulation and compromises performance during exercise (5). Exercise program organizers and leaders should ensure that replacement fluids are available and easily accessible, and program participants should be reminded to drink before, during, and after physical activity (5).

In most people, especially those older than 60 years, drinking alleviates thirst sensations well before sufficient fluid is consumed to replace sweat losses and return hydration levels to normal. Generalized recommendations regarding the amount of drinking necessary to replace sweat losses during exercise are of limited value because sweating varies greatly among individuals as a function of the environment, relative exercise intensity, and duration of exercise. However, a simple suggestion is for exercise program participants to drink 2 cups of fluid 2 hours before exercise; during exercise, they should attempt to drink fluids at a rate matching sweat losses (5). Exercisers should be advised to weigh themselves before and after each exercise session and that weight lost during the exercise session represents lost body water that must be replaced. Each pound of weight lost should be replaced with 16 oz of fluid.

Fluid replacement beverages should be served cooled (59 to 72°F) and palatable to encourage consumption. With few exceptions, water is the replacement drink of choice. Electrolyte losses are usually small during brief exercise sessions, and persons consuming a normal diet easily replenish electrolytes when the next meal is eaten. Exercisers on restricted salt diets should consult with their physicians regarding the effects of exercise on their salt balance. Unless the exercise bout lasts in excess of 60 to 90 minutes, there is little advantage in supplementing carbohydrates.

Disease and the effects of drugs may increase susceptibility to heat illness. For example, hypertension, cardiovascular disease, diabetes-associated neuropathies, and aging can all alter cardiovascular, skin blood flow and sweating responses to exercise heat stress, leading to impairments in temperature regulation (6). Obesity impairs heat dissipation, exacerbating physiologic strain during exercise-heat stress, presumably accounting for the increased risk of heat illness in obese persons (7). Drug therapies for these and other disorders, including diuretics, β-blockers, α-agonists, and vasodilators, as well as licit and illicit recreational drugs (e.g., alcohol), can alter vasomotor and cardiovascular responses to heat stress, exacerbate dehydration, and interfere with the ability to dissipate heat and maintain safe body temperatures during exercise. A prior history of heat illness or difficulty acclimating to heat may also forecast future problems. Clinicians and exercise professionals need to consider these limitations when recommending exercise programs for hot weather.

Fitness facilities and other organizations offering exercise programs must formulate a standardized heat stress management plan to be instituted during hot and/or humid weather. A comprehensive heat stress management plan would establish procedures for the following:

- Screening and surveillance of at-risk participants
- Environmental assessment, using WBGT as a criterion
- WBGT criteria for modifying or canceling exercise
- Facilitating heat acclimatization of participants
- Providing easy access to fluids and promoting hydration
- Increasing awareness of heat illness signs and symptoms
- Integrating heat illness into emergency procedures plan

Cold, Wind, and Rain

Winter weather presents less of an immediate health risk than summer for healthy people in terms of exercising. Many people avoid the cold altogether by exercising indoors during winter, but those who choose to continue with outdoor exercise are not usually at great risk because exercise causes the body to generate large amounts of heat. However, people participating in exercise programs, patients, and even the popular press and media often ask health and fitness professionals, "Is it too cold to exercise?" Indeed, there are certain circumstances under which people exercising outdoors might be at risk of cold injuries unless precautions are taken.

The two most serious potential cold-weather injuries arise due to excessive body heat loss during prolonged exposure to cold. These injuries are hypothermia (subnormal body core temperature) and frostbite (freezing of body tissues, typically skin of the periphery). Cold ambient temperatures favor body heat loss, and wind can exacerbate the heat loss (4). The wind chill index (WCI), which purports to integrate the potential stress arising from both factors, has achieved popular acceptance and is widely reported (8). The WCI estimates the combined cooling effects of wind and air temperature (8) and is typically used in tables to depict temperatures of "calm" air having equivalent cooling rates as different combinations of air temperature and wind speed.

Wind chill equivalent tables are widely available, and most are divided into three ranges of wind chill conditions, each of progressively worsening risk of freezing tissue injuries. Most tables indicate that there is little risk of injury when wind chill is above −25°F, but the danger increases below that temperature, and when wind chill equivalent temperatures are below −70°F, the danger of frostbite and other freezing tissue injuries is markedly increased. Lacking any better tool, these tables still are useful guidelines concerning the conduct or cancellation of outdoor activities; however, as with the WBGT, limitations to this approach should be appreciated. The wind chill concept is sound, but the equation for calculating WCI appears flawed in its physical and physiologic rationale (9). Wind chill tables overestimate the effect of increasing wind on the risk of tissue freezing, while underestimating the effect of decreasing air temperature (9). Further, the danger zones indicated in wind chill tables estimate risk of tissue freezing only for the exposed skin of sedentary persons. Thus, persons exercising in windproof clothing are at less risk of frostbite than the wind chill tables would suggest. Finally, wind chill tables provide no meaningful estimate of the risk of hypothermia.

Body heat production during moderate to strenuous exercise is sufficiently high enough to prevent hypothermia in air temperatures, including wind chill, as low as −25°F. Exercise program participants should avoid overdressing by wearing layers and clothes under a windproof outer shell. Heat production during aerobic exercise can often be high enough that clothing selected for comfort before exercise must be removed during exercise or overheating and sweating will result. However, once exercise stops, metabolic heat production declines, and clothing must be replaced or the individual must return indoors to maintain normal heat balance.

Water has a much higher thermal capacity than air. If clothing becomes wet due to accumulation of sweat or rain, the risk of hypothermia may be drastically increased, especially when exercise stops and metabolic heat production declines. When clothing becomes wet, its insulative value is compromised, and wetting of the skin facilitates heat loss by conduction, convection, and evaporation. During water immersion, conductive and convective heat transfer can be 70-fold greater than in air of the same temperature (4), depending on the water depth and amount of body surface immersed. Thus, even when water temperatures are relatively mild (e.g., 75 to 80°F), long-distance swimmers, triathletes, and fishermen or hunters who wade streams can lose considerable amounts of body heat.

Another question frequently directed at health and fitness professionals during winter concerns the possible consequences of inhaling cold air during exercise. The effects of cold air breathing during exercise are usually negligible. Upper airway temperatures, which remain unchanged during exercise under temperate conditions, fall substantially when extremely cold air (< -25°F) is breathed during strenuous exercise, but temperatures of the lower respiratory tract and deep body temperatures are unaffected (10). Pulmonary function during exercise is unaffected by breathing cold air in healthy athletes (11) and nonathletes (12). In allergy-prone athletes, breathing cold air during heavy exercise may cause bronchospasm, but this bronchospasm may actually be triggered by facial cooling rather than cooling of respiratory passages (13). Chronic breathing of cold air can increase respiratory passage secretions and decrease mucociliary clearance, and any resulting airway congestion may impair pulmonary mechanics during exercise (14).

While healthy persons can usually tolerate exercise in cold weather without problems, older people and persons having cardiovascular and circulatory disorders may need to use greater caution. Cold exposure, even when mild, stimulates the sympathetic nervous system, which, in turn, mediates systemic responses including elevations in total peripheral resistance, arterial pressure, myocardial contractility, and cardiac work during both rest and exercise (15). This probably explains why patients with coronary artery disease exercising outdoors often experience angina pectoris and ST-segment depression at lower exercise intensities in cold rather than warm weather (15). Some evidence suggests that, compared with those of younger persons, older persons' vasomotor adjustments in response to cold exposure may become slower and less effective in curtailing skin blood flow, but the increase in blood pressure is more pronounced in otherwise healthy persons over 50 years old (6). Particular caution should be advised for outdoor activities like chopping wood and snow shoveling (16,17), which require significant upper body use, since use of upper body muscle groups can greatly exacerbate blood pressure responses during exercise (15). Mortality due to coronary artery disease is well known to increase in winter, but to what extent this reflects the effects of cold exposure on unaccustomed physical activity remains unclear (15).

HIGH ALTITUDE

In the mountains, wind, snow, and rain frequently contribute to cold stress, while strenuous activity, heavy clothing, and increased solar radiation can contribute to heat stress. However, the unique physiologic stressor encountered when one ascends to high altitudes is hypoxia. Air, unlike water, is compressible. Therefore, at sea level, compression of air by the atmosphere above causes air density and barometric pressure to be greater than at higher elevations, where there is less atmosphere above compressing the air. Even in pressurized cabins, commercial airline passengers are exposed to barometric pressure reductions equivalent to altitudes of 5000 to 8000 feet. Because the fractional concentration of oxygen in the atmosphere (F_IO_2) remains constant at 0.2093, the decreasing barometric pressure with increasing altitude is also associated with a decreasing pressure of oxygen in the inspired air (P_IO_2).

One of the more noticeable effects that low-altitude residents experience when they ascend to high altitude is an increased pulmonary ventilation, particularly during exercise (18). This accounts for the common sensation of breathlessness at high altitude. The response, highly variable among individuals, becomes more pronounced after several days spent living at high altitude.

Despite increased ventilation, arterial oxygenation (i.e., P_aO_2, and S_aO_2) usually falls when low-altitude residents ascend to 5000 feet or higher above sea level (18). The resulting decrease in blood oxygen content necessitates an increased cardiac output, achieved by tachycardia, to sustain oxygen delivery required for a given level of muscular activity. Maximal cardiac output, however, remains the same at sea level and is, therefore, achieved at lower exercise intensities at high altitude. As a result, $\dot{V}O_{2max}$ is lower at high altitude than sea level. The increased cardiovascular strain of exercise and the reduced $\dot{V}O_{2max}$ at high altitude compromise work capacity and endurance. These impairments usually become noticeable at about 5000 feet above sea level (even lower for some very fit athletes) and worsen with increasing elevation. After 5 to 10 days of acclimatization at high altitude, cardiovascular adjustments lessen the physiologic strain of exercise, enabling some improvement in endurance and work capacity, but short of a full recovery to sea level performance.

When unacclimatized persons ascend rapidly to elevations 8000 feet above sea level and higher, many experience high-altitude illnesses, which can also limit exercise capacity (19). The most common of these is acute mountain sickness (AMS), which is characterized by severe headache, nausea and other gastrointestinal disturbances, and insomnia. In susceptible people these symptoms arise after 6 to 12 hours at altitude and usually abate after 3 to 7 days of acclimatization. Less common, but much more serious and even life threatening, are high-altitude pulmonary edema (HAPE) and high-altitude cerebral edema (HACE). Exercise at altitude usually exacerbates the symptoms of these illnesses and may, at least in the case of pulmonary edema, increase the likelihood that the illness will develop. The definitive treatment for all these illnesses is descent to lower altitude. Preventative measures include a gradual ascent to altitude, with overnight stops at intermediate altitudes and, especially when ascending higher than 8000 feet above sea level, avoidance of vigorous exercise for the first 2 or 3 days after arrival to allow for some acclimatization.

The higher cardiac output elicited during submaximal exercise on arrival at high altitude increases cardiac work and myocardial oxygen requirements, necessitating an increase in coronary blood flow relative to sea level exercise (15). In addition, blood pressure is increased when low-altitude residents ascend to high altitude and continues rising during the first week of acclimatization. Even healthy persons experience greater cardiovascular strain during exercise at altitude, contributing to their decreased exercise capacity. In persons with coronary artery disease, the greater cardiac work and coronary blood flow requirement during exercise at high altitudes can cause the onset of angina and/or ischemic ST-segment depression to occur at lower exercise intensities than at sea level (15). Hypertensive patients may experience a disproportionate elevation in blood pressure at rest and during exercise at high altitude (15).

For the first 1 to 3 days after sea level residents ascend to high altitude, use of the same THR as prescribed for sea level exercise will limit cardiac strain because it will necessitate a reduction in exercise intensity. However, with the development of altitude acclimatization during longer visits to high altitude, the initial tachycardia observed on arrival abates considerably. This effect of altitude acclimatization may require a downward adjustment in the prescribed THR for some individuals.

References

1. Armstrong LE, Epstein Y, Greenleaf JE, et al. American College of Sports Medicine position stand. Heat and cold illnesses during distance running. Med Sci Sports Exerc 1996;28:i–x.
2. National Institute for Occupational Safety and Health. Criteria for a recommended standard. Occupational exposure to hot environments. Washington, DC: US Department of Health and Human Services, DHHS NIOSH Publ. No. 86-113, 1986.
3. TB Med 507. Prevention, treatment and control of heat injury. Washington, DC: Department of the Army, 1980.
4. Gonzalez RR. Biophysics of heat exchange and clothing: applications to sports physiology. Med Exerc Nutr Health 1995;4:290–305.
5. Convertino VA, Armstrong LE, Coyle EF, et al. Exercise and fluid replacement. Med Sci Sports Exerc 1996;28:i–vii.
6. Kenney WL. Thermoregulation at rest and during exercise in healthy, older adults. Exerc Sports Sci Rev 1997;25:41–76.
7. Chung NK, Pin CH. Obesity and the occurrence of heat disorders. Mil Med 1996;161:739–742.
8. Siple PA, Passel CR. Measurements of dry atmospheric cooling in sub freezing temperatures. Proc Am Philosoph Soc 1945;89:177–199.
9. Danilesson U. Windchill and the risk of tissue freezing. J Appl Physiol 1996;81:2666–2673.
10. Jaeger JJ, Deal EC, Roberts DE, et al. Cold air inhalation and esophageal temperature in exercising humans. Med Sci Sports Exerc 1980;12:365–369.
11. Helenius IJ, Tikkanen HO, Haahtela T. Exercise-induced bronchospasm at low temperature in elite runners. Thorax 1990;51:628–629.
12. Chapman KR, Allen LJ, Romet TT. Pulmonary function in normal subjects following exercise at cold ambient temperatures. Eur J Appl Physiol 1990;60:228–232.
13. Koskela H, Tukainen H. Facial cooling, but not nasal breathing of cold air, induces bronchoconstriction: a study in asthmatic and healthy subjects. Eur Respir J 1995;8:2088–2093.
14. Giesbrecht GG. The respiratory system in a cold environment. Aviat Space Environ Med 1995;66:890–902.
15. Pandolf KB, Young AJ. Altitude and cold. In: Pollock ML, Schmidt DH, eds. Heart Disease and Rehabilitation. Champaign, IL: Human Kinetics, 1995:309–326.

16. Franklin BA, Hogan P, Bonzheim K, et al. Cardiac demands of heavy snow shoveling. JAMA 1995;273:880–882.
17. Franklin BA, Bonzheim K, Gordon S, et al. Snow shoveling: a trigger for acute myocardial infarction and sudden coronary death. Am J Cardiol 1996;77:855–858.
18. Young AJ, Young PM. Human acclimatization to high terrestrial altitude. In: Pandolf KB, Sawka MN, Gonzalez RR, eds. Human Performance Physiology and Environmental Medicine at Terrestrial Extremes. Indianapolis, IN: Benchmark, 1988:497–543.
19. Malkonian MK, Rock PB. Medical problems related to altitude. In: Pandolf KB, Sawka MN, Gonzalez RR, eds. Human Performance Physiology and Environmental Medicine at Terrestrial Extremes. Indianapolis, IN: Benchmark, 1988:545–563.

APPENDIX F
American College of Sports Medicine Certifications

This appendix details information about American College of Sports Medicine (ACSM) certification programs, as well as a complete listing of the current knowledge, skills, and abilities (KSAs) that comprise the foundations of these certification examinations. The goals of the ACSM Committee for Certification and Education through the process of certifying clinical and health/fitness personnel are to 1) enhance professionalism within the fitness, clinical, and health care arenas, and 2) increase public access to appropriate exercise services.

ACSM CERTIFICATIONS AND THE PUBLIC

The first of the ACSM Clinical Track certifications was initiated nearly 25 years ago in conjunction with publication of the first edition of the *Guidelines for Exercise Testing and Prescription*. That era was marked by rapid development of exercise programs for stable coronary artery disease (CAD) patients. ACSM sought a means to disseminate accurate information on this health care initiative through expression of consensus from its members in basic science, clinical practice, and education. Thus, these early clinical certifications were viewed as an aid to the establishment of safe and scientifically based exercise services within the framework of cardiac rehabilitation.

Over the past 25 years, exercise has gained widespread favor as an important component in programs of rehabilitative care or health maintenance for an expanding list of chronic diseases and disabling conditions. The growth of public interest in the role of exercise in health promotion has been equally impressive. In addition, federal government policy makers have revisited questions of medical efficacy and financing for exercise services in rehabilitative care of selected patients. Over the past several years, recommendations from the U.S. Public Health Service and the U.S. Surgeon

General have increasingly acknowledged a central role for regular physical activity in the prevention of disease and promotion of health.

The development of the Health/Fitness Track certifications in the 1980s reflected ACSM's intent to increase the availability of qualified professionals to provide scientifically sound advice and supervision regarding appropriate physical activities for health maintenance in the apparently healthy adult population.

Since 1975, nearly 20,000 certificates have been awarded. With this exponential growth, ACSM has taken steps to ensure that its competency-based certifications will continue to be regarded as the premier program in the exercise field. A periodical dealing with professional practice issues targeted to those who are certified, *ACSM Certified News,* is one example. Implementation of continuing education requirements for maintenance of certification is another. Continuing education credits can be accrued through ACSM-sponsored educational programs such as ACSM workshops (Exercise Leader®, Health/Fitness Instructor_{SM}, and Exercise Specialist®), regional chapter and annual meetings, and other educational programs approved by the ACSM Professional Education Committee. These enhancements are intended to support continuing professional growth of those who have made a commitment to service in this rapidly growing health and fitness field. ACSM also acknowledges the expectation from successful candidates that the public will be informed of the high standards, values, and professionalism implicit in meeting these certification requirements. Most recently, the College has formally organized its volunteer committee structure and national office staff to give added emphasis to informing the public, professionals, and government agencies about issues of critical importance to ACSM. Informing these constituencies about the meaning and value of ACSM certification is one important priority that will be given attention in this initiative.

ACSM Certification Programs

The ACSM certifications are categorized by "tracks." The Health/Fitness Track is designed primarily for those individuals who provide leadership in fitness assessment and exercise programming of a preventive nature for apparently healthy individuals and individuals with controlled disease in corporate, commercial, and community settings. The Clinical Track is designed for professionals who may work with high-risk or diseased individuals as well as apparently healthy individuals.

Certification at a given level requires the candidate to have a knowledge and skills base commensurate with that specific level of certification. In addition, higher levels of certification incorporate the knowledge and skills associated with other designated certification levels as illustrated in Figure F-1. Candidates are expected to understand not only the KSAs of their specific level, but also the KSAs of the additional certification levels listed in Figure F-1. In addition, each level of certification has minimum requirements for experience, level of education, or other certifications. Minimum

Clinical Track		Health/Fitness Track		
Program Director (PD)	Exercise Specialist (ES)	Health/ Fitness Director (HFD)	Health/ Fitness Instructor (HFI)	Exercise Leader (EL)
PD	ES	HFD	HFI	EL
ES	HFI	HFI	EL	
HFI	EL	EL		
EL				

FIGURE F-1. Each level of certification is responsible for the knowledge, skills, and abilities (KSAs) for all levels of certification listed below it, inclusive. *For attaining and maintaining every level of ACSM certification, concurrent cardiopulmonary resuscitation (CPR) is a requirement.*

requirements and recommended competencies are listed for each level of certification.

Health/Fitness Track

There are three levels of certification within the Health/Fitness Track: ACSM Health/Fitness Director®, ACSM Health/Fitness Instructor$_{SM}$, and ACSM Exercise Leader®.

ACSM HEALTH/FITNESS DIRECTOR®

The ACSM Health/Fitness Director® (HFD) is the highest level of certification in the Health/Fitness Track. The HFD certification provides professionals with recognition of their practical experience and demonstrated competence as an administrative leader of health and fitness programs in the corporate, commercial, or community setting in which apparently healthy individuals and individuals with controlled disease participate in health promotion and fitness-related activities. The professional responsibilities of an HFD encompass an advanced knowledge of applied exercise physiology, exercise programming, emergency procedures and safety, program administration, staff training and supervision, as well as overall facility and program management.

Minimum Requirements A 2-year, 4-year, or Masters degree in a health-related field from a regionally accredited college or university (verification by transcript or copy of the degree) *plus* a minimum of 2 years (full time) or 4000 hours of experience as a fitness manager or director
OR
Current ACSM Health/Fitness Instructor$_{SM}$ certification plus 2 years (full time) or 4000 hours of experience as a fitness manager or director
AND
Current cardiopulmonary resuscitation (CPR) certification.

Recommended Competencies

1. Demonstrate competence in the KSAs required of the ACSM Health/Fitness Director®, ACSM Health/Fitness Instructor$_{SM}$, and ACSM Exercise Leader® as listed in the sixth edition of *ACSM's Guidelines for Exercise Testing and Prescription*.
2. Demonstrate the practical skills in basic business organization and finance.
3. Demonstrate the ability to organize and administer health and fitness programs for a wide range of apparently healthy persons (low risk) or those with controlled disease as well as experience in the supervision and administration of health and fitness programs.

ACSM HEALTH/FITNESS INSTRUCTOR$_{SM}$

The ACSM Health/Fitness Instructor$_{SM}$ (HFI) is a professional qualified to assess, design, and implement individual and group exercise and fitness programs for apparently healthy individuals and individuals with controlled disease. The HFI is skilled in evaluating health behaviors and risk factors, conducting fitness assessments, writing appropriate exercise prescriptions, and motivating individuals to modify negative health habits and maintain positive lifestyle behaviors for health promotion.

Minimum Requirements   A 2-year, 4-year, or Masters degree in a health-related field from a regionally accredited college or university (verification by transcript or copy of the degree)
OR
Current enrollment as a junior or higher in a degree granting health-related field from a regionally accredited college or university
OR
A minimum of 900 hours of practical experience in a fitness setting
AND
Current cardiopulmonary resuscitation (CPR) certification.

Recommended Competencies

1. Demonstrate competence in the KSAs required of the ACSM Health/Fitness Instructor$_{SM}$, and ACSM Exercise Leader® as listed in the sixth edition of *ACSM's Guidelines for Exercise Testing and Prescription*.
2. Have work-related experience within the health and fitness field.
3. Have adequate knowledge of and skill in risk factor and health status identification, fitness appraisal, and exercise prescription.
4. Demonstrate ability to incorporate suitable and innovative activities that improve functional capacity.
5. Demonstrate ability to effectively educate and/or counsel individuals regarding lifestyle modification.
6. Have the ability to organize and administer health and fitness programs for a wide range of apparently healthy individuals (low risk) or those with controlled disease.

ACSM EXERCISE LEADER®

The ACSM Exercise Leader® (EL) is a professional involved in group exercise leadership. Using a variety of teaching techniques, the EL is proficient in leading and demonstrating safe and effective methods of exercise by applying the fundamental principles of exercise science. The EL is familiar with all forms of group exercise including traditional low, high, mixed, and step aerobics; slide, stationary indoor cycling, interval, circuit, water, muscle conditioning, and flexibility training.

Minimum Requirements   Fitness certification from a nationally recognized organization
OR
Completed or current enrollment in exercise-related college courses at a regionally accredited college or university
OR
300 hours of group exercise instruction experience
AND
Current cardiopulmonary resuscitation (CPR) certification.

Recommended Competencies

1. Demonstrate competence in the KSAs required of the ACSM Exercise Leader® as listed in the sixth edition of *ACSM's Guidelines for Exercise Testing and Prescription.*
2. Demonstrate practical skills and abilities associated with group exercise leadership.
3. Demonstrate the ability to positively motivate the group and to communicate and interact effectively with members of the group.
4. Possess adequate knowledge of how the body responds to, and is affected by, exercise.
5. Demonstrate the ability to safely apply the principles of exercise and training to group fitness programs.
6. Demonstrate the ability to answer basic questions related to exercise science and to refer others to appropriate sources of information.

Clinical Track

There are two levels of certification within the Clinical Track: Program Director$_{SM}$ and Exercise Specialist®.

PROGRAM DIRECTOR$_{SM}$

The ACSM Program Director$_{SM}$ (PD) is the highest level of certification in the Clinical Track. This certification is directed toward professionals whose primary responsibilities are developing and directing safe and effective clinical exercise programs. The PD certification requires a significant increase in breadth and depth of knowledge and experience beyond that of an Exercise Specialist®.

Minimum Requirements Postbaccalaureate degree (or equivalent) training in exercise science, medicine, or an allied health field *plus* 2 years of clinical experience
AND
A minimum of 1 year of recent experience in a position of administrative authority working with a clinical exercise program
AND
Current certification in Basic Life Support (BLS)
AND
Written recommendation from current certified ACSM Program Director$_{SM}$.

Recommended Competencies

1. Demonstrate competence in the KSAs for the ACSM Program Director$_{SM}$, Exercise Specialist®, Health/Fitness Instructor$_{SM}$, and Exercise Leader® as listed in the sixth edition of the *ACSM's Guidelines for Exercise Testing and Prescription.*
2. Have ability to organize and administer preventive and rehabilitative exercise programs for healthy and diseased populations.

EXERCISE SPECIALIST®

The successful ACSM Exercise Specialist® (ES) candidate must demonstrate competence in graded exercise testing, exercise prescription, exercise leadership, patient counseling, and education in clinical exercise programs.

Minimum Requirements Baccalaureate degree in an allied health field or the equivalent (2-year degree plus a minimum of 2 years experience in cardiac rehabilitation/clinical exercise testing environment)
AND
Minimum of 600 hours of practical experience in a clinical exercise program (e.g., cardiac/pulmonary) including exercise testing
AND
Current cardiopulmonary resuscitation (CPR) certification.

Recommended Competencies

1. Demonstrate competence in the KSAs required of the ACSM Exercise Specialist®, Health/Fitness Instructor$_{SM}$, and Exercise Leader® as listed in the sixth edition of the *ACSM's Guidelines for Exercise Testing and Prescription.*

HOW TO OBTAIN INFORMATION AND APPLICATION MATERIALS

The certification programs of ACSM are subject to continuous review and revision. Content development is entrusted to a committee of professional volunteers with expertise in science, medicine, and program management. Expertise in design and procedures for competency assessment is also represented on this committee. Administration of certification is the responsibility of the ACSM National Center. Inquiries concerning certifications, application requirements, fees, and examination test sites and dates may be made to

ACSM Certification Resource Center
1-800-486-5643
E-mail: www.lww.com/acsmcrc

KNOWLEDGE, SKILLS, AND ABILITIES (KSAS) UNDERLINING ACSM CERTIFICATIONS

Minimal competencies for each certification level are outlined below. Certification examinations are constructed based upon these KSAs. A companion ACSM publication, *Resource Manual for Guidelines for Exercise Testing and Prescription*, third edition, may be used to gain further insight pertaining to the topics identified here. Neither the *Guidelines for Exercise Testing and Prescription* nor the *Resource Manual* provide all of the information upon which the ACSM Certification examinations are based. However, the *Resource Manual* may prove to be beneficial as a review of specific topics and as a general outline of many of the integral concepts to be mastered by those seeking certification.

Numbering System

The system for numbering KSAs has been changed. It is designed to more specifically denote the *level of certification* (the first number in sequence) and the *content matter* (the second number in the sequence) of the KSA. The system is as follows.

Level of Certification

The first number in the sequence denotes the certification level of the KSA. KSAs numbered "1._" are specific to Exercise Leader; KSAs numbered "2._" are specific to Health/Fitness Instructor, and so on. The first numbers denote level of certification as follows:

1._ Exercise Leader
2._ Health/Fitness Instructor
3._ Health/Fitness Director
4._ Exercise Specialist
5._ Program Director

Content Matter

The second number in the sequence denotes the content matter of the KSA. KSAs numbered "_.1" are related to Anatomy and Biomechanics; KSAs numbered "_.2" are related to Exercise Physiology. The second numbers denote content matter as follows:

_.1 Anatomy and Biomechanics
_.2 Exercise Physiology
_.3 Human Development and Aging
_.4 Pathophysiology and Risk Factors
_.5 Human Behavior and Psychology
_.6 Health Appraisal and Fitness Testing
_.7 Safety and Injury Prevention
_.8 Exercise Programming
_.9 Nutrition and Weight Management
_.10 Program and Administration/Management
_.11 Electrocardiography

Example   A KSA numbered "1.3._" is a KSA for an Exercise Leader that relates to Human Development and Aging. A KSA numbered "4.4._" is for an Exercise Specialist that relates to Pathophysiology and Risk Factors.

This numbering system allows exact determination of KSAs specific to the level of certification and the content matter.

ANATOMY AND BIOMECHANICS

1.1.0	Knowledge of anatomy as it relates to exercise and health.
1.1.0.1	Knowledge of the basic structures of bone, skeletal muscle, and connective tissues.
1.1.0.2	Knowledge of the basic anatomy of the cardiovascular system and respiratory system.
1.1.0.3	Ability to identify the major bones and muscles. Major muscles include, but are not limited to, the following: trapezius, pectoralis major, latissimus dorsi, biceps, triceps, rectus abdominis, internal and external obliques, erector spinae, gluteus maximus, quadriceps, hamstrings, adductors, abductors, and gastrocnemius.
1.1.0.4	Knowledge of the definition of the following terms: supination, pronation, flexion, extension, adduction, abduction, hyperextension, rotation, circumduction, agonist, antagonist, and stabilizer.
1.1.0.5	Ability to identify the joints of the body.
1.1.1	Knowledge of biomechanical aspects of exercise participation.
1.1.1.1	Knowledge to identify the plane in which each muscle action occurs.
1.1.1.2	Knowledge of the interrelationships among center of gravity, base of support, balance, stability, and proper spinal alignment.
1.1.1.3	Ability to describe the following curvatures of the spine: lordosis, scoliosis, and kyphosis.

1.1.1.4	Knowledge of and skill to demonstrate exercises designed to enhance muscular strength and/or endurance of specific major muscle groups.
1.1.1.5	Knowledge of and skill to demonstrate exercises for enhancing musculo-skeletal flexibility.
1.1.1.6	Knowledge to describe the myotatic stretch reflex.
1.1.1.7	Knowledge to identify the primary action and joint range of motion for each major muscle group.

2.1.0	Knowledge of functional anatomy and biomechanics.
2.1.0.1	Knowledge of the structure and ability to describe movements for the major joints of the body.
2.1.0.2	Ability to locate the anatomic landmarks for palpation of peripheral pulses.
2.1.0.3	Ability to locate the brachial artery and correctly place the cuff and stethoscope in position for blood pressure measurement.
2.1.0.4	Ability to locate common sites for measurement of skinfold thicknesses and circumferences (for determination of body composition and waist-hip ratio).
2.1.1	Knowledge of biomechanical principles that underlie performance of the following activities: walking, jogging, running, swimming, cycling, weight lifting, and carrying or moving objects.

3.1.0	Ability to describe modifications in exercise prescription for individuals with functional disabilities and musculoskeletal injuries.
3.1.1	Ability to describe the relationship between biomechanical efficiency, oxygen cost of activity (economy), and performance of physical activity.

4.1.0	Knowledge of anatomy as it relates to exercise testing and programming.
4.1.0.1	Ability to locate anatomic landmarks for palpitation of radial, brachial, carotid, femoral, popliteal, and tibialis arteries.
4.1.0.2	Ability to locate the appropriate sites for the limb and chest leads for resting, standard, and exercise (Mason Likar) electrocardiograms (ECGs), as well as commonly used bipolar systems (e.g., CM-5).
4.1.0.3	Knowledge of coronary anatomy.
4.1.0.4	Knowledge of basic joint movements, muscle actions, and points of insertions as it relates to exercise programming.
4.1.1	Knowledge of the biomechanical factors associated with various disease states, neuromuscular disorders, and orthopedic limitations.
4.1.1.1	Knowledge of common gait abnormalities as they relate to exercise testing and programming.
4.1.1.2	Knowledge of neuromuscular disorders (e.g., Parkinson's disease, multiple sclerosis) as they relate to modifications of exercise testing and programming.
4.1.1.3	Knowledge of orthopedic limitations (e.g., gout, foot drop, specific joint problems) as they relate to modifications of exercise testing and programming.

5.1.1	Knowledge of standard auscultatory regions in the chest for listening to heart sounds, murmurs, and lung sounds.

5.1.1.1 Ability to list regions of auscultatory interest (e.g., aortic, pulmonic, tricuspid, mitral areas).

5.1.1.2 Knowledge of heart sounds and murmurs (e.g., first heart sound, second heart sound, gallop sounds, midsystolic clicks, systolic ejection murmurs, diastolic murmurs).

5.1.1.3 Knowledge of lung sounds (e.g., rales, crackles).

EXERCISE PHYSIOLOGY

1.2.0 Basic knowledge of exercise physiology as it relates to exercise prescription.

1.2.1 Ability to define aerobic and anaerobic metabolism.

1.2.2 Knowledge of the role of aerobic and anaerobic energy systems in the performance of various activities.

1.2.3 Knowledge of the following terms: ischemia, angina pectoris, tachycardia, bradycardia, arrhythmia, myocardial infarction, cardiac output, stroke volume, lactic acid, oxygen consumption, hyperventilation, systolic blood pressure, diastolic blood pressure, and anaerobic threshold.

1.2.4 Knowledge of the role of carbohydrates, fats, and proteins as fuels for aerobic and anaerobic metabolism.

1.2.5 Knowledge of the components of fitness: cardiorespiratory fitness, muscular strength, muscular endurance, flexibility, and body composition.

1.2.6 Knowledge to describe normal cardiorespiratory responses to static and dynamic exercise in terms of heart rate, blood pressure, and oxygen consumption.

1.2.7 Knowledge of how heart rate, blood pressure, and oxygen consumption responses change with adaptation to chronic exercise training.

1.2.8 Knowledge of the physiological adaptations associated with strength training.

1.2.9 Ability to identify and apply to both groups and individuals methods used to monitor exercise intensity, including heart rate and rating of perceived exertion.

1.2.10 Knowledge of the physiological principles related to warm-up and cool-down.

1.2.11 Knowledge of the common theories of muscle fatigue and delayed onset muscle soreness (DOMS).

2.2.0 Knowledge of exercise physiology including the role of aerobic and anaerobic metabolism, muscle physiology, cardiovascular physiology, and respiratory physiology at rest and during exercise. In addition, demonstrate an understanding of the components of physical fitness, the effects of aerobic and strength and/or resistance training on the fitness components and the effects of chronic disease.

2.2.1 Knowledge of the physiological adaptations that occur at rest and during submaximal and maximal exercise following chronic aerobic and anaerobic exercise training.

2.2.2 Knowledge of the differences in cardiorespiratory response to acute graded exercise between conditioned and unconditioned individuals.

2.2.3 Knowledge of the structure of the skeletal muscle fiber and the basic mechanism of contraction.

2.2.4 Knowledge of the characteristics of fast and slow twitch fibers.

2.2.5	Knowledge of the sliding filament theory of muscle contraction.
2.2.6	Knowledge of twitch, summation, and tetanus with respect to muscle contraction.
2.2.7	Ability to discuss the physiological principles involved in promoting gains in muscular strength and endurance.
2.2.8	Ability to define muscular fatigue as it relates to task, intensity, duration, and the accumulative effects of exercise.
2.2.9	Knowledge of the relationship between the number of repetitions, intensity, number of sets, and rest with regard to strength training.
2.2.10	Knowledge of the basic properties of cardiac muscle and the normal pathways of conduction in the heart.
2.2.11	Knowledge of the response of the following variables to acute exercise: heart rate, stroke volume, cardiac output, pulmonary ventilation, tidal volume, respiratory rate, and arteriovenous oxygen difference.
2.2.12	Knowledge of the differences in the cardiorespiratory responses to static exercise compared with dynamic exercise, including possible hazards and contraindications.
2.2.13	Ability to describe how each of the following differs from the normal condition: premature atrial contractions and premature ventricular contractions.
2.2.14	Knowledge of blood pressure responses associated with acute exercise, including changes in body position.
2.2.15	Knowledge of and ability to describe the implications of ventilatory threshold (anaerobic threshold) as it relates to exercise training and cardiorespiratory assessment.
2.2.16	Knowledge of and ability to describe the physiological adaptations of the respiratory system that occur at rest and during submaximal and maximal exercise following chronic aerobic and anaerobic training.
2.2.17	Ability to describe how each of the following differs from the normal condition: dyspnea, hypoxia, and hypoventilation.
2.2.18	Knowledge of and ability to discuss the physiological basis of the major components of physical fitness: flexibility, cardiovascular fitness, muscular strength, muscular endurance, and body composition.
2.2.19	Ability to explain how the principle of specificity relates to the components of fitness.
2.2.20	Ability to explain the concept of detraining or reversibility of conditioning and its implications in fitness programs.
2.2.21	Ability to discuss the physical and psychological signs of overtraining and to provide recommendations for these problems.
2.2.22	Ability to describe the physiological and metabolic responses to exercise associated with chronic disease (heart disease, hypertension, diabetes mellitus, and pulmonary disease).

3.2.0	Knowledge of the muscular, cardiorespiratory, and metabolic responses to decreased exercise intensity.

4.2.0	Knowledge of exercise physiology as it relates to exercise testing and training.
4.2.0.1	Ability to describe the physiological effects of bed rest and discuss the appropriate physical activities that might be used to counteract these changes.
4.2.0.2	Ability to describe the normal and abnormal cardiorespiratory responses at rest and exercise.
4.2.0.3	Ability to describe the principle of specificity of training as it relates to the mode of exercise testing and training.

4.2.0.4	Ability to list the cardiorespiratory responses associated with postural changes.
4.2.0.5	Knowledge of acute and chronic adaptations to exercise for apparently healthy individuals (low risk) and for those with cardiovascular, pulmonary, and metabolic diseases.
4.2.0.6	Ability to describe normal and abnormal chronotropic and inotropic responses to exercise testing and training.
4.2.1	Knowledge of activities that are primarily aerobic and anaerobic.
4.2.1.1	Ability to describe the aerobic and anaerobic metabolic demands of exercise for individuals with cardiovascular, pulmonary, and/or metabolic diseases undergoing exercise testing or training and the implications of such exercise.
4.2.1.2	Ability to identify the metabolic equivalent (MET) requirements of various occupational, household, sport/exercise, and leisure time activities.
4.2.2	Knowledge of the unique hemodynamic responses of arm versus leg exercise and of static versus dynamic exercise.
4.2.2.1	Ability to describe the differences in the physiological responses to various modes of ergometry (e.g., treadmill, cycle and arm ergometers) as they relate to exercise testing and training.
4.2.2.2	Ability to discuss the effects of isometric exercise in individuals with cardiovascular, pulmonary, and/or metabolic diseases or with low functional capacity.
4.2.3	Knowledge of the determinants of myocardial oxygen consumption and the effects of exercise training on those determinants.
4.2.3.1	Ability to explain maximal oxygen (O_2) consumption and how it is measured.
4.2.3.2	Ability to list and explain the variables measured during cardiopulmonary exercise testing (e.g., heart rate, blood pressure, rate of perceived exertion, ventilation, oxygen consumption, ventilatory threshold, pulmonary circulation) and their potential relationship to cardiovascular, pulmonary, and metabolic disease.
4.2.3.3	Ability to list and plot the normal resting and exercise values associated with increasing exercise intensity (and how they may differ for diseased population) for the following: heart rate, stroke volume, cardiac output, double product, arteriovenous O_2 difference, O_2 consumption, systolic and diastolic blood pressure, minute ventilation, tidal volume, breathing frequency, Vd/Vt, $\dot{V}_E/\dot{V}O_2$, and $\dot{V}_E/\dot{V}CO_2$.

5.2.0	Ability to discuss the mechanisms by which functional capacity and cardiovascular, pulmonary, metabolic, endocrine, and neuromuscular adaptations occur in response to exercise testing and training in healthy and various diseased states.

HUMAN DEVELOPMENT AND AGING

1.3.0	Knowledge of the benefits and risks associated with exercise training in prepubescent and postpubescent youth.
1.3.1	Knowledge of the benefits and precautions associated with resistance and endurance training in older adults.
1.3.2	Ability to describe specific leadership techniques appropriate for working with participants of all ages.

2.3.0	Knowledge of the changes that occur during growth and development from childhood to old age.
2.3.0.1	Ability to modify cardiovascular and resistance exercises based on age and physical condition.
2.3.0.2	Knowledge of and ability to describe the changes that occur in maturation from childhood to adulthood for the following: skeletal muscle, bone structure, reaction time, coordination, heat and cold tolerance, maximal oxygen consumption, strength, flexibility, body composition, resting and maximal heart rate, and resting and maximal blood pressure.
2.3.0.3	Knowledge of the effect of the aging process on the musculoskeletal and cardiovascular structure and function at rest, during exercise, and during recovery.
2.3.0.4	Ability to characterize the differences in the development of an exercise prescription for children, adolescents, and older participants.
2.3.0.5	Knowledge of and ability to describe the unique adaptations to exercise training in children, adolescents, and older participants with regard to strength, functional capacity, and motor skills.
2.3.0.6	Knowledge of common orthopedic and cardiovascular considerations for older participants and the ability to describe modifications in exercise prescription that are indicated.

4.3.0	Knowledge of selecting appropriate testing and training modalities according to the age and functional capacity of the individual.
4.3.0.1	Ability to select an appropriate test protocol according to the age and functional capacity of the individual.
4.3.1	Ability to describe the importance of and appropriate methods for resistance training in older individuals.

5.3.0	Ability to explain differences in overall policy and procedures for the inclusion of different age groups in an exercise program.
5.3.1	Ability to discuss facility and equipment adaptations necessary for different age groups.

Pathophysiology/Risk Factors

1.4.0	Knowledge of cardiovascular, respiratory, metabolic, and musculoskeletal risk factors that may require further evaluation by medical or allied health professionals before participation in physical activity.
1.4.0.1	Ability to determine those risk factors that may be favorably modified by physical activity habits.
1.4.0.2	Knowledge to define the following terms: total cholesterol (TC), high-density lipoprotein cholesterol (HDL-C), TC/HDL-C ratio, low-density lipoprotein cholesterol (LDL-C), triglycerides, hypertension, and atherosclerosis.

1.4.0.3   Knowledge of plasma cholesterol levels for adults as recommended by the National Cholesterol Education Program (NCEP II).

2.4.0   Knowledge of the pathophysiology of atherosclerosis and how this process is influenced by physical activity.
2.4.1   Knowledge of the risk factor concept of CAD and the influence of heredity and lifestyle on the development of CAD.
2.4.2   Knowledge of the atherosclerotic process, the factors involved in its genesis and progression, and the potential role of exercise training in treatment.
2.4.3   Ability to discuss in detail how lifestyle factors, including nutrition, physical activity, and heredity, influence lipid and lipoprotein profiles.
2.4.4   Knowledge of cardiovascular risk factors or conditions that may require consultation with medical personnel before testing or training, including inappropriate changes in resting or exercise heart rate and blood pressure, new onset discomfort in chest, neck, shoulder, or arm, changes in the pattern of discomfort during rest or exercise, fainting or dizzy spells, and claudication.
2.4.5   Knowledge of respiratory risk factors or conditions that may require consultation with medical personnel before testing or training, including asthma, exercise-induced bronchospasm, extreme breathlessness at rest or during exercise, bronchitis, and emphysema.
2.4.6   Knowledge of metabolic risk factors or conditions that may require consultation with medical personnel before testing or training, including body weight more than 20% above optimal, BMI > 30, thyroid disease, diabetes or glucose intolerance, and hypoglycemia.
2.4.7   Knowledge of musculoskeletal risk factors or conditions that may require consultation with medical personnel before testing or training, including acute or chronic back pain, osteoarthritis, rheumatoid arthritis, osteoporosis, tendonitis, and low back pain.

3.4.0   Ability to define atherosclerosis, the factors causing it, and the interventions that may potentially delay or reverse the atherosclerotic process.
3.4.1   Ability to describe the causes of myocardial ischemia and infarction.
3.4.2   Ability to describe the pathophysiology of hypertension, obesity, hyperlipidemia, diabetes, chronic obstructive pulmonary diseases, arthritis, osteoporosis, chronic diseases, and immunosuppressive disease.
3.4.3   Ability to describe the effects of the above diseases and conditions on cardiorespiratory and metabolic function at rest and during exercise.

4.4.0   Ability to risk stratify individuals with cardiovascular, pulmonary, and metabolic diseases, using appropriate materials and understanding the prognostic indicators for high-risk individuals.
4.4.1   Ability to list the effects of cardiovascular, pulmonary, and metabolic diseases on performance and safety during exercise testing and training.
4.4.2   Knowledge of the common procedures used for radionuclide imaging (e.g., thallium, technetium, sestamibi, single photon emission computed tomography (SPECT), planar).
4.4.3   Ability to define myocardial ischemia and ability to identify the methods used to measure ischemic response.
4.4.4   Ability to describe the cardiorespiratory and metabolic responses in myocardial dysfunction and ischemia at rest and during exercise.

4.4.5	Knowledge of the differences between typical, atypical, and vasospastic angina.
4.4.6	Knowledge of the pathophysiology of the healing myocardium and the potential complications after acute myocardial infarction (MI) (extension, expansion, rupture)
4.4.7	Knowledge of the purpose of coronary angiography.
4.4.8	Knowledge of the indications for use of streptokinase, tissue plasminogen activase, and other thrombolytic agents.
4.4.9	Ability to describe PTCA and other catheter revascularization techniques (e.g., atherectomy, stent placement) as an alternative to medical management or coronary artery bypass surgery (CABS).
4.4.10	Ability to demonstrate an understanding of the indications and limitations for medical management and interventional techniques in different subsets of individuals with CAD and CABS.
4.4.11	Ability to describe the cardiorespiratory and metabolic responses that accompany or result from pulmonary diseases at rest and during exercise.
4.4.12	Ability to describe reversible airway (obstructive) and restrictive lung diseases and their effect on exercise testing and training.
4.4.13	Ability to describe the signs and symptoms of peripheral vascular diseases and their effect on exercise.
4.4.14	Ability to describe the metabolic responses at rest and during exercise and potential complications in individuals with type 1 or type 2 diabetes.
4.4.15	Ability to describe the influence of exercise on weight reduction, hyperlipidemia, hypertension, and diabetes.
4.4.16	Knowledge of the effects of variation in ambient temperature, humidity, carbon dioxide, ozone, and altitude on functional capacity for normal individuals and those with cardiovascular, pulmonary, and metabolic diseases.
4.4.17	Skill in adapting the exercise prescription appropriately in environmental extremes for normal individuals and those with cardiovascular, pulmonary, and metabolic diseases.

5.4.0	Knowledge of the atherosclerotic process, including current hypotheses regarding onset and rate of progression and/or regression.
5.4.1	Knowledge of the lipoprotein classifications and their relationship to atherosclerosis or other diseases.
5.4.2	Ability to identify and explain the mechanisms by which exercise may contribute to preventing or rehabilitating individuals with cardiovascular, pulmonary, and metabolic diseases.
5.4.3	Knowledge and ability to describe coronary angiography, radionuclide imaging, echocardiography imaging, and pharmacologic studies, including the type of information obtained, sensitivity, specificity, predictive value, and associated risks and indications for use.

HUMAN BEHAVIOR AND PSYCHOLOGY

1.5.0	Ability to identify and define at least five behavioral strategies to enhance exercise and health behavior change (i.e., reinforcement, goal setting, social support).

1.5.1 Ability to list and define the five important elements that should be included in each counseling session.

1.5.2 Knowledge of specific techniques to enhance motivation (e.g., posters, recognition, bulletin boards, games, competitions). Define extrinsic and intrinsic reinforcement and give examples of each.

1.5.3 Knowledge of the stages of motivational readiness.

1.5.4 Ability to list and describe three counseling approaches that may assist less motivated clients to increase their physical activity.

2.5.0 Ability to list and describe the specific strategies aimed at encouraging the initiation, adherence, and return to participation in an exercise program.

2.5.1 Knowledge of symptoms of anxiety and depression that may necessitate referral.

2.5.2 Knowledge of the potential symptoms and causal factors of test anxiety (i.e., performance, appraisal threat during exercise testing) and how it may affect physiological responses to testing.

3.5.0 Knowledge of and ability to apply basic cognitive-behavioral intervention such as shaping, goal setting, motivation, cueing, problem solving, reinforcement strategies, and self-monitoring.

3.5.1 Knowledge of the selection of an appropriate behavioral goal and the suggested method to evaluate goal achievement for each stage of change.

4.5.0 Ability to identify and explain five behavioral strategies as they apply to lifestyle modifications, such as exercise, diet, stress, and medication management.

4.5.1 Ability to describe signs and symptoms of maladjustment and/or failure to cope during an illness crisis and/or personal adjustment crisis (e.g., job loss) that might prompt a psychological consult or referral to other professional services.

4.5.2 Ability to describe the general principles of crisis management and factors influencing coping and learning in illness states.

4.5.3 Ability to describe the psychological issues to be confronted by the patient and by family members of patients who have cardiorespiratory disease and/or who have had an acute MI or cardiac surgery.

4.5.4 Knowledge of the psychological issues associated with an acute cardiac event versus those associated with chronic cardiac conditions.

4.5.5 Knowledge of the psychological stages involved with the acceptance of death and dying and ability to recognize when it is necessary for a psychological consult or referral to a professional resource.

5.5.0 Ability to demonstrate an understanding of the need for psychosocial consultation and referral of individuals who exhibit signs of psychological distress.

5.5.1 Knowledge of community resources for psychosocial support and behavior modification and outline an example of a referral system.

5.5.2 Knowledge of the observable signs and symptoms of anxiety or depressive symptoms secondary to cardiopulmonary disorders.

Health Appraisal and Fitness Testing

1.6.1	Knowledge of the importance of a health/medical history.
1.6.2	Knowledge of the value of a medical clearance prior to exercise participation.
1.6.3	Skill to measure pulse rate accurately both at rest and during exercise.

2.6.0	Knowledge, skills, and abilities to assess the health status of individuals and the ability to conduct fitness testing.
2.6.0.1	Ability to obtain a health history and risk appraisal that includes past and current medical history, family history of cardiac disease, orthopedic limitations, prescribed medications, activity patterns, nutritional habits, stress and anxiety levels, and smoking and alcohol use.
2.6.0.2	Ability to describe the categories of participants who should receive medical clearance prior to administration of an exercise test or participation in an exercise program.
2.6.0.3	Ability to identify relative and absolute contraindications to exercise testing or participation.
2.6.0.4	Ability to discuss the limitations of informed consent and medical clearance prior to exercise testing.
2.6.0.5	Ability to obtain informed consent.
2.6.0.6	Ability to explain the purpose and procedures for monitoring clients prior to, during, and after cardiorespiratory fitness testing.
2.6.0.7	Skill in instructing participants in the use of equipment and test procedures.
2.6.0.8	Ability to describe the purpose of testing, select an appropriate submaximal or maximal protocol, and conduct an assessment of cardiovascular fitness on the cycle ergometer or the treadmill.
2.6.0.9	Skill in accurately measuring heart rate, blood pressure, and obtaining rating of perceived exertion (RPE) at rest and during exercise according to established guidelines.
2.6.0.10	Ability to locate and measure skinfold sites, skeletal diameters, and girth measurements used for estimating body composition.
2.6.0.11	Ability to describe the purpose of testing, select appropriate protocols, and conduct assessments of muscular strength, muscular endurance, and flexibility.
2.6.0.12	Skill in various techniques of assessing body composition.
2.6.0.13	Knowledge of the advantages/disadvantages and limitations of the various body composition techniques.
2.6.0.14	Ability to interpret information obtained from the cardiorespiratory fitness test and the muscular strength and endurance, flexibility, and body composition assessments for apparently healthy individuals and those with stable disease.
2.6.0.15	Ability to identify appropriate criteria for terminating a fitness evaluation and demonstrate proper procedures to be followed after discontinuing such a test.
2.6.0.16	Ability to modify protocols and procedures for cardiorespiratory fitness tests in children, adolescents, and older adults.
2.6.0.17	Knowledge of common drugs from each of the following classes of medications and describe the principal action and the effects on exercise testing and prescription:
2.6.0.17.1	Antianginals
2.6.0.17.2	Antihypertensives

2.6.0.17.3	Antiarrhythmics
2.6.0.17.4	Bronchodilators
2.6.0.17.5	Hypoglycemics
2.6.0.17.6	Psychotropics
2.6.0.17.7	Vasodilators
2.6.0.18	Ability to identify the effects of the following substances on exercise response: antihistamines, tranquilizers, alcohol, diet pills, cold tablets, caffeine, and nicotine.
2.6.0.19	Skill in techniques for calibration of a cycle ergometer and a motor-driven treadmill.

3.6.0	Knowledge of the use and value of the results of the fitness evaluation and exercise test for various populations.
3.6.1	Ability to design and implement a fitness testing/health appraisal program that includes, but is not limited to, staffing needs, physician interaction, documentation, equipment, marketing, and program evaluation.
3.6.2	Ability to recruit, train, and evaluate appropriate staff personnel for performing exercise tests, fitness evaluations, and health appraisals.
3.6.3	Ability to identify and describe the principal action, mechanisms of action, and major side effects from each of the following classes of medications:
3.6.3.1	Antianginals
3.6.3.2	Antihypertensives
3.6.3.3	Antiarrhythmics
3.6.3.4	Bronchodilators
3.6.3.5	Hypoglycemics
3.6.3.6	Psychotropics
3.6.3.7	Vasodilators

4.6.0	Knowledge and skills necessary for interpreting medical history and physical examination findings as they relate to health appraisal and exercise testing.
4.6.0.1	Ability to obtain a routine medical history prior to health appraisal and exercise testing.
4.6.0.2	Ability to identify individuals for whom physician supervision is recommended during maximal and submaximal exercise testing.
4.6.0.3	Ability to identify appropriate individuals who require exercise testing prior to exercise training.
4.6.1	Knowledge and skills necessary to conduct pretest procedures.
4.6.1.1	Knowledge of basic equipment and facility requirements for exercise testing.
4.6.1.2	Ability to obtain a standard and modified (Mason-Likar) 12-lead ECG on a participant in different body positions.
4.6.1.3	Ability to minimize resting ECG artifact.
4.6.1.4	Ability to accurately record a right and left arm blood pressure in different body positions.
4.6.1.5	Ability to instruct the test participant in the use of the RPE scale and other appropriate subjective scales, such as the dyspnea and angina scales.
4.6.1.6	Ability to gain informed consent.
4.6.1.7	Knowledge of the absolute and relative contraindications to an exercise test.
4.6.2	Knowledge and skills necessary for administering an exercise test.
4.6.2.1	Ability to calibrate testing equipment and explain procedures for calibration (e.g., a motor-driven treadmill, mechanical cycle ergometer, arm ergometer, electrocardiograph, and aneroid and mercury sphygmomanometers).

4.6.2.2	Knowledge of procedures and protocols for the exercise test, including the selection of the exercise test protocol in terms of modes of exercise, starting levels, increments of work, ramping versus standard protocols, length of stages, and frequency of measures.
4.6.2.3	Knowledge of appropriate techniques of measurement of physiological and subjective responses (e.g., symptoms, ECG, blood pressure, heart rate, RPE and other scales, oxygen saturation, and oxygen consumption measures) at appropriate intervals during the test.
4.6.2.4	Knowledge of how age, weight, level of fitness, and health status are considered in the selection of an exercise test protocol.
4.6.2.5	Knowledge of the technical factors that may indicate test termination (e.g., loss of ECG signal, loss of power).
4.6.2.6	Knowledge of the clinical factors that may indicate test termination (e.g., termination criteria).
4.6.2.7	Knowledge of immediate postexercise procedures and ability to list various approaches to cool-down.
4.6.2.8	Ability to record, organize, and perform necessary calculations of test data for summary presentation.
4.6.3	Knowledge and skills necessary to interpret the exercise test.
4.6.3.0	Knowledge of the prognostic implications of the exercise ECG and hemodynamic responses in light of the current medication status of the participant as well as any comorbidities.
4.6.3.1	Ability to provide objective recommendations to an individual regarding such factors as physical conditioning, return to work, and performance of selected activities for daily living (such as driving, stair climbing, sexual activity) based on exercise test results and clinical status.
4.6.4	Knowledge and skills necessary for administering an exercise test with special populations or test considerations.
4.6.4.1	Knowledge of exercise testing procedures for various clinical populations including those individuals with cardiovascular, pulmonary, and metabolic diseases in terms of exercise modality, protocol, physiological measurements, and expected outcomes.
4.6.4.2	Knowledge of the appropriate end points for exercise testing for various clinical populations.
4.6.4.3	Ability to describe silent ischemia and its implications for exercise testing and training.
4.6.4.4	Knowledge of techniques for measurement of oxygen consumption at appropriate intervals during an exercise test for special populations (e.g., congestive heart failure, valvular heart disease, coronary artery disease).
4.6.4.5	Ability to explain indications for combining exercise testing with radionuclide imaging.
4.6.4.6	Knowledge of the differences in test protocol and procedures when the exercise test involves the addition of various methodologies to increase the sensitivity and/or specificity of the test, such as radionuclide imaging or echocardiography.
4.6.4.7	Knowledge of testing procedures and protocol for children and the elderly with or without various clinical conditions.
4.6.5	Knowledge in recognizing medications commonly encountered during exercise testing and training and knowledge of the indications and effects on the ECG, heart rate, and blood pressure at rest and during exercise.
4.6.5.1	Antianginals
4.6.5.2	Antihypertensives
4.6.5.3	Antiarrythmics
4.6.5.4	Bronchodilators
4.6.5.5	Hypoglycemics
4.6.5.6	Psychotropics
4.6.5.7	Vasodilators

4.6.5.8	Anticoagulant and antiplatelet drugs (warfarin, aspirin, ticlopidine, clopidogrel, etc.)
4.6.5.9	Lipid-lowering agents
4.6.6	Knowledge and ability to administer and interpret basic resting spirometric tests and measures including forced expiratory volume in 1 second ($FEV_{1.0}$), FVC, and MVV.

5.6.0	Knowledge of the various diagnostic and treatment modalities currently used in the management of cardiovascular disease.
5.6.1	Knowledge of the diagnostic and prognostic value of the results of the graded exercise test for various populations.

Safety, Injury Prevention, and Emergency Care

1.7.0	Knowledge of and skill in obtaining basic life support and cardiopulmonary resuscitation certification.
1.7.1	Knowledge of appropriate emergency procedures (i.e., telephone procedures, written emergency procedures, personnel responsibilities) in the group exercise setting.
1.7.2	Knowledge of basic first aid procedures for exercise-related injuries, such as bleeding, strains/sprains, fractures, and exercise intolerance (dizziness, syncope, heat injury).
1.7.3	Knowledge of basic precautions taken in a group exercise setting to ensure participant safety.
1.7.4	Ability to identify the physical and physiological signs and symptoms of overtraining.
1.7.5	Ability to list the effects of temperature, humidity, altitude, and pollution on the physiological response to exercise.
1.7.6	Knowledge of the following terms: shin splints, sprain, strain, tennis elbow, bursitis, stress fracture, tendonitis, patellar femoral pain syndrome, low back pain, plantar fasciitis, and rotator cuff tendonitis.
1.7.7	Skill to demonstrate exercises used for people with low back pain.
1.7.8	Knowledge of hypothetical concerns and potential risks that may be associated with the use of exercises such as straight leg sit-ups, double leg raises, full squats, hurdlers stretch, yoga plough, forceful back hyperextension, and standing bent-over toe touch.

2.7.0	Skill in demonstrating appropriate emergency procedures during exercise testing and/or training.
2.7.1	Knowledge of safety plans, emergency procedures, and first aid techniques needed during fitness evaluations, exercise testing, and exercise training.
2.7.2	Ability to identify the components that contribute to the maintenance of a safe environment.
2.7.3	Knowledge of the health/fitness instructor's responsibilities, limitations, and the legal implications of carrying out emergency procedures.
2.7.4	Ability to describe potential musculoskeletal injuries (e.g., contusions,

sprains, strains, fractures), cardiovascular/pulmonary complications (e.g., tachycardia, bradycardia, hypotension/hypertension, tachypnea) and metabolic abnormalities (e.g., fainting/syncope, hypoglycemia/hyperglycemia, hypothermia/hyperthermia).

2.7.5 Knowledge of the initial management and first aid techniques associated with open wounds, musculoskeletal injuries, cardiovascular/pulmonary complications, and metabolic disorders.

2.7.6 Knowledge of the components of an equipment maintenance/repair program and how it may be used to evaluate the condition of exercise equipment to reduce the potential risk of injury.

3.7.0 Ability to identify the process to train the exercise staff in cardiopulmonary resuscitation.

3.7.1 Ability to design and evaluate emergency procedures for a preventive exercise program and an exercise testing facility.

3.7.2 Ability to train staff in safety procedures, risk reduction strategies, and injury care techniques.

3.7.3 Knowledge of the legal implications of documented safety procedures, the use of incident documents, and ongoing safety training.

4.7.0 Knowledge in responding with appropriate emergency procedures to situations which might arise before, during, and after administration of an exercise test and/or exercise session.

4.7.1 Ability to list and describe the use of emergency equipment and personnel that should be present in an exercise testing laboratory and rehabilitative exercise training setting.

4.7.2 Knowledge of verifying operating status of and maintaining emergency equipment.

4.7.3 Ability to describe emergency procedures that may arise during exercise testing or training, including (but not limited to):

4.7.3.1 Cardiac arrest
4.7.3.2 Hypoglycemia and hyperglycemia
4.7.3.3 Bronchospasm
4.7.3.4 Sudden onset hypotension
4.7.3.5 Serious (including possibly life-threatening) arrhythmias (VT, Vfib, etc.)
4.7.3.6 ICD discharge
4.7.3.7 TIA
4.7.3.8 MI
4.7.3.9 Coronary thrombosis

4.7.4 Ability to identify the emergency drugs that should be available in exercise testing sessions and training sessions and to describe the mechanisms of action.

4.7.5 Ability to possess necessary emergency skills similar to or associated with current Advanced Cardiac Life Support (ACLS) policies and procedures.

5.7.0 Ability to diagram an emergency response system and discuss minimum standards for equipment and personnel required in settings for rehabilitative exercise programs.

5.7.1 Ability and knowledge to discuss the concepts of informed consent, risk management, negligence, and standards of care as they relate to exercise testing and training.

5.7.2   Ability and knowledge to discuss procedures for training and drilling staff on emergency response.

Exercise Programming

1.8.0   Knowledge of the recommended intensity, duration, frequency, and type of physical activity necessary for development of cardiorespiratory fitness in an apparently healthy population.

1.8.1   Ability to differentiate between the amount of physical activity required for health benefits and the amount of exercise required for fitness development.

1.8.2   Ability to describe exercises designed to enhance muscular strength and/or endurance of specific major muscle groups.

1.8.3   Knowledge of the principles of overload, specificity, and progression and how they relate to exercise programming.

1.8.4   Skill to teach and demonstrate appropriate exercises used in the warm-up and cool-down of a variety of group exercise classes.

1.8.5   Ability to teach the components of an exercise session (i.e., warm-up, aerobic stimulus phase, cool-down, muscular strength/endurance, flexibility).

1.8.6   Knowledge of the following terms: progressive resistance, isotonic/isometric, concentric, eccentric, atrophy, hypertrophy, sets, repetitions, plyometrics, Valsalva maneuver.

1.8.7   Skill to teach class participants how to monitor intensity of exercise using heart rate and rating of perceived exertion.

1.8.8   Skill to teach participants how to use RPE and heart rate to adjust the intensity of the exercise session.

1.8.9   Ability to calculate training heart rates using two methods: percent of age-predicted maximum heart rate and heart rate reserve (Karvonen).

1.8.10   Skill to teach and demonstrate appropriate modifications in specific exercises for the following groups: older adults, pregnant and postnatal women, obese persons, and persons with low back pain.

1.8.11   Ability to recognize proper and improper technique in the use of resistive equipment such as stability balls, weights, bands, resistance bars, and water exercise equipment.

1.8.12   Ability to recognize proper and improper technique in the use of cardiovascular conditioning equipment (e.g., steps, cycles, slides).

1.8.13   Skill to teach and demonstrate appropriate exercises for improving range of motion of all major joints.

1.8.14   Ability to modify exercises in the group setting for apparently healthy persons of various fitness levels.

1.8.15   Ability to teach a progression of exercises for all major muscle groups to improve muscular strength and endurance.

1.8.16   Knowledge to describe the various types of interval, continuous, and circuit training programs.

1.8.17   Knowledge to describe various ways a leader can take a position relative to the group to enhance visibility, participant interactions, and communication.

1.8.18   Ability to communicate effectively with exercise participants in the group exercise session.

1.8.19   Knowledge to describe partner resistance exercises that can be used in a group class setting.

1.8.20	Ability to demonstrate techniques for accommodating various fitness levels within the same class.
1.8.21	Knowledge of the properties of water that affect the design of a water exercise session.
1.8.22	Knowledge of basic music fundamentals, including downbeat, 8 count, and 32 count.
1.8.23	Skill to effectively use verbal and nonverbal cues in the group exercise setting, including anticipatory, motivational, safety, and educational.
1.8.24	Skill to demonstrate the proper form, alignment, and technique in typical exercises used in the warm-up, stimulus, muscle conditioning and cool-down phases of the group session.
1.8.25	Ability to evaluate specific exercises in terms of safety and effectiveness for various participants.
1.8.26	Ability to demonstrate a familiarity with a variety of group exercise formats (e.g., traditional, step, slide, muscle conditioning, flexibility, indoor cycling, water fitness, walking).

2.8.0	Knowledge, skills, and abilities to prescribe and administer exercise programs for apparently healthy individuals, individuals at higher risk, and individuals with known disease.
2.8.0.1	Ability to design, implement, and evaluate individualized and group exercise programs based on health history and physical fitness assessments.
2.8.0.2	Ability to modify exercises based on age and physical condition.
2.8.0.3	Knowledge, skills, and abilities to calculate energy cost, $\dot{V}O_2$, METs, and target heart rates and apply the information to an exercise prescription.
2.8.0.4	Ability to convert weights from pounds (lb) to kilograms (kg) and speed from miles per hour (mph) to meters per minute ($m \cdot min^{-1}$).
2.8.0.5	Ability to convert METs to $\dot{V}O_2$ expressed as $mL \cdot kg^{-1} \cdot min^{-1}$, $L \cdot min^{-1}$, and/or $mL \cdot kg\ FFW^{-1} \cdot min^{-1}$.
2.8.0.6	Ability to calculate the energy cost in METs and kilocalories for given exercise intensities in stepping exercise, cycle ergometry, and during horizontal and graded walking and running.
2.8.0.7	Knowledge of approximate METs for various sport, recreational, and work tasks.
2.8.0.8	Ability to prescribe exercise intensity based on $\dot{V}O_2$ data for different modes of exercise, including graded and horizontal running and walking, cycling, and stepping exercise.
2.8.0.9	Ability to explain and implement exercise prescription guidelines for apparently healthy clients, increased risk clients, and clients with controlled disease.
2.8.0.10	Ability to adapt frequency, intensity, duration, mode, progression, level of supervision, and monitoring techniques in exercise programs for patients with controlled chronic disease (heart disease, diabetes mellitus, obesity, hypertension), musculoskeletal problems, pregnancy and/or postpartum, and exercise-induced asthma.
2.8.0.11	Ability to understand the components incorporated into an exercise session and the proper sequence (i.e., preexercise evaluation, warm-up, aerobic stimulus phase, cool-down, muscular strength and/or endurance, and flexibility).
2.8.0.12	Skill in the use of various methods for establishing and monitoring levels of exercise intensity, including heart rate, RPE, and METs.
2.8.0.13	Knowledge of special precautions and modifications of exercise programming for participation at altitude, different ambient temperatures, humidity, and environmental pollution.
2.8.0.14	Ability to design resistive exercise programs to increase or maintain muscular strength and/or endurance.

2.8.0.15 Ability to evaluate flexibility and prescribe appropriate flexibility exercises for all major muscle groups.

2.8.0.16 Knowledge of the importance of recording exercise sessions and performing periodic evaluations to assess changes in fitness status.

2.8.0.17 Knowledge of the advantages and disadvantages of implementation of interval, continuous, and circuit training programs.

2.8.0.18 Ability to design training programs using interval, continuous, and circuit training programs.

2.8.0.19 Ability to discuss the advantages and disadvantages of various commercial exercise equipment in developing cardiorespiratory fitness, muscular strength, and muscular endurance.

2.8.0.20 Knowledge of the types of exercise programs available in the community and how these programs are appropriate for various populations.

4.8.0 Knowledge of the implications (benefits versus risks) of exercise for individuals with CAD risk factors and for individuals with established stable cardiovascular, pulmonary, metabolic, and/or orthopedic disorders.

4.8.1 Knowledge, skills, and abilities necessary to establish and supervise individualized exercise prescriptions based on medical information and exercise test data, including intensity, duration, frequency, progression, precautions, and type of physical activity for a variety of chronic disease and disability conditions, including, but not limited to:

4.8.1.1 CAD/MI
4.8.1.2 PTCA/stent
4.8.1.3 CHF
4.8.1.4 Heart transplantation
4.8.1.5 COPD
4.8.1.6 Asthma
4.8.1.7 Bronchitis
4.8.1.8 Stroke/TIA
4.8.1.9 Diabetes
4.8.1.10 Hypertension
4.8.1.11 Obesity
4.8.1.12 Renal disease/transplantation
4.8.1.13 Common orthopedic and neuromuscular conditions

4.8.2 Ability to modify exercise (type of physical activity, intensity, duration, progression) according to the current health status.

4.8.3 Knowledge of basic mechanisms of action of medications that may affect exercise testing and the exercise prescription, including:

4.8.3.1 β-Adrenergic blockers
4.8.3.2 Diuretics
4.8.3.3 Calcium channel blockers
4.8.3.4 Antihypertensives
4.8.3.5 Antihistamines
4.8.3.6 Antihyperglycemics
4.8.3.7 Psychotropics
4.8.3.8 Alcohol
4.8.3.9 Diet pills
4.8.3.10 Cold tablets
4.8.3.11 Caffeine
4.8.3.12 Nicotine

4.8.4 Ability to discuss warm-up and cool-down phenomena with *specific reference* to angina and ischemic ECG changes, arrhythmias, and blood pressure changes, and with *general reference* to cardiovascular, pulmonary, and metabolic diseases.

4.8.5	Ability to discuss the appropriate use of static and dynamic exercise for individuals with cardiovascular, pulmonary, and metabolic disease.
4.8.6	Knowledge in the design of a strength and flexibility program for the following individuals or groups:
4.8.6.1	Cardiovascular disease, pulmonary disease, metabolic disease, or musculoskeletal disorders
4.8.6.2	Elderly
4.8.6.3	Children
4.8.7	Ability to discuss modifications in monitoring of exercise intensity for various disease groups (cardiovascular, pulmonary, and metabolic diseases).
4.8.8	Ability to discuss possible adverse responses to exercise in various patient groups (cardiovascular, pulmonary, and metabolic diseases) and what precautions may be taken to prevent them.
4.8.9	Knowledge of the relative and absolute contraindications to exercise training as related to the current health status of the patient.
4.8.10	Ability to devise a supervised exercise program for the first 6 weeks after hospitalization and for the following 3 months for the following conditions:
4.8.10.1	MI
4.8.10.2	Angina
4.8.10.3	Congestive heart failure
4.8.10.4	PTCA
4.8.10.5	CABG
4.8.10.6	Stents and other catheter revascularization techniques
4.8.10.7	Chronic pulmonary disease
4.8.10.8	Transplants
4.8.11	Ability to identify characteristics that correlate or predict poor compliance to exercise programs, and strategies to increase exercise adherence.
4.8.12	Ability to identify and describe the role of various allied health professionals and the indications and procedures for referral necessary in a multidisciplinary rehabilitation program.
4.8.13	Knowledge of the concept of "Activities of Daily Living" (ADLs) and its importance in the overall rehabilitation of the individual.
4.8.14	Knowledge prescribing exercise using nontraditional exercise modalities (e.g., bench stepping, elastic bands, isodynamic exercise, water aerobics) for individuals with cardiovascular, pulmonary, or metabolic diseases, or those with orthopedic limitations.

5.8.0	Ability to discuss the level of supervision and level of monitoring recommended for various chronic disease conditions during exercise testing and training using risk stratification.

Nutrition and Weight Management

1.9.0	Knowledge to define the following terms: obesity, overweight, percent fat, lean body mass, anorexia nervosa, bulimia, and body fat distribution.
1.9.1	Knowledge of the relationship between body composition and health.
1.9.2	Knowledge of the effects of diet plus exercise, diet alone, and exercise alone as methods for modifying body composition.

1.9.3   Knowledge of the importance of an adequate daily energy intake for healthy weight management.

1.9.4   Ability to differentiate between fat-soluble and water-soluble vitamins.

1.9.5   Ability to describe the importance of maintaining normal hydration before, during, and after exercise.

1.9.6   Knowledge of the USDA Food Pyramid.

1.9.7   Knowledge of the importance of calcium and iron in women's health.

1.9.8   Ability to describe the myths and consequences associated with inappropriate weight loss methods (e.g., saunas, vibrating belts, body wraps, electric simulators, sweat suits, fad diets).

1.9.9   Knowledge of the number of kilocalories in one gram of carbohydrate, fat, protein, and alcohol.

1.9.10   Knowledge of the number of kilocalories equivalent to losing 1 pound of body fat.

2.9.0   Knowledge, skills, and abilities to provide information concerning nutrition and the role of diet and exercise on body composition and weight control.

2.9.0.1   Ability to describe the health implications of variation in body fat distribution patterns and the significance of the waist to hip ratio.

2.9.0.2   Knowledge of the guidelines for caloric intake for an individual desiring to lose or gain weight.

2.9.0.3   Knowledge of common nutritional ergogenic aids, the purported mechanism of action, and any risk and/or benefits (e.g., carbohydrates, protein/amino acids, vitamins, minerals, sodium bicarbonate, creatine, bee pollen).

2.9.0.4   Knowledge of nutritional factors related to the female athlete triad syndrome (i.e., eating disorders, menstrual cycle abnormalities, and osteoporosis).

2.9.0.5   Knowledge of the NIH Consensus statement regarding health risks of obesity, Nutrition for Physical Fitness Position Paper of the American Dietetic Association, and the ACSM Position Stand on proper and improper weight loss programs.

2.9.0.6   Knowledge of NCEP II guidelines for lipid management.

PROGRAM AND ADMINISTRATION/MANAGEMENT

2.10.0   Knowledge, skills, and ability to administer and deliver health/fitness programs.

2.10.0.1   Knowledge of the health/fitness instructor's supportive role in administration and program management within a health/fitness facility.

2.10.0.2   Ability to administer fitness-related programs within established budgetary guidelines.

2.10.0.3   Ability to develop marketing materials for the purpose of promoting fitness-related programs.

2.10.0.4   Ability to use various sales techniques for prospective program clients/participants.

2.10.0.5   Ability to describe and use the documentation required when a client shows signs or symptoms during an exercise session and should be referred to a physician.

2.10.0.6   Ability to create and maintain records pertaining to participant exercise adherence, retention, and goal setting.

2.10.0.7   Ability to develop and administer educational programs (e.g., lectures, workshops) and educational materials.

2.10.0.8   Knowledge of management of a fitness department (e.g., working within a budget, training exercise leaders, scheduling, running staff meetings).

2.10.0.9   Knowledge of the importance of tracking and evaluating member retention.

3.10.0.0   Ability to manage personnel effectively.

3.10.0.1   Ability to describe a management plan for the development of staff, continuing education, marketing and promotion, documentation, billing, facility management, and financial planning.

3.10.0.2   Ability to describe the decision-making process related to budgets, market analysis, program evaluation, facility management, staff allocation, and community development.

3.10.0.3   Ability to describe the development, evaluation, and revision of policies and procedures for programming and facility management.

3.10.0.4   Ability to describe how the computer can assist in data analysis, spreadsheet report development, and daily tracking of customer utilization.

3.10.0.5   Ability to define and describe the total quality management (TQM) and continuous quality improvement (CQI) approaches to management.

3.10.0.6   Ability to interpret applied research in the areas of exercise testing, exercise programming, and educational programs to maintain a comprehensive and current state-of-the-art program.

3.10.0.7   Ability to develop a risk factor screening program, including procedures, staff training, feedback, and follow-up.

3.10.1   Knowledge of administration, management and supervision of personnel.

3.10.1.1   Ability to describe effective interviewing, hiring, and employee termination procedures.

3.10.1.2   Ability to describe and diagram an organizational chart and show the relationships between a health/fitness director, owner, medical advisor, and staff.

3.10.1.3   Knowledge of and ability to describe various staff training techniques.

3.10.1.4   Knowledge of and ability to describe performance reviews and their roll in evaluating staff.

3.10.1.5   Knowledge of the legal obligations and problems involved in personnel management.

3.10.1.6   Knowledge of compensation, including wages, bonuses, incentive programs, and benefits.

3.10.1.7   Knowledge of methods for implementing a sales commission system.

3.10.1.8   Ability to describe the significance of a benefits program for staff and demonstrate an understanding in researching and selecting benefits.

3.10.1.9   Ability to write and implement thorough and legal job descriptions.

3.10.1.10   Knowledge of personnel time management techniques.

3.10.2   Knowledge of administration, management, and development of a budget and of the financial aspects of a fitness center.

3.10.2.1   Knowledge of the principles of financial management.

3.10.2.2   Knowledge of basic accounting principles such as accounts payable, accounts receivable, accrual, cash flow, assets, liabilities, and return on investment.

3.10.2.3   Ability to identify the various forms of a business enterprise such as sole proprietorship, partnership, corporation, and S-corporation.

3.10.2.4   Knowledge of the procedures involved with developing, evaluating, revising, and updating capital and operating budgets.

3.10.2.5   Ability to manage expenses with the objective of maintaining a positive cash flow.

3.10.2.6   Ability to understand and analyze financial statements, including income statements, balance sheets, cash flows, budgets, and pro forma projections.

3.10.2.7   Knowledge of program-related break-even and cost/benefit analysis.

3.10.2.8   Knowledge of the importance of short-term and long-term planning.

3.10.3	Knowledge of the principles of marketing and sales.
3.10.3.1	Ability to identify the steps in the development, implementation, and evaluation of a marketing plan.
3.10.3.2	Knowledge of the components of a needs assessment/market analysis.
3.10.3.3	Knowledge of various sales techniques for prospective members.
3.10.3.4	Knowledge of techniques for advertising, marketing, promotion, and public relations.
3.10.3.5	Ability to describe the principles of developing and evaluating product and services, and establishing pricing.
3.10.4	Knowledge of the principles of day-to-day operation of a fitness center.
3.10.4.1	Knowledge of the principles of pricing and purchasing equipment and supplies.
3.10.4.2	Knowledge of facility layout and design.
3.10.4.3	Ability to establish and evaluate an equipment preventive maintenance and repair program.
3.10.4.4	Ability to describe a plan for implementing a housekeeping program.
3.10.4.5	Ability to identify and explain the operating policies for preventive exercise programs, including data analysis and reporting, confidentiality of records, relationships with health care providers, accident and injury reporting, and continuing education of participants.
3.10.4.6	Knowledge of the legal concepts of tort, negligence, liability, indemnification, standards of care, health regulations, consent, contract, confidentiality, malpractice, and the legal concerns regarding emergency procedures and informed consent.
3.10.4.7	Ability to implement capital improvements with minimal disruption of client or business needs.
3.10.4.8	Ability to coordinate the operations of various departments, including, but not limited to, the front desk, fitness, rehabilitation, maintenance and repair, day care, housekeeping, pool, and management.
3.10.5	Knowledge of management and principles of member service and communication.
3.10.5.1	Skills in effective techniques for communicating with staff, management, members, health care providers, potential customers, and vendors.
3.10.5.2	Knowledge of and ability to provide strong customer service.
3.10.5.3	Ability to develop and implement customer surveys.
3.10.5.4	Knowledge of the strategies for management conflict.
3.10.6	Knowledge of the principles of health promotion and ability to administer health promotion programs.
3.10.6.1	Knowledge of health promotion programs (e.g., nutrition and weight management, smoking cessation, stress management, back care, body mechanics, and substance abuse).
3.10.6.2	Knowledge of the specific and appropriate content and methods for creating a health promotion program.
3.10.6.3	Knowledge of and ability to access resources for various programs and delivery systems.
3.10.6.4	Knowledge of the concepts of cost-effectiveness and cost-benefit as they relate to the evaluation of health promotion programming.
3.10.6.5	Ability to describe the means and amounts by which health promotion programs might increase productivity, reduce employee loss time, reduce health care costs, and improve profitability in the workplace.

5.10.0	Knowledge and ability to administer a clinical exercise program, including personnel, finance, risk management, program development, outcomes measurement, and continuous quality improvement.
5.10.1	Knowledge of general human resource policy and procedures, including job descriptions, leave policies, disabilities, discipline, and job performance evaluations.

5.10.2	Ability to diagram and explain an organizational chart and show staff relationships between an exercise program director, governing body, exercise leader, exercise specialist, registered nurse, physical therapist, medical director or advisor, and a participant's personal physician.
5.10.3	Ability to identify and explain operating policies for preventive and rehabilitative exercise programs.
5.10.4	Ability to describe the role of the medical director and referring physician in the program design and implementation, and to describe the responsibility of the program director to these individuals.
5.10.5	Ability to describe and explain strategies for enhancing the understanding of the role of rehabilitation on the part of the public, health care policy makers, health care providers, and the medical community.
5.10.6	Ability to discuss the role of the rehabilitative staff in the development and implementation of the comprehensive patient care plan.
5.10.7	Ability to justify the inclusion of a comprehensive rehabilitation program in the health care setting.
5.10.8	Ability to describe the concept of risk stratification and its application to program administration.
5.10.9	Ability to identify and explain operating policies and procedures for clinical exercise programs including data analysis and reporting, reimbursement of service fees, confidentiality of records, relationships between program and referring physicians, continuing education of participants and family, legal liability, and accident or injury reporting.
5.10.10	Ability to assume fiscal (financial) responsibility for clinical programs.
5.10.11	Knowledge and ability to implement and monitor a comprehensive continuous quality improvement process.
5.10.12	Knowledge of the relationship between insurance reimbursement and services fees.
5.10.13	Knowledge of awareness of health care reform and the potential impact upon preventive and rehabilitative exercise programs.
5.10.14	Knowledge of marketing and public relation functions for a rehabilitative exercise program.
5.10.15	Ability to identify ways to increase physician and nonphysician referrals into a comprehensive rehabilitative exercise program.

ELECTROCARDIOGRAPHY

4.11.0	Knowledge and skills necessary to identify resting and exercise ECG changes associated with the following abnormalities:
4.11.0.1	Bundle branch blocks and bifascicular blocks
4.11.0.2	Atrioventricular blocks
4.11.0.3	Sinus bradycardia and tachycardia
4.11.0.4	Sinus arrest
4.11.0.5	Supraventricular premature contractions and tachycardia
4.11.0.6	Ventricular premature contractions (including frequency, form, couplets, salvos, tachycardia)
4.11.0.7	Atrial flutter and fibrillation
4.11.0.8	Ventricular fibrillation
4.11.0.9	Myocardial ischemia, injury, and infarction
4.11.1	Knowledge and skills necessary to define the limits or considerations for initiating and terminating exercise testing or training based on the ECG abnormalities listed above.

4.11.2   Knowledge and skills necessary to identify myocardial ischemia, injury, and infarction.

4.11.2.1   Ability to identify ECG changes that correspond to ischemia in various myocardial regions (e.g., inferior, posterior, anteroseptal, anterior, anterolateral, lateral).

4.11.2.2   Ability to differentiate between Q-wave and non–Q-wave infarction.

4.11.2.3   Ability to identify ECG changes that typically occur due to hyperventilation, electrolyte abnormalities, and drug therapy.

4.11.3   Knowledge and skills necessary to identify cardiac arrhythmias and conduction defects during exercise.

4.11.3.1   Knowledge of the potential causes of various cardiac arrhythmias.

4.11.3.2   Knowledge of the significance of arrhythmia occurrence during rest, exercise, and recovery.

4.11.3.3   Ability to identify potentially hazardous arrhythmias or conduction defects observed on the ECG at rest, during exercise, and recovery.

4.11.3.4   Knowledge of appropriate procedures in the event of such arrhythmias or conduction defects.

4.11.4   Knowledge of the important ECG patterns at rest and during exercise in healthy persons and in patients with cardiovascular, pulmonary, and metabolic diseases.

4.11.4.0   Ability to identify resting ECG changes associated with diseases other than coronary artery disease (such as hypertensive heart disease, cardiac chamber enlargement, pericarditis, pulmonary disease, metabolic disorders).

4.11.4.1   Ability to identify the significance of important ECG abnormalities in the designation of the exercise prescription and in activity selection.

4.11.5   Knowledge of the indications and methods for ECG monitoring during exercise testing and during exercise sessions.

4.11.6   Knowledge of the causes and means of reducing false positive and false negative exercise ECG responses.

4.11.7   Knowledge of ECG patterns and responses of pacemakers and programmable cardioverter defibrillators.

5.11.0   Knowledge of the implications of various ECG patterns for exercise testing, exercise programming, prognosis, and risk stratification.

5.11.1   Knowledge of the diagnostic and prognostic significance of ischemic ECG responses and arrhythmias at rest, during exercise, or recovery.

5.11.2   Knowledge of Baye's theorem as it relates to pretest likelihood of CAD and the predictive value of positive or negative diagnostic exercise ECG results.

5.11.3   Knowledge of the role of the ECG during exercise testing as it relates to radionuclide imaging and echocardiography imaging.

APPENDIX G
Editor's Note

In January 2000, the ACSM Committee on Certification and Education approved the renaming of the ACSM Exercise Leader® to the ACSM Group Exercise Leader$_{SM}$ to more accurately reflect the KSAs for this certification level. Please note that in the ACSM's Guidelines for Exercise Testing and Prescription, sixth edition, references to the ACSM Exercise Leader also refer to the ACSM Group Exercise Leader. This change will be incorporated into the next edition of ACSM's Guidelines for Exercise Testing and Prescription.

INDEX

Page numbers in *italics* denote figures, those followed by a "t" denote tables, and those followed by a "b" denote boxes.